MOSBY'S HANDBOOK OF
Pharmacology in nursing

MOSBY'S HANDBOOK OF
Pharmacology in nursing

BRUCE D. CLAYTON, B.S., Pharm.D.

Associate Professor and Vice Chairman
Department of Pharmacy Practice,
College of Pharmacy, University of
Nebraska Medical Center,
Omaha, Nebraska

THIRD EDITION

The C. V. Mosby Company

ST. LOUIS   TORONTO   1984

Editor: Julie Cardamon
Assistant editor: Bess Arends
Manuscript editor: Rebecca A. Reece
Book design: Gail Morey Hudson
Cover design: Diane Beasley
Production: Judy England, Barbara Merritt

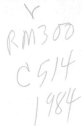

THIRD EDITION

The C.V. Mosby Company
11830 Westline Industrial Drive, St. Louis, Missouri 63146

Library of Congress Cataloging in Publication Data

Clayton, Bruce D., 1947-
  Mosby's handbook of pharmacology in nursing.

  Rev. ed. of: Handbook of practical pharmacology
Sheila A. Ryan, Bruce D. Clayton. 2nd ed. 1980.
  Bibliography: p.
  Includes index.
    1. Pharmacology—Handbooks, manuals, etc.
2. Chemotherapy—Handbooks, manuals, etc. 3. Nursing—
Handbooks, manuals, etc. I. Ryan, Sheila A., 1945-
Handbook of practical pharmacology. II. Title.
[DNLM: 1. Drug therapy—Nursing texts. 2. Pharmacology—
Nursing texts. QV 4 C622m]
RM300.C514 1984   615'.1   83-13304
ISBN 0-8016-4243-4

TS/D/D   9   8   7   6   5   4   3   03/A/367

Nurse consultant board

JAN 30 1987

To

Francine

for her unfailing support and encouragement

and to

Sarah and Beth

the lights of our lives

Preface
to the third edition

As with the first edition, the response to the second edition has been most gratifying. The success of the first two editions (*Handbook of Practical Pharmacology*), in addition to the support and suggestions offered by reviewers, colleagues, and students, has prompted the development of a third edition, *Mosby's Handbook of Pharmacology in Nursing*, with expanded content.

Although those familiar with previous editions of this manual will recognize the format of the present edition, several major chapters and sections have been added. Over 100 new drugs have been included, bringing the total to more than 400 single-entity agents and over 90 combination products.

Significant effort has been made to expand on the descriptions of therapeutic and adverse effects of drugs and the patient parameters that should be monitored to improve therapeutic effect and reduce the incidence of adverse activity. Major additions have been made to the chapters on antibiotics, cardiovascular agents, analgesics, biologic agents, and psychoactive agents. New sections have been created on the calcium ion antagonists, beta-adrenergic blocking agents, theophylline derivatives, and nonsteroidal antiinflammatory agents. The chapter on diabetic agents has been completely revised to conform to the new nomenclature of the National Diabetes Data Group and contains descriptions of the newer, more purified insulins. New chapters have been written on agents used in obstetrics and in the treatment of parkinsonism and hyperlipidemia. The appendixes have been expanded to include techniques of medication administration by eye, ear, nose, rectal, and parenteral routes.

I wish to extend a word of thanks to the many students and colleagues who offered suggestions for improvement of this edition. Linda Beckius deserves recognition for her excellent secretarial assistance.

Special recognition must go to Francine E. Clayton for her patience, support, and secretarial assistance in the preparation of the third edition. Special thanks is extended to the John D. Clayton family and the Francis H. Purdy family for their support and encouragement.

Bruce D. Clayton

Preface
to the first edition

No single aspect of patient care demands greater accuracy than drug therapy. The continuing exchange of updated knowledge concerning the more than 7000 principal drugs in today's medical arsenal increases the need for accurate, readily available information. This practical, convenient pocket reference, a thorough compilation of information about the most commonly used single-entity drugs currently on the market, emphasizes the need for knowledge and understanding of precautions and potential drug interactions during administration.

Drugs discussed in the book are categorized in chapters according to their primary pharmacologic activity. Most chapters provide an introduction that briefly discusses pathologic conditions for which the agents are used, how treatment should be approached, and what adjunctive measures should be employed to provide patient comfort and improve therapeutic effectiveness of the agent.

Monographs of drugs are arranged alphabetically by generic name within each chapter. More information about these monographs is contained in the Note to the reader. The individual monograph of each drug lists the generic name and a representative sample of trade names. Under each generic name is the *American Hospital Formulary Service* number that refers the reader to more detailed information about that drug. The category to which the drug belongs follows the AHFS number.

The first section of each monograph includes primary action and use. Knowledge of the mechanism of action is essential to ensure proper utilization of the drug. The actions discussed include the more important mechanisms sufficient for understanding uses and particular side effects, although the discussions in no way reflect the depth of a primary reference text. The most common and frequent usages for each drug have been included, but no attempt has been made to list historical or investigational uses.

The characteristics section represents a search of the literature for physiologic parameters of the drug. These parameters provide a more complete understanding and thus more effective monitoring of both therapeutic activity and adverse effects. Such characteristics include half-life; extent of protein binding; rates of absorption; onset, peak, and duration of action; sites of metabolism and excretion; and requirements of dosage supplementation in patients undergoing dialysis.

The section on dosage administration in each monograph is more complete than in many other references. It discusses dosage adjustments for neonatal, pediatric, and adult patients in relation to sites of administration and indications for use, while placing emphasis on techniques and rates of administration. Flow rate charts are provided for those drugs administered by continuous infusion to provide accuracy in calculations and to allow closer correlation with dosage and patient response.

One of the most valuable and important units of each monograph is that on special remarks and cautions. This section provides more clinically pertinent information about observation and interpretation of drug response. It does not belabor long lists of side effects that are experienced infrequently or that are based only on theoretical considerations. It includes reminders of information that the patient needs for improved understanding and compliance, warnings about interferences with laboratory tests, and use of the drug during pregnancy and lactation.

The concluding section of each monograph provides the health professional with information on significant interactions with other therapeutic agents. Drug interactions are a frequent cause of adverse effects, decreased compliance, and prolonged hospitalizations. Continual awareness of the possibility of interactions and observation for these complications are the responsibility of all health professionals.

No clinically oriented reference would be complete without charts that summarize frequently used data on administration, dosage adjustments, and monitoring. Hence, the appendixes include tables on mathematical conversions, correlation of body surface area with height and weight, pediatric dosage adjustment charts, and tables on excretion of drugs in breast milk and discoloration of excreta secondary to drug metabolism.

Safe monitoring of therapeutic agents carries enormous implications for every health professional. We believe that this book will serve as a review to help ensure the safe administration of medications. Students and practitioners in the health sciences will find this a useful and convenient source of accurate, readily applicable information.

Sheila A. Ryan
Bruce D. Clayton

Acknowledgments

Use of the *American Hospital Formulary Service*
> Permission to use the pharmacologic-therapeutic classification system of the *American Hospital Formulary Service* has been granted by the American Society of Hospital Pharmacists. The Society is not responsible for the accuracy of transpositions, or additions, or excerpts from the original context. For complete information concerning all drugs, consult the two-volume *American Hospital Formulary Service*. Permission to use excerpts from the *American Hospital Formulary Service* has been granted by the American Society of Hospital Pharmacists. The Society is not responsible for the accuracy of transpositions or excerpts from the original context. This material is copyrighted by the American Society of Hospital Pharmacists, Inc. All rights reserved.

Use of therapeutic, toxic, and lethal blood level data in the section on characteristics in each monograph
> Done, A.K.: The toxic emergency, Emergency Medicine **7**:193-201, May 1975.

Use of dialysis information in the section on characteristics in each monograph
> Bennett, W.M., and others: A guide to drug therapy in renal failure, J.A.M.A. **230**:1544, Dec. 16, 1974. Copyright 1974, American Medical Association.

Note to the reader

Trade name

The trade names represent an arbitrary selection and imply no preference for any brand name or manufacturer.

AHFS

This number directs the user to the *American Hospital Formulary Service* a source of more complete information on the drug.

Action and use

The mechanisms of action provide an overview and are not meant to include minor or proposed mechanisms. The uses are those generally accepted in medical practice today; however, the dosages and uses suggested do not necessarily have specific approval by the Food and Drug Administration. The manufacturer's product information should be consulted for approval.

Characteristics

A wide degree of clinical variation may alter these parameters. Metabolic and excretory data are based on patients with normal renal and hepatic function. Therapeutic blood level data may vary between laboratories and the specificity of the assay methods used. Toxic and lethal blood level data are often based on a few cases, and toxic effects may be intensified by the ingestion of other drugs.

The qualitative effect of dialysis on drug removal is indicated by a *no* or a *yes*. A *no* indicates that dosage adjustment is not indicated after either peritoneal dialysis (P) or hemodialysis (H). A *yes* indicates that enough drug is removed in the dialysate to require an extra maintenance dose to ensure adequate therapeutic blood levels. It must be emphasized that even though dosage adjustment may not be required, dialysis may still be beneficial in case of poisoning.

Administration and dosage

Dosages given are for adults, children, and neonates. The severity of the disease as well as the age and state of health of the patient may alter the dosages. Administration charts are provided for those drugs administered by continuous infusion to provide accuracy in calculations and to allow closer correlation with dosage and patient response. The "Notes" contain particular warnings that relate to administration.

Nurse and patient considerations

Information provided in this section includes:

The more clinically pertinent side effects. Other sources should be consulted for a complete list of adverse effects.

Advice that should be given to help promote patient understanding and compliance and to prevent complications in therapy. Data provided on laboratory test interferences. The data often refer to tests run by specific methods, many of which are infrequently used. Consult your laboratory for their methods of assay.

Use of drugs during pregnancy and lactation. Most drugs are not approved for use in pregnancy, and many have restrictions concerning pediatric use resulting from a lack of studies in these patient populations. Consult appropriate texts for use if the benefits of therapy outweigh the risks incurred by such therapy.

Drug interactions

Those listed are the more common, potentially significant interactions. If a reaction is suspected, consult texts that provide more complete information.

Contents

Antimicrobial agents

Antimicrobial agents
GENERAL INFORMATION

Antimicrobial agents are chemicals that eliminate living organisms pathogenic to the host (that is, the patient). Methods of classifying these agents include (1) mechanism of action (inhibition of protein synthesis, activity on the cell membrane, alternation of nucleic acid metabolism), (2) spectrum of activity (gram-positive organisms, gram-negative organisms, rickettsia, tuberculosis), (3) similarity in chemical structure (penicillins, cephalosporins, aminoglycosides, sulfonamides), and (4) the source (living organisms—bacteria, fungi, or chemical synthesis).

Selection of the antimicrobial agent must be based on organism sensitivity, patient variation, and relative toxicity of the agents being considered. If at all possible, the infecting organism should be isolated and identified. Culture and sensitivity tests should be completed, and appropriate antibiotic therapy based on the sensitivity results as well as on the clinical judgment of the physician should be initiated.

Host (patient) factors that may alter the response of the infection and therapy include the patient's age, other diseases (diabetes mellitus, malignancy), organ impairment (renal, hepatic, neurologic, immune deficiency), pregnancy, allergy, and concomitant drug therapy.

Nurse and patient considerations

Hypersensitivity reactions may develop after exposure to any antimicrobial agent. The severity of allergic reaction ranges from mild rash to fatal anaphylaxis. Allergic reactions may develop within 30 min of administration (anaphylaxis, laryngeal edema, shock, dyspnea, skin reactions) or may occur several days after discontinuance of therapy (skin rashes, drug fever, hemolysis, nephritis, agranulocytosis). All patients must be questioned for previous allergic reactions, and allergy-prone patients must be observed closely.

Antimicrobial agents by any route may predispose a patient to superinfection from nonsusceptible microorganisms. Superinfections occur most frequently with the use of broad-spectrum antibiotics and with agents causing diminished host resistance, such as corticosteroids and antineoplastic agents. Stomatitis, glossitis, itching, and vulvovaginitis are often caused by the candidal species of fungi. Viral infections, such as with the herpes strain, may also occur, especially in the perioral area.

Orally administered antimicrobial agents frequently cause gastrointestinal symptoms of nausea, vomiting, and diarrhea. These adverse effects are often dose related and result from changes in normal flora, irritation, and superinfection.

Patients receiving irrigant solutions over a prolonged period or topical applications to large body surface areas must be observed for toxic effects caused by systemic absorption. Systemic symptomatology may also develop from oral or rectal administration of "nonabsorbable" antibiotics, especially when the intestinal mucosa is inflamed.

The importance of rest as an adjunct to therapy should be emphasized to the patient. Patients should also understand the unique use of the drug for a particular organism and hence be instructed to neither save nor share medication. The drug should be continued during the entire prescribed period and not discontinued after symptomatic relief.

Penicillins
GENERAL INFORMATION

The penicillins were the first true antibiotic agents isolated and used by mankind against bacteria. In 1928, Fleming observed that penicillium mold that had contaminated laboratory bacterial culture specimens was inhibiting the growth of the bacteria. Eleven years later, in 1939, work began on the extraction and biosynthesis of penicillin from cultures of the fungus *Penicillium notatum.*

Penicillin G is the naturally occurring parent of this class of antibiotics. Semisynthetic compounds are made from modification of the parent molecule to alter the spectrum of activity, increase acid stability for oral use, enhance absorption, and increase resistance against penicillinase, an enzyme produced by certain bacteria that destroy penicillin (see Tables 1-1 and 1-2).

The mechanism of action of the penicillins is interference with cell wall formation. Penicillin is more effective against actively dividing organisms than resting, mature cells.

Nurse and patient considerations

Before therapy is initiated, inquiry must be made concerning possible allergy to penicillin. Hypersensitivity reactions ranging from maculopapular rash, urticaria, eosinophilia, and serum sickness to anaphylaxis have occurred in up to 10% of patients receiving penicillin. Patients with a history of hives, asthma, hay fever, and other allergies to drugs must be observed particularly closely.

Dermatologic reactions of varying character and distri-
Text continued on p. 8.

Table 1-1. Penicillin derivatives

| Generic name | Route of administration | | | Penicillinase resistant | Used against |
	PO	IM	IV		
Penicillin G	X	X	X	No	*Streptococcus* species, *Neisseria* species, *Pneumococcus* species, some *Staphylococcus* species, *Treponema pallidum*
Penicillin V	X			No	
Phenethicillin	X			No	
Oxacillin	X	X	X	Yes	*Staphylococcus aureus*
Cloxacillin	X			Yes	
Dicloxacillin	X			Yes	
Methicillin		X	X	Yes	
Nafcillin	X	X	X	Yes	
Ampicillin	X	X	X	No	As for penicillin G; *Haemophilus influenzae, Escherichia coli, Proteus mirabilis, Salmonella* and *Shigella* species, *Neisseria meningitidis*
Amoxacillin	X			No	
Bacampicillin	X			No	
Cyclacillin	X			No	
Hetacillin	X			No	
Carbenicillin	X	X	X	No	As for ampicillin; *Pseudomonas* species, *Enterobacter* species, *Proteus* species (indole positive)
Ticarcillin		X	X	No	
Mezlocillin		X	X	No	As for ampicillin; *Pseudomonas* species, *Enterobacter* species, *Klebsiella, Serratia,* and *Bacteroides* species, *Clostridium difficile*
Piperacillin		X	X	No	
Azlocillin			X	No	*Pseudomonas aeruginosa*

Table 1-2. Comparison of penicillinase-resistant penicillins*

Penicillin	Peak levels (min)	Duration (hr)	Protein binding (%)	Half-life (min)	Excretion	Dialysis H	Dialysis P	Dosage† Neonate	Dosage† Child	Dosage† Adult
Cloxacillin sodium (Tegopen)	30-60 (PO)	<4	88-96	30	10% active metabolites in urine; small amounts in bile; remainder unchanged in urine	No	No	—	PO: <20 kg: 50 to 100 mg/kg every 6 hr; >20 kg: 250-500 mg every 6 hr	PO: 250-500 mg every 6 hr
Dicloxacillin sodium (Dynapen, Pathocil, Veracillin)	60 (PO); 30-60 (IM)	<4; 4-6	96-98	40	Small amounts in bile; the rest unchanged in urine	No	No	—	PO: <40 kg: 12.5-25 mg/kg/day divided into 4 doses; >40 kg: 125-250 mg every 6 hr	PO: 125-250 mg every 6 hr; >1 g every 6 hr IM: 250-500 mg every 6 hr

*For Nurse and patient considerations see p. 3; for Drug interactions see p. 8; for discussion of methicillin see p. 16.
†Food interferes with absorption of PO dosage forms. Administer at least 1 hr before or 2 hr after meals.

Continued.

Table 1-2. Comparison of penicillinase-resistant penicillins*—cont'd

AHFS 8:12.16

Penicillin	Peak levels (min)	Duration (hr)	Protein binding (%)	Half-life (min)	Excretion	Dialysis H	Dialysis P	Dosage† Neonate	Dosage† Child	Dosage† Adult
									IM: >40 kg: 25-50 mg/kg/day divided into 4 doses; >40 kg: 250-500 mg every 6 hr	
Nafcillin (Unipen)	30-60 (PO, IM)	<4	65-90	60	30% unchanged in urine	No	No	PO: 30-40 mg/kg/day divided into 4 doses IM: 20 mg/kg/day divided into 2 doses	PO: 50 mg/kg/day divided into 4 doses IM: 50 mg/kg/day divided into 2 doses IV: 50 mg/kg/day divided into 6 doses	PO: 250 mg to 1 g every 4-6 hr IM: 500 mg every 4-6 hr IV: 500 mg to 1 g every 4 hr

| Oxacillin so-dium (Prostaph-lin) | 30 (PO sus-pension); 60 (PO capsules); 30 (IM) | <4 | <4 | <4 | 85-94 | 30 | Metabolite and unchanged drug in urine | No | No | IM and IV: 25 mg/kg/day in 4 divided doses | PO: <20 kg: 50 mg/kg/day divid-ed into 4 doses; >20 kg: 500 mg every 4-6 hr IM and IV: <20 kg: 50-100 mg/kg/day divided into 4-6 doses; >20 kg: 250-500 mg every 4-6 hr | PO: 500 mg every 4-6 hr IM and IV: 250 mg to 1 g every 4-6 hr |

bution are the most common allergic reactions to penicillin, although any manifestation of hypersensitivity, including anaphylaxis, is possible. Skin rashes and serum sickness may be controlled by antihistamines (diphenhydramine) or corticosteroids (hydrocortisone, prednisone). When reactions do occur, discontinue use of the antibiotic, unless a life-threatening infection is being treated. If major allergic manifestations develop (laryngeal edema, anaphylactic shock), treat with epinephrine, oxygen, intravenous steroids, and airway intubation if necessary.

The most common side effects of orally administered penicillins are nausea, vomiting, epigastric distress, and diarrhea.

Adverse effects of parenteral therapy include:

1. Neurologic: greater than 60 million units/day of penicillin G or 10 g/day of carbenicillin may produce hallucinations, hyperreflexia, seizures, and delirium. Preexisting neurologic disease or renal dysfunction may predispose a patient to these adverse effects.

2. Electrolyte imbalances: patients receiving large parenteral doses of sodium or potassium penicillin or carbenicillin may display electrolyte disturbances resulting in cardiac arrhythmias, hyperreflexia, convulsions, and coma. Patients with impaired renal function are more prone to these serious side effects.

3. Hematologic: penicillin hypersensitivity may include development of a positive Coombs' test and hemolytic anemia, particularly after high doses (20 million units) and a long duration of therapy. Other hematologic side effects include thrombocytopenia, thrombocytopenic purpura, and agranulocytosis. These are usually readily reversible on discontinuance of therapy.

4. Renal: *interstitial nephritis* manifested by oliguria, proteinuria, hematuria, casts, azotemia, pyuria, cylindruria, fever, and sometimes (very rarely) a rash is seen with all penicillins, but especially methicillin and oral ampicillin. It is most frequently reported in severely ill patients who are receiving high parenteral doses of penicillins and who may have impaired renal function. It is a hypersensitivity reaction.

Drug interactions

Penicillin is a bactericidal antibiotic. It requires actively growing cells to be effective. When it is used concomitantly with bacteriostatic antibiotics, its effectiveness may be decreased or destroyed. Examples of bacteriostatic antibiotics are chloramphenicol, erythromycin, and tetracyclines.

Probenecid inhibits the excretion of penicillin by increasing blood levels and prolonging activity. This combination may be used to advantage in the treatment of gonorrhea and other infections where high and prolonged blood levels are indicated.

Excessive antacids may delay or diminish absorption of penicillin.

Hypersensitivity reactions may result from a cross-sensitivity to cephalosporins.

See specific penicillin monographs for interactions pertaining to that antibiotic.

Amoxicillin
(Amoxil, Larotid, Polymox)

AHFS 8:12.16
CATEGORY Penicillin
antibiotic

Action and use

Amoxicillin is a semisynthetic, broad-spectrum derivative with an antibacterial activity similar to that of ampicillin. It does have greater activity against *Shigella* organisms and is more completely absorbed, allowing 3 doses daily versus 4 doses daily with ampicillin.

Characteristics

Amoxicillin is stable in gastric acid and rapidly absorbed on PO administration. Peak serum level: 2 hr. Protein binding: 20% to 25%. Half-life: 60 min. Excretion: 60% unchanged in urine after 8 hr. Dialysis: yes, H; no, P.

Administration and dosage
Adult

PO—250 to 500 mg every 8 hr.
IM—Not available.
IV—Not available.

Pediatric

1. Drops (50 mg/ml):
   a. Under 6 kg (13 lb): 0.5 to 1 ml every 8 hr.
   b. Between 6 and 8 kg (13 to 18 lb): 1 to 2 ml every 8 hr.
2. PO suspension (125 mg/5 ml or 250 mg/5 ml):
   a. Between 8 and 20 kg (18 to 44 lb): 20 to 40 mg/kg/24 hr in divided doses every 8 hr.
   b. Over 20 kg (44 lb): follow adult dosages.

After reconstitution, amoxicillin drops or suspension may be added to milk, formula, water, or fruit juice to enhance ease of administration.

> **Nurse and patient considerations**
>
> * See General information on penicillin (p. 3).
> * Since a parenteral dosage form is not available, amoxicillin is not indicated in the initial treatment of severe, life-threatening infections.

Drug interactions

See General information on penicillin (p. 3).

Ampicillin
(Principen, Omnipen, Penbritin, Polycillin)

AHFS 8:12.16
CATEGORY Penicillin antibiotic

Action and use

Ampicillin is a semisynthetic, broad-spectrum penicillin antibiotic effective against gram-positive cocci as well as many groups of gram-negative bacteria. Its primary indication is in the treatment of susceptible gram-negative bacteria including *Escherichia coli, Haemophilus influenzae, Proteus mirabilis,* and species of *Shigella* and *Neisseria.*

Characteristics

Peak plasma level: 5 min (IV), 1 hr (IM), 2 hr (PO). Protein binding: 20% to 25%. Half-life: 90 min. Excretion: 35% of PO dose active in urine, 70% of IM dose active in urine. Dialysis: yes, H; no, P.

Administration and dosage
Adult

PO—250 to 500 mg every 6 hr for respiratory tract, soft tissue, and skin infections. 500 mg every 6 hr for gastrointestinal and urinary tract infections. The presence of food diminishes the absorption of ampicillin.

IM—Same as PO.

IV—Same as PO. Septicemia or bacterial meningitis: 8 to 14 g/day in divided doses every 3 to 4 hr. Ampicillin must be given ai a rate no faster than 100 mg/min to prevent convulsive seizures. Dilute the powder with sterile water or any other parenteral fluid for injection.

Pediatric
Neonates

IV 1. First 7 days after birth: 25 mg/kg/12 hr.
2. After 7 days: 33 to 50 mg/kg/8 hr.
3. After 30 days: 33 to 50 mg/kg/6 hr.

Children under 40 kg (88 lb)

PO—50 to 200 mg/kg/24 hr in divided doses.
IM or IV—As for PO.

Children over 40 kg (88 lb)

PO—1 to 2 g/24 hr in divided doses.
IM or IV—For severe infections 8 to 14 g/24 hr in divided
doses.

Nurse and patient considerations

* See General information on penicillin (p. 3).
* When ampicillin is administered to a patient with
mononucleosis, there is an 80% to 90% incidence of
skin rash.

Drug interactions

See General information on penicillin (p. 3).

Ampicillin may rapidly inactivate gentamicin. They
probably should not be mixed together or administered concurrently.

Allopurinol (Zyloprim) and ampicillin used concurrently may manifest a 23% incidence of rash.

Ampicillin may interfere with oral contraceptive therapy. See General information on oral contraceptives (p.
499).

Azlocillin
(Azlin)

AHFS 8:12.16
CATEGORY Penicillin antibiotic

Action and use

Azlocillin is a semisynthetic penicillin (ureido) derivative closely related in chemical structure and activity to carbenicillin, ticarcillin, mezlocillin, and piperacillin. It is indicated for the treatment of lower respiratory tract, urinary
tract, skin, and bone and joint infections and septicemia
caused by *Pseudomonas aeruginosa*. It should be used in

combination with an aminoglycoside antibiotic (gentamicin, tobramycin, amikacin) for the treatment of patients receiving immunosuppressant therapy, patients with cystic fibrosis, or those patients with severe, life-threatening infections.

Characteristics

Duration: dose and rate dependent. Protein binding: 30% to 46%, dependent on serum concentration. Half-life: 36 to 78 min, dose dependent. Metabolism: miminal. Excretion: 50% to 60% excreted unchanged in urine. Dialysis: yes, H. Breast milk: yes.

Administration and dosage

IV—Reconstitute each gram with at least 10 ml of usual parenteral fluids and vigorous shaking.
  1. Direct injection: The reconstituted solution may be injected directly into a vein or IV tubing over at least 5 min. Chest pain is caused by rapid injection. Observe also for phlebitis.
  2. Infusion: The reconstituted solution is further diluted to 50 to 100 ml with an appropriate parenteral fluid. Administer by direct infusion over 30 min.

DOSAGE SCHEDULES
Adult

IV 1. Normal renal function
    a. Urinary tract infection (uncomplicated): 2 g every 6 hr.
    b. Urinary tract infection (complicated): 3 g every 6 hr.
    c. Lower respiratory tract, skin, bone and joint infections, septicemia: 3 g every 4 hr or 4 g every 6 hr.
    d. Life-threatening infections: 4 g every 4 hr.
  2. Impaired renal function: see chart below.

| | *Creatinine clearance (ml/min)* | | |
	<10	*10-30*	*>30*
Urinary tract infection (uncomplicated)	1.5 g every 12 hr	1.5 g every 12 hr	As above
Urinary tract infection (complicated)	2 g every 12 hr	1.5 g every 8 hr	As above
Systemic infection	3 g every 12 hr	2 g every 8 hrs	As above

Pediatric

Neonates. No dosage recommendations.

Children. Administer 75 mg/kg every 4 hr, not to exceed 24 g/day. Infuse over at least 30 min.

Nurse and patient considerations

* See General information on penicillin (p. 3).
* Since resistant organisms may develop, susceptibility testing should be performed before and during the course of therapy.
* Patients with impaired renal function tend to accumulate azlocillin. As noted above, these patients should receive lower doses. The clinician should monitor coagulation tests and platelet function tests and observe for signs of hemorrhage and neurotoxicity.
* Azlocillin sodium has a sodium content of 2.17 mEq/g of azlocillin and should be considered in patients where sodium restriction is necessary.
* High urine concentrations of azlocillin may produce false-positive protein reactions (pseudoproteinuria) with the following test methods: sulfosalicylic acid and boiling test, acetic acid test, biuret reaction, and nitric acid test. The bromphenol blue (Albustix, Multistix) reagent strip test is reliable.

Drug interactions

See General information on penicillin (p. 3).

Azlocillin has been reported to inactivate aminoglycosides (tobramycin, gentamicin) when mixed together; therefore give IV at different times or give the aminoglycoside IM and the azlocillin IV.

Bacampicillin
(Spectrobid)

AHFS unlisted
CATEGORY Penicillin antibiotic

Action and use

Bacampicillin itself is inactive but is hydrolyzed to ampicillin during absorption from the gastrointestinal tract. Since it is more completely absorbed, lower total daily doses are required and serum levels are sustained with administration only every 12 hr. See Ampicillin (p. 10).

Characteristics

Peak plasma level: 0.9 hr. Protein binding: 20% to 25% (as ampicillin). Half-life: 1.1 hr. Excretion: 75% of PO dose active in urine. Dialysis: yes, H; no, P. Breast milk: yes.

Administration and dosage
Adult

PO—400 to 800 mg every 12 hr. Tablets may be taken with meals.
IM—Not available.
IV—Not available.

Pediatric (to 25 kg [55 lb])

PO—25 to 50 mg/kg/day in 2 equally divided doses every 12 hr. Suspension should be given on an empty stomach.

Nurse and patient considerations

* See General information on penicillins (p. 3).
* Since a parenteral dosage form is not available, bacampicillin is not indicated in the initial treatment of severe, life-threatening infections.
* See Nurse and patient considerations for ampicillin (p. 11).

Drug interactions

See General information on penicillin (p. 3).
See Drug interactions for ampicillin (p. 11).
Do not administer bacampicillin to patients receiving disulfiram (Antabuse) therapy.

Carbenicillin, indanyl sodium and disodium
(Geocillin, Geopen, Pyopen)

AHFS 8:12.16
CATEGORY Penicillin antibiotic

Action and use

Carbenicillin is a semisynthetic penicillin derivative. It is the first antibiotic of this class to be effective against *P. aeruginosa*. Carbenicillin is indicated in the treatment of severe systemic infections and chronic urinary tract infections caused by susceptible strains of *Proteus*, *E. coli*, and *Pseudomonas*.

Characteristics

Peak levels: 15 to 30 min (IV), 30 to 120 min (IM). Protein binding: 50% to 60%. Half-life: 60 min. Excretion: 75% to 85% unchanged in urine. Dialysis: yes, H; no, P.

Administration and dosage
Adult

PO—Indanyl sodium salt: 382 to 764 mg 4 times daily for chronic urinary tract infections.

IM—Disodium salt: not more than 2 g of the drug should be administered in each IM injection. For IM use only the powder may be diluted with 0.5% lidocaine solution (without epinephrine) or bacteriostatic water containing 0.9% benzyl alcohol to reduce pain on injection.

IV—Disodium salt: 250 to 500 mg/kg/day to 20 to 30 g/day for *Proteus* or *E. coli,* 30 to 40 g/day for *Pseudomonas*. To keep vein irritation to a minimum, dilute the powder to 1 g/20 ml and administer as slowly as possible. Dilution may be completed with any of the major IV fluids, NS, D-5, D-10, or LR. Rapid IV infusion may produce neurotoxicity manifested by hallucinations, inability to think clearly, and seizures.

Pediatric
Neonates. For severe *Pseudomonas, E. coli, Proteus,* and *H. influenzae* infections, administer IM or by a 15 min IV infusion.

1. Under 2 kg:
    a. First 7 days after birth: 100 mg/kg/12 hr.
    b. After 7 days: 100 mg/kg/8 hr.
2. Over 2 kg:
    a. First 7 days after birth: 100 mg/kg/12 hr.
    b. After 7 days: 100 mg/kg/6 hr.

Children

IV 1. Severe systemic *Pseudomonas* infections: 400 to 500 mg/kg/24 hr in divided doses.
2. Severe systemic *E. coli* or *Proteus* infections: 300 to 400 mg/kg/24 hr in divided doses.

Nurse and patient considerations

* See General information on penicillin (p. 3).
* Since resistant organisms may develop, susceptibility testing should be performed before and during the course of therapy.

* PO administration often produces an unpleasant taste sometimes accompanied by nausea, dry mouth, and furry tongue.
* Patients with impaired renal function tend to accumulate carbenicillin. These patients should receive lower doses, and the clinician should monitor coagulation tests and observe for signs of hemorrhage and neurotoxicity. If the patient's creatinine clearance is less than 5 ml/min, therapeutic urine levels will not be achieved.
* Carbenicillin disodium has a large sodium content, 5 to 6 mEq/g and should therefore be used with caution in patients on sodium-restricted diets; their cardiac and electrolyte status should be monitored closely.

Drug interactions

See General information on penicillin (p. 3).

Carbenicillin has been reported to inactivate aminoglycosides (gentamicin, tobramycin, others) in vitro; therefore give IV at different times or give the gentamicin IM and the carbenicillin IV.

Methicillin
(Staphcillin, Celbenin)

AHFS 8:12.16
CATEGORY Penicillin
antibiotic

Action and use

Methicillin is a penicillinase-resistant derivative of penicillin. It is used to treat moderate to severe infections caused by penicillinase-producing staphylococci.

Characteristics

Peak serum levels: 30 to 60 min (IM). Protein binding: 35% to 40%. Half-life: 30 min. Excretion: unchanged in urine. Dialysis: no, H, P.

Administration and dosage
Adult

IM—Dissolve 1 g of powder in 1.5 ml sterile water to make a solution of 500 mg/ml. Administer 1 to 2 g every 4 to 6 hr.

IV—Dilute 1 g/50 ml of saline solution and administer at a rate of 10 ml/min. Administer 1 to 2 g every 4 to 6 hr.

Pediatric
Neonates

IV 1. Under 2 kg: 25 mg/kg every 12 hr for the first 2
       weeks of age; every 8 hr after 2 weeks of age.
    2. Over 2 kg: 25 mg/kg every 8 hr for the first 2 weeks of
       age; every 6 hr from 2 to 4 weeks of age.
   For severe staphylococcal disease or meningitis, 50 mg/
kg administered IV on the above schedule is recommended.

Infants and older children. Administer 50 mg/kg every 6
   hr.

Nurse and patient considerations

* See General information on penicillin (p. 3).
* Methicillin is an irritant, and pain is a common
  complaint even on deep IM injection. Rotate sites of
  injection and observe for signs of inflammation.
* Although rare, methicillin may cause interstitial
  nephritis. The inflammation may result 1 to 4
  weeks after therapy is initiated and is fully reversible in the majority of cases after therapy is discontinued. Renal function should be monitored routinely and methicillin should be used with caution
  in patients with impaired renal function.
* Bone marrow suppression is more common with
  methicillin than with other penicillin derivatives.
  Agranulocytosis, thrombocytopenia, and anemia
  have occurred with usual doses of methicillin.
* One gram of methicillin contains 3 mEq (69 mg) of
  sodium.

Drug interactions

   See General information on penicillin (p. 3).

Mezlocillin
(Mezlin)

AHFS 8:12.16
CATEGORY Penicillin antibiotic

Action and use

   Mezlocillin is a semisynthetic penicillin (ureido) derivative closely related in chemical structure and activity to carbenicillin, ticarcillin, azlocillin, and piperacillin. Mezlocillin

and piperacillin have a wider spectrum of activity than other penicillins, especially against gram-negative organisms such as *Klebsiella, Citrobacter, Proteus, Enterobacter, Serratia,* and *Pseudomonas* species. Mezlocillin is also quite effective against gram-positive organisms including *Streptococcus faecalis.* It is inactive against penicillinase-producing strains of *Staphylococcus aureus.* Mezlocillin may be used to treat susceptible organisms causing complicated and uncomplicated urinary tract infections, septicemia, uncomplicated gonococcal urethritis, and lower respiratory tract, intraabdominal, gynecologic, and skin infections. In severe infections, especially those in which *P. aeruginosa* is suspected, mezlocillin should be administered in conjunction with an aminoglycoside (gentamicin, tobramycin) antibiotic.

Characteristics

Bioavailable fraction: 0.63 (IM). Protein binding: dose dependent, 27% to 46%. Half-life: 1 hr. Excretion: biliary—20% to 25%; renal—40% to 70% unchanged in urine. Dialysis: yes, H, P. Breast milk: yes.

Administration and dosage

IM—Reconstitute each gram with 3 to 4 ml of sterile water for injection or 3 to 4 ml of 0.5% or 1% lidocaine solution (without epinephrine). Not more than 2 g of mezlocillin should be administered in each IM injection. Inject slowly over 12 to 15 sec to minimize pain.

IV 1. Infusion: Each gram of mezlocillin should be reconstituted by vigorous shaking with at least 10 ml of usual parenteral fluids. The dissolved drug should be further diluted to 50 to 100 ml. Administer by direct infusion over 30 min.
   2. Injection: The reconstituted solution may be injected directly into a vein or IV tubing over 3 to 5 min. Observe for phlebitis.

DOSAGE SCHEDULES
Adult

1. Normal renal function:
   a. Urinary tract infection (uncomplicated): 1.5 to 2 g every 6 hr IM or IV.
   b. Urinary tract infection (complicated): 3 g every 6 hr IV.
   c. Lower respiratory tract, intraabdominal, gynecologic, skin infections, septicemia: 3 g every 4 hr IV or 4 g every 6 hr IV.

   d. Gonococcal urethritis (acute, uncomplicated): 1 to 2 g
      IM or IV with 1 g PO probenecid.
   e. Life-threatening infections: 4 g every 4 hr.
2. Impaired renal function: see chart below.

	Creatinine clearance (ml/min)		
	<10	10-30	>30
Urinary tract infection (uncomplicated)	1.5 g every 8 hr	1.5 g every 8 hr	As above
Urinary tract infection (complicated)	1.5 g every 8 hr	1.5 g every 6 hr	As above
Systemic infection	2 g every 8 hr	3 g every 8 hr	As above
Life-threatening infection	2 g every 6 hr	3 g every 6 hr	As above

Pediatric
Neonates

Body weight (g)	Age	
	≤7 Days	>7 Days
≤2000	75 mg/kg every 12 hr (150 mg/kg/day)	75 mg/kg every 8 hr (225 mg/kg/day)
>2000	75 mg/kg every 12 hr (150 mg/kg/day)	75 mg/kg every 6 hr (300 mg/kg/day)

Children (1 month to 12 years of age). Administer 50 mg/kg
   every 4 hr (300 mg/kg/day) by IV infusion over 30 min or
   by IM injection.

Nurse and patient considerations

* See General information on penicillin (p. 3).
* Since resistant organisms may develop, susceptibility testing should be performed before and during the course of therapy.
* Patients with impaired renal function tend to accumulate mezlocillin. As noted above, these patients should receive lower doses. The clinician should monitor coagulation tests and platelet function tests and observe for signs of hemorrhage and neurotoxicity.

✳ Mezlocillin sodium has a sodium content of 1.85 mEq/g of mezlocillin and should be considered in patients for whom sodium restriction is necessary.

✳ High urine concentrations of mezlocillin may produce false-positive protein reactions (pseudoproteinuria) with the following test methods: sulfosalicylic acid and boiling test, acetic acid test, biuret reaction, and nitric acid test. The bromphenol blue (Albustix, Multistix) reagent strip test is reliable.

Drug interactions

See General information on penicillin (p. 3).

Mezlocillin has been reported to inactivate aminoglycosides (tobramycin, gentamicin) when mixed together; therefore give IV at different times or give the aminoglycoside IM and the mezlocillin IV.

Penicillin G
(Pentids, Pfizerpen, Kesso-Pen-G)

AHFS 8:12.16
CATEGORY Penicillin antibiotic

Action and use

Penicillin G is a bactericidal antibiotic highly effective against many gram-positive streptococci, pneumococci, and nonpenicillinase-producing staphylococci. Other organisms include *Treponema pallidum* (syphilis), *Neisseria gonorrhoeae* (gonorrhea), *Neisseria meningitidis* (meningitis), and *Clostridium*. Most strains of *E. coli*, *Klebsiella*, *Proteus*, *Aerobacter*, and *Pseudomonas* are highly resistant to this form of penicillin.

Characteristics

Peak serum level: 15 to 30 min (IM), 30 to 60 min (PO). Protein binding: 50% to 60%; Half-life: 30 min. Excretion: 60% to 90% of an IM dose unchanged in urine, small amount of feces and milk. Dialysis: no, H, P.

Administration and dosage
Adult

PO—200,000 to 500,000 units every 6 to 8 hr. PO administration of penicillin G should be used only for those microorganisms highly sensitive to it. Penicillin G is partially inactivated by acidic gastric secretions.

Adsorption onto food further diminishes absorption. Administer 1 hr before or 2 hr after meals.

IM—300,000 to 4.8 million units depending on the microorganism and severity of infection being treated.

IV—1 million to 80 million units depending on the microorganism and severity of infection being treated.

Pediatric

Premature and full-term neonates. Administer 30,000 to 50,000 units/kg/12 hr IM or IV. For neonates with meningitis administer 75,000 to 125,000 units/kg/12 hr IV.

Children. Administer 25,000 to 50,000 units/kg/24 hr in 4 to 6 divided doses PO, IM, or IV. If PO administer ½ hr before meals or 2 hr after meals. For children with life-threatening infections such as meningitis, administer 200,000 to 400,000 units/kg/24 hr.

Nurse and patient considerations

* See General information on penicillin (p. 3).

* One million units of penicillin G potassium contain 1.7 mEq (66 mg) of potassium. One million units of penicillin G sodium contain 1.7 mEq (39 mg) of sodium. Electrolytes must be monitored closely when large doses of sodium or potassium penicillin G are administered IV.

Drug interactions

See General information on penicillin (p. 3).

Penicillin V (potassium phenoxymethyl penicillin)
(Compocillin-VK, Pen-Vee-K, V-Cillin K)

AHFS 8:12.16
CATEGORY Penicillin antibiotic

Action and use

Penicillin V is a natural penicillin derivative similar in spectrum and activity to penicillin G. It is, however, more stable in acid media and better absorbed following PO administration. Average blood levels following PO administration are 2 to 5 times higher than those following equal PO doses of penicillin G potassium. Penicillin V is used to treat mild to moderate streptococcal and pneumococcal infections of the upper respiratory tract, otitis media, scarlet fever, and mild, non-penicillinase-producing staphylococcal infections of the skin and soft tissues.

Characteristics

Peak serum levels: 30 to 60 min (PO). Protein binding: 55% to 80%. Half-life: 30 min. Excretion: mostly unchanged in urine, small amount in feces and milk. Dialysis: no, H, P.

Administration and dosage
Adult

PO—250 to 500 mg every 6 hr. Food has minimal effects on absorption; however, it is recommended that administration be 1 hr before or 2 hr after meals.
IM—Not available.
IV—Not available.

Pediatric (under 12 years of age)

PO—30 to 50 mg/kg/day in 3 to 4 divided doses.

> **Nurse and patient considerations**
> ∗ See General information on penicillin (p. 3).

Drug interactions

See general information on penicillin (p. 3).

Piperacillin
(Pipracil)

AHFS 8:12.16
CATEGORY Penicillin antibiotic

Action and use

Piperacillin is a semisynthetic penicillin (aminobenzyl) derivative closely related in chemical structure and activity to carbenicillin, ticarcillin, mezlocillin, and azlocillin. Piperacillin and mezlocillin have a wider spectrum of activity than other penicillins, especially against gram-negative organisms such as *Klebsiella, Citrobacter, Enterobacter, Serratia,* and *Proteus* species. Piperacillin is also quite effective against gram-positive organisms, including *S. faecalis*. It is inactive against penicillinase-producing strains of S. *aureus*.

Piperacillin may be used in the same types of infections for which mezlocillin is indicated, but it has the additional advantages of greater activity against *P. aeruginosa* and better penetration in bone and joint infections. In severe, systemic infections, especially those in which *P. aeruginosa* is suspected, piperacillin should be administered in conjunction with an aminoglycoside (gentamicin, tobramycin) antibiotic.

Characteristics

Bioavailable fraction: 0.7 to 0.8 (IM). Protein binding: 22%. Half-life: 1 hr. Metabolism: none. Excretion: biliary 10% to 25%; 50% to 90% unchanged in urine. Dialysis: yes, H, P. Breast milk: yes.

Administration and dosage

IM—Reconstitute each gram with 2 ml of sterile water for injection or 0.5% of 1% lidocaine solution (without epinephrine). Not more than 2 g of piperacillin should be administered in each IM injection. Inject slowly over 12 to 15 sec to minimize pain.

IV—Infusion: Each gram of piperacillin should be reconstituted with at least 5 ml of usual parenteral fluids. The dissolved drug should be further diluted to 50 to 100 ml. Administer by infusion over 30 min.

Injection: Each gram of piperacillin should be reconstituted by vigorous shaking with at least 5 ml of usual parenteral fluids. Inject directly into a vein or IV tubing over 3 to 5 min. Observe for phlebitis.

DOSAGE SCHEDULES
Adult

1. Normal renal function:
   a. Urinary tract infection (uncomplicated): 6 to 8 g every 6 to 12 hr IM or IV.
   b. Urinary tract infection (complicated): 8 to 16 g every 6 to 8 hr IV.
   c. Lower respiratory tract, intraabdominal, gynecologic, skin infections, septicemia: 12 to 18 g every 4 to 6 hr IV.
   d. Gonococcal urethritis (uncomplicated): 2 g IM with 1 g PO probenecid.
   e. Life-threatening infections: 4 g every 4 hr.
2. Impaired renal function: see chart on p. 24.

| | Creatinine clearance (ml/min) | | |
	< 20	20-40	> 40
Urinary tract infection (uncomplicated)	3 g every 12 hr	As above	As above
Urinary tract infection (complicated)	3 g every 12 hr	3 g every 8 hr	As above
Systemic infection	4 g every 12 hr	4 g every 8 hr	As above

Pediatric

Dosage schedules have not been developed for infants and children under 12 years of age.

Nurse and patient considerations

* See General information on penicillin (p. 3).
* Since resistant organisms may develop, susceptibility testing should be performed before and during the course of therapy.
* Patients with impaired renal function tend to accumulate piperacillin. These patients should receive lower doses. The clinician should monitor coagulation tests and platelet function tests and observe for signs of hemorrhage and neurotoxicity.
* Piperacillin has a sodium content of 1.98 mEq/g and should be considered in patients in whom sodium restriction is necessary.

Drug interactions

See General information on penicillin (p. 3).

Piperacillin has been reported to inactivate aminoglycosides (tobramycin, gentamicin) when mixed together; therefore give IV at different times or give the aminoglycoside IM and the piperacillin IV.

Ticarcillin disodium
(Ticar)

AHFS 8:12.16
CATEGORY Penicillin antibiotic

Action and use

Ticarcillin is a semisynthetic penicillin derivative closely related in chemical structure and activity to carbenicillin.

Ticarcillin (in combination with other antipseudomonal agents) is used primarily in the treatment of infections caused by *P. aeruginosa*. It may also be used to treat susceptible strains of *Proteus species* and *E. coli.* In the appropriate doses ticarcillin may be useful for the treatment of serious systemic, respiratory tract, urinary tract, or soft tissue or skin infections due to susceptible organisms.

Characteristics

Peak level: 60 min (IM). Duration: 4 to 6 hr (IM). Protein binding: 50% to 65%. Half-life: 70 min. Metabolism: liver. Excretion: 85% to 95% unchanged, 5% to 15% as penicilloic acid, in urine. Dialysis: yes, H, P.

Administration and dosage
Adult

IM—Reconstitute each gram with 2 ml of sterile water for injection. Not more than 2 g of the drug should be administered in each IM injection. For IM use only the powder may be diluted with 1% lidocaine solution (without epinephrine) or bacteriostatic water containing 0.9% benzyl alcohol to reduce pain on injection.

IV 1. Normal renal function: 200 to 350 mg/kg/day in divided doses for systemic, respiratory, and soft tissue infections; 1 g every 6 hr for urinary tract infections.

2. Impaired renal function: loading dose of 3 g followed by subsequent doses (see chart below).

Creatinine clearance rate (CCR)(ml/min)	Dosage
>60	3 g every 4 hr
30 to 60	2 g every 4 hr
10 to 30	2 g every 8 hr
<10	2 g every 12 hr (or 1 g IM every 6 hr)

In patients with hepatic dysfunction and a creatinine clearance of less than 10 ml/min administer 2 g/day IV or 1 g every 12 hr IM.

Each gram of ticarcillin should be reconstituted with at least 4 ml of sterile water for injection. The reconstituted solution may be added to usual IV solutions and administered by continuous or intermittent drip. A suggested method is to give one sixth the total daily dose as a 2 hr infusion every 4 hr.

Pediatric
Neonates

1. Under 2 kg: initially 100 mg/kg IM or as a 10 to 20 min IV infusion. Follow every 8 hr with IV infusions of 75 mg/kg during the first week after birth, then increase to 75 mg/kg every 4 to 6 hr.
2. Over 2 kg: initially 100 mg/kg IM or as a 10 to 20 min IV infusion. Follow every 4 to 6 hr with IV infusions of 75 mg/kg during the first 2 weeks after birth, then increase to 100 mg/kg every 4 hr.

Children. For systemic, respiratory, and soft tissue infections, administer IM or IV as for adults. For urinary tract infections in children under 40 kg administer 50 to 100 mg/kg/day IM or IV in divided doses every 6 to 8 hr. For urinary tract infections in children over 40 kg (88 lb) administer as for adults.

Nurse and patient considerations

* See General information on penicillin (p. 3).
* Since resistant organisms may develop, susceptibility testing should be performed before and during the course of therapy.
* Patients with impaired renal function tend to accumulate ticarcillin. As noted above, and these patients should receive lower doses. The clinician should monitor coagulation tests and platelet function and observe for signs of hemorrhage and neurotoxicity.
* Ticarcillin disodium has a high sodium content (5 to 6.5 mEq/g) and should therefore be used with caution in patients on sodium-restricted diets; their cardiac and electrolyte status should be monitored closely.

Drug interactions

See General information on penicillin (p. 3).

Ticarcillin has been reported to inactivate gentamicin and tobramycin when mixed together; therefore give IV at different times or give the gentamicin or tobramycin IM and the carbenicillin IV.

Cephalosporins
GENERAL INFORMATION

The cephalosporins are structurally and pharmacologically related to the penicillins. The parent compound, cephalosporin C, was produced from the fungus *Cephalosporium acremonium,* which was first collected from a sewer effluent on the island of Sardinia in 1945.

The mechanism of action of cephalosporins is inhibition of mucopeptide synthesis in the bacterial cell wall. The drugs are both bacteriostatic and bactericidal, depending on the concentration of the drug present. Cephalosporins are usually resistant to penicillinase; however, strains that may produce destructive enzymes called cephalosporinases are becoming more common.

Cephalosporins may be divided into groups or generations, based on their chemical structure and biologic activity. They are highly effective in the therapy of a variety of mild to severe infections caused by both gram-positive and gram-negative microorganisms. See Table 1-3 for a comparison of cephalosporins.

Nurse and patient considerations

Before cephalosporin therapy is initiated, inquiry must be made concerning allergic reactions to cephalosporins and penicillin. Hypersensitivity reactions ranging from maculopapular rash, urticaria, eosinophilia, and serum sickness to anaphylaxis have occurred in about 5% of patients receiving cephalosporins. Patients who are allergy prone, especially to drugs, must be observed particularly closely.

Dermatologic reactions of varying character and distribution are the most common allergic reactions to cephalosporins, although any manifestation of hypersensitivity, including anaphylaxis, is possible. Skin rashes and serum sickness may be controlled by antihistamines (diphenhydramine) or corticosteroids (hydrocortisone, prednisone). When reactions do occur, discontinue use of the antibiotic, unless a life-threatening infection is being treated. If major allergic manifestations develop (laryngeal edema, anaphylactic shock), treat with epinephrine, oxygen, intravenous steroids, and airway intubation if necessary.

Adverse effects that have occurred with all cephalosporins include oral thrush, gastrointestinal symptoms (especially diarrhea), genital and anal pruritus, genital candidiasis, vaginitis, and vaginal discharge.

A false-positive reaction for glucose in the urine may occur with Clinitest tablets, but not with Tes-Tape.

Transient elevations of SGOT, SGPT, BUN, serum cre-

Table 1-3. Comparison of the cephalosporins

Cephalosporin	Peak level	Protein binding (%)	Half-life (min)	Excretion	Dialysis H	Dialysis P	Neonate	Child	Adult
FIRST GENERATION									
Cephadroxil (Duricef)	1.5 hr (PO)	20	63-119	Excreted unchanged in urine	Yes	Yes	Not recommended	PO: 10-15 mg/kg 3-4 times daily	PO: 1-2 g 1-2 times daily
Cefazolin (Ancef, Kefzol)	(See p. 32)								
Cephalothin (Keflin)	(See p. 39)								
Cephapirin (Cefadyl)	30 min (IM)	45-50	20-50	70% excreted unchanged in urine	Yes	Yes	—	IM or IV: 40-80 mg/kg/day in 4 divided doses	IM or IV: 500 mg to 1 g every 4 to 6 hr
Cephradine (Anspor, Velosef)	60 min (PO); 1-2 hr (IM)	0-20	40-120	Excreted unchanged in urine	Yes	Yes	—	PO: 25-50 mg/kg/day in 4 divided doses; IM or IV: 50-100 mg/kg/day in 4 divided doses	PO: 250-500 mg every 6 hr; IM or IV: 500 mg to 1 g every 6 hr; do not exceed 8 g/day

SECOND GENERATION

Cefaclor (Ceclor)	30-60 min	25	Excreted unchanged in urine	Yes	Yes	Not recommended	PO: 20-40 mg/kg/day in 3 divided doses; do not exceed 1 g/day	PO: 250-500 mg every 8 hr; do not exceed 4 g/day
Cefamandole (Mandol)	(See p. 31)							
Cefoxitin (Mefoxin)	20-30 min	50-80	41-65	Excreted unchanged in urine	Yes	No	Not recommended under 3 months of age	IM or IV: 80-160 mg/kg/day in 4 to 6 divided doses; do not exceed 12 g/day	IM or IV: 1-2 g every 6 to 8 hr; do not exceed 12 g/day

THIRD GENERATION

Cefoperazone (Cefobid)	—	(See p. 34)
Cefotaxime (Claforan)	—	(See p. 36)
Moxalactam (Moxam)	—	(See p. 40)

atinine, and alkaline phosphatase levels have been observed. Nephrotoxicity, as evidenced by proteinuria, hematuria, casts, decreased creatinine clearance, and decreased urine output, has also occurred.

Neutropenia, leukopenia, thrombocytopenia, and positive direct and indirect Coombs' tests have been reported. These are all readily reversible on discontinuation.

Hypoprothrombinemia, with and without bleeding, has been reported. These rare reports occur most frequently in elderly, debilitated, or other compromised patients with a borderline deficiency of vitamin K. Treatment with broad-spectrum antibiotics eliminates enough gastrointestinal flora to cause a further reduction in vitamin K synthesis. The hypoprothrombinemia is readily reversed by administration of vitamin K, 5 to 10 mg.

Phlebitis and thrombophlebitis are recurrent problems associated with intravenous administration of cephalosporins. Use small IV needles and larger veins and alternate infusion sites if possible to minimize irritation.

Cephalosporins readily cross the placental barrier and are probably secreted in human breast milk. Safe use in pregnancy has not been established.

Drug interactions

The cephalosporins are primarily bactericidal antibiotics. They require actively growing cells to be effective. When used concomitantly with bacteriostatic antibiotics, their effectiveness may be decreased or destroyed. Examples of bacteriostatic antibiotics are chloramphenicol, erythromycin, and the tetracyclines.

Probenecid reduces the renal clearance of the cephalosporins, thereby increasing the plasma concentration. This interaction is potentially more significant with those cephalosporins not metabolized (cephalexin, cefazolin, cefoxitin, cephradine, cefadroxil) before excretion. Probenecid does not significantly affect the elimination of moxalactam or cefoperazone.

The possibility of nephrotoxicity may be enhanced by administration of cephalosporins with aminoglycosides (gentamicin, tobramycin, neomycin, kanamycin) and potent diuretics (furosemide, ethacrynic acid).

Alcohol consumed within 48 to 72 hr after ingestion of cefamandole, cefoperazone, and moxalactam may produce a disulfiram-like reaction of alcohol intolerance. Patients become flushed, tremulous, dyspneic, tachycardic, and hypotensive. The use of all alcohol, including medicinal agents with an alcohol base, must be avoided.

Cefamandole naftate
(Mandol)

AHFS 8:12.06
CATEGORY Cephalosporin
antibiotic

Action and use

Cefamandole is a second generation, semisynthetic cephalosporin antibiotic. It is indicated in the treatment of serious infections of the respiratory tract, skin and skin structure, urinary tract, and bone and joints and septicemia caused by susceptible organisms. In addition to providing coverage against those organisms susceptible to first generation cephalosporins (see Cephalothin [p. 39]), cefamandole is more active against gram-negative aerobes such as *H. influenzae,* indole-positive *Proteus, Klebsiella,* and *Enterobacter* species and anaerobes including *Clostridium, Peptococcus, Peptostreptococcus,* and *Bacteroides* species.

Characteristics

Bioavailable fraction: 0.85 to 0.89. Peak serum levels: 30 to 120 min (IM); 10 min (IV). Protein binding: 67% to 74%. Half-life: 60 min (IM); 30 min (IV). Excretion: unchanged in urine. Dialysis: yes, H, P. Breast milk: yes.

Administration and dosage
Adult

IM or IV 1. Normal renal function: 0.5 to 1 g every 4 to 8 hr, not to exceed 12 g/24 hr. IV infusion rate: 3 to 5 min.

2. Impaired renal function: a loading dose of 1 to 2 is given, followed by a dosage adjustment based on creatinine clearance (see chart below).

Creatinine clearance (ml/min)	Mild to moderate infections	Severe infections
50-80	0.75-1.5 g every 6 hr	1.5 g every 4 hr or 2 g every 6 hr
25-50	0.75-1.5 g every 8 hr	1.5 g every 6 hr or 2 g every 8 hr
10-25	0.5-1 g every 8 hr	1 g every 6 hr or 1.25 g every 8 hr
<2	0.25-0.5 g every 12 hr	0.5 g every 8 hr or 0.75 g every 12 hr

Pediatric
Neonates. The use of cephalosporins is not recommended in these patients

Children (over 1 month of age)
IV—Administer 50 to 100 mg/kg/day in 3 to 6 divided doses. In severe infections, pediatric dosages may be increased to 150 mg/kg/day, not to exceed recommendations for adults.

Nurse and patient

* Pain, tenderness, and induration are common following repeated IM injections. Rotate injection sites and observe for inflammation. Thrombophlebitis is a relatively common complication of IV therapy. Observe for it. Some studies indicate that in-line filters may be successful in reducing venous irritation.

* See General information on cephalosporins (p. 27).

Drug interactions

Alcohol consumed within 48 to 72 hr after administration of cefamandole may produce a disulfiram-like reaction of alcohol intolerance. Clinically, patients become flushed, tremulous, dyspneic, tachycardic, and hypotensive. The use of all alcohol, including medicinal agents with an alcohol base, must be avoided in these patients.

See General information on cephalosporins (p. 27).

Cefazolin sodium
(Kefzol, Ancef)

AHFS 8:12.06
CATEGORY Cephalosporin antibiotic

Action and use

Cefazolin sodium is a first generation cephalosporin with an action and a spectrum similar to cephalothin, with the following exceptions. It is effective in treating susceptible gram-negative and gram-positive organisms of the respiratory and genitourinary tract and staphylococcal infections of bones and joints. It is not recommended for use in gram-negative skin and soft tissue infections, endocarditis, meningitis, or peritonitis.

Characteristics

Peak plasma levels: 60 min (IM). Protein binding: 75% to 80%. Half-life: 100 min. Excretion: 80% unchanged in urine in 24 hr. Dialysis: no, H, P.

Administration and dosage
Adult

PO—Not available.

IM—250 mg to 1 g every 6 to 8 hr.

IV—250 mg to 1.5 g every 6 to 8 hr. Dilute 500 mg to 1 g of reconstituted cefazolin in a minimum of 10 ml of sterile water for injection. Inject slowly over 5 min through the tubing or directly into the vein. Cefazolin is stable after reconstitution for 24 hr at room temperature and for 96 hr if stored under refrigeration.

NOTE: As a result of minimal metabolism and major excretion via the kidneys, dosage adjustment is required in patients with impaired renal function.

Pediatric
Neonates. Safety for use in premature infants and infants under 1 month of age has not been established. The use of cefazolin is not recommended in these patients.

Children

IM or IV
1. Mild to moderate infections: 25 to 50 mg/kg/24 hr (10 to 20 mg/16 to 24 hr) in divided doses.
2. Life-threatening infections: to 100 mg/kg/24 hr in divided doses.

Nurse and patient considerations

* See General information on cephalosporins (p. 27).
* A specific advantage of cefazolin over other parenteral cephalosporins is the relative pain-free IM injection.

Drug interactions

See General information on cephalosporins (p. 27).

Cefoperazone sodium
(Cefobid)

AHFS 8:12.06
CATEGORY Cephalosporin
antibiotic

Action and use

Cefoperazone is a third generation semisynthetic cephalosporin derivative. The third generation cephalosporins are somewhat less active against gram-positive cocci than the first and second generation cephalosporins. They are, however, more active against gram-negative organisms such as *E. coli, Klebsiella, N. gonorrhoeae,* indole-positive *Proteus,* and *H. influenzae.* They are also the first cephalosporins to have some activity against *P. aeruginosa.*

Cefoperazone may be used to treat serious urinary tract, skin and skin structure, lower respiratory tract, intraabdominal, and gynecologic infections. It may also be used to treat septicemia caused by susceptible organisms. It is not indicated in bone and joint infections or meningitis.

When compared with moxalactam and cefotaxime, cefoperazone does have the advantages of greater activity against *P. aeruginosa* (although it is not the drug of choice), high biliary concentrations, and 2 times daily dosage, and no adjustment in dosage is necessary in renal failure.

Characteristics

Peak serum levels: 1.5 hr (IM). Protein binding: 87% to 93%. Half-life: 1.6 to 2.6 hr; severe hepatic dysfunction—3 to 7.1 hr. Metabolism: minimal. Excretion: biliary—60% to 85%; renal—15% to 36% by glomerular filtration. Dialysis: yes, H; no, P. Breast milk: yes.

Administration and dosage
Adult

IM—As for IV. Not recommended in septicemia, shock, or life-threatening infections. Reconstitute with sterile water for injection or 0.5% lidocaine hydrochloride injection (without epinephrine). Reconstitution with lidocaine is recommended if the final concentration is greater than 250 mg/ml.

IV   1. Reconstitute with 3 to 5 ml of parenteral diluent/g of cefoperazone.
   2. Infusion: Dilute with 20 to 40 ml of parenteral fluid/g and administer over 15 to 30 min.

DOSAGE SCHEDULE

Administer 1 to 2 g every 12 hr. For severe infections, increase the total daily dosage to 6 to 12 g, divided into 3 or 4 equal dosages. Dosage adjustment for renal impairment alone is not necessary. Adjustment is necessary in patients with both severe hepatic and renal dysfunction.

Pediatric

Dosage recommendations have not been established.

Nurse and patient considerations

* Hypersensitivity reactions have been reported to occur in about 2% of patients receiving cefoperazone.
* The most frequently occurring adverse effect (5%) has been diarrhea or loose stools. Most cases have been mild to moderate in severity and self-limiting. Antibiotic-associated pseudomembranous colitis caused by toxin-producing clostridia has rarely been reported. If significant diarrhea develops (more than 5 bowel movements/day), the drug should be discontinued. The use of opiates, meperidine (Demerol), loperamide (Imodium), or diphenoxylate with atropine (Lomotil) may prolong and/or worsen the condition. Large doses of kaolin-pectin (Kaopectate) may be effective in diminishing the diarrhea. Oral vancomycin has been quite effective in controlling the overgrowth of clostridia.
* Cefoperazone has a sodium content of 1.5 mEq/g and should be considered in patients for whom sodium restriction is necessary.
* See General information on cephalosporins (p. 27).

Drug interactions

Alcohol consumed within 48 to 72 hr after administration of cefoperazone may produce a disulfiram-like reaction of alcohol intolerance. Clinically, patients become flushed, tremulous, dyspneic, tachycardic, and hypotensive. The use of all alcohol, including medicinal agents with an alcohol base, must be avoided in these patients. See General information on cephalosporins. (p. 27).

Cefotaxime sodium
(Claforan)

AHFS 8:12.06
CATEGORY Cephalosporin
antibiotic

Action and use

Cefotaxime is a third generation semisynthetic cephalosporin derivative. The third generation cephalosporins are somewhat less active against gram-positive cocci than the first and second generation cephalosporins. They are, however, more active against gram-negative organisms such as *E. coli, Klebsiella, Neisseria,* indole-positive *Proteus,* and *H. influenzae.* They are also the first cephalosporins to have some activity against *P. aeruginosa;* however, they should not be considered drugs of choice for this pathogen.

Cefotaxime may be used to treat genitourinary tract, bone and joint, skin and skin structure, lower respiratory tract, intraabdominal, and gynecologic infections. It may also be used to treat meningitis and septicemia caused by susceptible organisms. Cefotaxime has certain advantages over moxalactam, another third generation cephalosporin. Cefotaxime has greater activity against gram-positive cocci and gram-negative cocci, *Acinetobacter, E. coli, Klebsiella, Proteus,* and *Serratia.* It is also considerably more active against penicillinase-producing *N. gonorrhea* than moxalactam.

Characteristics

Peak serum levels: 30 min. (IM). Protein binding: 13% to 38%. Metabolism: blood—desacetylcefotaxime (active); liver—desacetylcefotaxime lactone (inactive). Half-lives: cefotaxime-biphasic (normal renal function)—alpha-phase, 0.2 to 0.4 hr, beta-phase, 0.9 to 1.7 hr; severe renal failure—beta-phase, 1.4 to 11.5 hr, desacetylcefotaxime (normal renal function)—beta-phase, 1.4 to 1.9 hr; severe renal failure—8.2 to 56.8 hr. Excretion: renal—40% to 60% as unchanged drug and 24% as desacetylcefotaxime within 24 hr. Dialysis: yes, H; no, P. Breast milk: yes.

Administration and dosage
Adult

IM—As for IV. Not recommended in septicemia, shock, or life-threatening infections.

IV—Direct. Inject directly into vein or freely flowing parenteral solution over 3 to 5 min. Intermittent infusion. Dilute to 50 to 100 ml and administer over 20 to 30 min. A solution of 1 g cefotaxime in 14 ml of sterile water for injection is isotonic.

DOSAGE SCHEDULES

1. Normal renal function (not to exceed 12 g daily):
   a. Gonorrhea: 1 g IM (single dose).
   b. Respiratory and urinary tract infection (uncomplicated): 1 g every 12 hr IM or IV.
   c. Moderate to severe infections: 1 to 2 g every 6 to 8 hrs IM or IV.
   d. Septicemia: 2 g every 6 to 8 hrs IV
   e. Life-threatening infections: 2 g every 4 hr IV
2. Impaired renal function (creatinine clearance <20 ml/min/1.73 m^2). Reduce the dosage by one-half.

Pediatric

Ages 0 to 1 week. Administer 50 mg/kg every 12 hr IV.

Ages 1 to 4 weeks. Administer 50 mg/kg every 8 hr IV.

Ages 1 month to 12 years (<50 kg). Administer 50 to 180 mg/kg every 4 to 6 hr IM or IV.

Ages 5 to 12 years (>50 kg). Administer adult doses.

Nurse and patient considerations

∗ Hypersensitivity reactions have been reported to occur in about 2% of patients receiving cefotaxime.
∗ The most frequently occurring adverse effects (5%) have been at the site of injection. Patients complain of pain, induration, and tenderness at the IM injection site, and IV administration causes phlebitis.
∗ Adverse gastrointestinal effects are reported in about 2% of patients receiving cefotaxime. Symptoms include anorexia, abdominal pain, nausea, vomiting, diarrhea, and colitis. Antibiotic-associated pseudomembranous colitis caused by toxin-producing clostridia has rarely been reported. If significant diarrhea develops (more than 5 bowel movements/day), the drug should be discontinued. The use of opiates, meperidine (Demerol), loperamide (Imodium), or diphenoxylate with atropine (Lomotil) may prolong and/or worsen the condition. Large doses of kaolin-pectin (Kaopectate) may be effective in diminishing the diarrhea. Oral vancomycin has been quite effective in controlling the overgrowth of clostridia.

* Contrary to reports concerning most other cephalosporins, cefotaxime does not appear to cause false-positive results with urine glucose tests using the cupric sulfate method (Clinitest).
* Cefoperazone has a sodium content of 2.2 mEq/g and should be considered in patients for whom sodium restriction is necessary.
* See General information on cephalosporins (p. 27).

Drug Interactions

See General information on cephalosporins (p. 27).

Cephalexin monohydrate
(Keflex)

AHFS 8:12.06
CATEGORY Cephalosporin
antibiotic

Action and use

Cephalexin is a first generation, semisynthetic antibiotic for PO administration. It is used for patients treated initially with a parenteral cephalosporin who require continued antibiotic therapy but whose improved clinical status no longer warrants parenteral administration.

Characteristics

Peak plasma levels: 1 hr. Protein binding: 10% to 15%. Half-life: 1 hr. Metabolism: none. Excretion: more than 90% unchanged within 8 hr in urine. Dialysis: yes, H, P.

Administration and dosage
Adult

PO—250 mg to 1 g every 6 hr.

Pediatric

PO—25 to 50 mg/kg/24 hr in divided doses.

Nurse and patient considerations

* See General information on cephalosporins (p. 27).
* Mild diarrhea is a common side effect of cephalexin. Nausea, vomiting, and abdominal pain also occur.

Drug interactions

See General information on cephalosporins (p. 27).

Cephalothin sodium
(Keflin)

AHFS 8:12.06
CATEGORY Cephalosporin
antibiotic

Action and use

Cephalothin is a first generation semisynthetic cephalosporin derivative. The first generation cephalosporins are fairly active against gram-positive cocci such as *Streptococcus pneumoniae*, groups A and B streptococci, non-penicillinase-producing *S. aureus,* and *Staphylococcus epidermidis*. The first generation derivatives are less active against gram-negative organisms including *E. coli,* Klebsiella *Pneumoniae, P. mirabilis,* and *Shigella*. They are inactive against enterococci such as *S. faecalis, Bacteroides,* other *Proteus* species, *Providencia, Pseudomonas,* and *Serratia* species.

Cephalothin is indicated in the treatment of respiratory and urinary tract, soft tissue and skin, gastrointestinal tract, bone and joint, and septicemic infections caused by susceptible organisms. It is not considered a drug of choice for meningitis.

Characteristics

Peak plasma level: 30 min (IM). Protein binding: 56% to 60%. Half-life: 40 min. Metabolism: 20% to 30% to a weakly active metabolite. Excretion: 60% to 80% unchanged, 20% to 30% as weakly active metabolite, in urine. Dialysis: yes, H, P.

Administration and dosage
Adult

PO—Not available.

IM—500 mg to 1 g every 4 to 6 hr.

IV—Mild to moderate infections: 500 mg to 1 g every 4 to 6 hr; life-threatening infections: 1 g to 2 g every 4 to 6 hr. Dosage adjustment is required in impaired renal function.

RATE—1 g diluted in 10 ml of diluent and administered over 5 min. Solutions stored at room temperature should be used within 6 hr after reconstitution. The concentrated solution will darken, especially at room temperature.

Pediatric

IM OR IV—80 to 160 mg/kg/24 hr (40 to 80 mg/lb) in divided doses.

RATE—As for adult dosages.

Nurse and patient considerations

* Pain, tenderness, and induration is common following repeated IM injections. Rotate injection sites and observe for inflammation. Thrombophlebitis is a relatively common complication of IV therapy. It is associated with doses of more than 6 g daily for longer than 3 days. Some studies indicate that inline filters may be successful in reducing venous irritation.
* See General information on cephalosporins (p. 27).

Drug interactions

See General information on cephalosporins (p. 27).

Moxalactam disodium
(Moxam)

AHFS 8:12.28
CATEGORY Cephalosporin-like antibiotic

Action and use

Moxalactam is a semisynthetic beta-lactam antibiotic. It is not a true cephalosporin but is similar in chemical structure and is classified as a third generation cephalosporin along with cefotaxime and cefoperazone.

The third generation cephalosporins are somewhat less active against gram-positive cocci than the first and second generation cephalosporins. They are, however, more active against gram-negative organisms such as *E. coli, Klebsiella, Neisseria,* indole-positive *Proteus,* and *H. influenzae.* They are also the first cephalosporins to have some activity against *P. aeruginosa;* however, they should not be considered drugs of choice for this pathogen.

Moxalactam may be used to treat serious urinary tract, bone and joint, skin and skin structure, lower respiratory tract, and intraabdominal infections. It also may be used to treat meningitis and septicemia caused by susceptible organisms. Moxalactam currently offers few advantages over cefotaxime. Moxalactam does show more activity against *Enterobacter* organisms, is effective in the treatment of gram-negative meningitis, and is more resistant to destruction by beta-lactamases than cephalosporins.

Characteristics

Peak serum levels: 30 to 120 min (IM). Protein binding: 45% to 60%. Half-life: normal renal function—2 to 3.5 hr;

severe renal failure—14 hr. Metabolism: no. Excretion: 60% to 97% unchanged in urine in 24 hr by glomerular filtration, no tubular secretion. Dialysis: yes, H; no, P. Breast milk: unknown, but probable.

Administration and dosage
Adult

IM—As for IV. Not recommended in septicemia, shock, or life-threatening infections.

IV—Direct. Inject directly into vein or freely flowing parenteral solution over 3 to 5 min.

Intermittent infusion. Dilute to 50 to 100 ml and administer over 20 to 30 min. A solution of 1 g moxalactam in 20 ml of sterile water for injection is isotonic.

DOSAGE SCHEDULE

1. Normal renal function (not to exceed 12 g daily):
   a. Mild skin infection and uncomplicated pneumonia: 500 mg every 8 hr IM or IV.
   b. Mild to moderate infections: 500 mg to 2 g every 12 hr.
   c. Urinary tract infection (uncomplicated): 250 mg every 12 hr.
   d. Urinary tract infection (complicated): 500 mg every 8 to 12 hr IM or IV.
   e. Life-threatening infections: up to 4 g every 8 hr.
2. Impaired renal function:
   IM or IV—A loading dose of 1 to 2 g is given, followed by a dosage adjustment based on creatinine clearance (see chart below).

Creatinine clearance (ml/min)	Mild to moderate infections	Severe infections
50-80	0.5-1 g every 8 hr	3 g every 8 hr
25-50	0.25-1 g every 12 hr	3 g every 12 hr
2-25	0.25-0.5 g every 8 hr	1.25 g every 12 hr
<2	0.25-0.5 g every 12 hr	1 g every 24 hr

Pediatric

Ages 0 to 1 week. Administer 50 mg/kg every 12 hr IV.

Ages 1 to 4 weeks. Administer 50 mg/kg every 8 hr IV.

Ages 1 month to 1 year. Administer 50 mg/kg every 6 hr IV.

Ages 1 to 14 years. Administer 50 mg/kg every 6 to 8 hr IV.

Maximum dosage is 200 mg/kg, up to 12 g daily.

Nurse and patient considerations

* Hypersensitivity reactions have been reported to occur in about 3% of patients receiving moxalactam. There is also a 5% incidence of cross-sensitivity to patients with a history of allergy to penicillins and/or cephalosporins.
* Adverse gastrointestinal effects are reported in about 3% of patients who received moxalactam. Symptoms include anorexia, abdominal pain, nausea, vomiting, diarrhea, and colitis. Antibiotic-associated pseudomembranous colitis caused by toxin-producing clostridia has rarely occurred. If significant diarrhea develops (more than 5 bowel movements per day), the drug should be discontinued. The use of opiates, meperidine (Demerol), loperamide (Imodium), or diphenoxylate with atropine (Lomotil) may prolong and/or worsen the condition. Large doses of kaolin-pectin (Kaopectate) may be effective in diminishing the diarrhea. Oral vancomycin has been quite effective in controlling the overgrowth of clostridia.
* Moxalactam does *not* appear to cause false-positive results with urine glucose tests using the cupric sulfate method (Clinitest).
* Moxalactam has a sodium content of 3.8 mEq/g and should be considered in patients where sodium restriction is necessary.
* See General information on cephalosporins (p. 27).

Drug interactions

Alcohol consumed within 48 to 72 hr after administration of moxalactam may produce a disulfiram-like reaction of alcohol intolerance. Clinically, patients become flushed, tremulous, dyspneic, tachycardic, and hypotensive. The use of all alcohol, including medicinal agents with an alcohol base, must be avoided in these patients.

See General information on cephalosporins (p. 27).

Aminoglycosides
GENERAL INFORMATION

Aminoglycoside antibiotics are an important class of antibacterial agents used in moderate to severe infections. The aminoglycosides act directly on the 30 S ribosomal subunit of bacterial cells, causing mutations of the genetic code required for normal protein synthesis. High concentrations of aminoglycosides are bactericidal, while low concentrations are bacteriostatic. Resting cells are less susceptible to the drug than are multiplying bacteria. Aminoglycosides are primarily effective against gram-negative bacterial infections. As a result of the widespread use of aminoglycosides, resistant strains of microorganisms have rapidly emerged. Combination therapy with other antibiotics with an alternate mechanism of action is often used to inhibit the emergence of resistant strains.

Nurse and patient considerations

A relatively common, dose-related side effect of the aminoglycosides is ototoxicity. It may affect the vestibular branch of the eighth cranial nerve, resulting in dizziness, vertigo, tinnitus, and roaring in the ears. Damage to the cochlear branch of the eighth cranial nerve may result in deafness. Instruct the patient to report any of these toxic effects. Withhold the next dose pending consultation with the physician. Audiometric studies are recommended during prolonged or with increased dosage therapy.

Other neurologic dysfunctions include peripheral neuritis causing tingling and numbness usually around the mouth and of the hands and neuromuscular blockade that may result in respiratory depression and/or paralysis.

Renal damage is a potential toxic effect of aminoglycoside therapy. Nephrotoxicity may be manifested by oliguria, granular casts in the urine, proteinuria, and increased BUN and serum creatinine levels. Input and output, as well as a progressive decrease in daily urine volume or changes in visual characteristics, should be reported.

Skin rashes, eosinophilia, fever, blood dyscrasias, stomatitis, and anaphylaxis are among the hypersensitivity reactions that may follow the administration of aminoglycosides.

Blood dyscrasias are rare, but may include neutropenia, agranulocytosis, aplastic anemia, and thrombocytopenia with purpura.

Other rare adverse effects include loss of hair, increased salivation, hypotension, hypertension, anorexia, weight loss, and joint pain.

Transient hepatosplenomegaly has occurred with elevated serum transaminase levels and hyperbilirubinemia.

Drug interactions

Cephalosporins may enhance the nephrotoxic potential of the aminoglycosides.

Ethacrynic acid (Edecrin) and furosemide (Lasix) may enhance the ototoxicity of aminoglycosides.

Aminoglycoside antibiotics, alone and in combination with skeletal muscle relaxants (succinylcholine, tubocurarine, pancuronium bromide) may produce respiratory paralysis. This interaction has occurred 48 hr postoperatively and is independent of the route of administration. Calcium and reversible cholinesterase inhibitors (neostigmine—Prostigmin, edrophonium—Tensilon) have been effective in reversing the paralysis.

Amikacin sulfate
(Amikin)

AHFS 8:12.28
CATEGORY Aminoglycoside antibiotic

Action and use

Amikacin is an aminoglycoside antibiotic used in the short-term treatment of serious infections caused by susceptible bacteria. Clinical studies indicate that amikacin may be effective against *P. aeruginosa, E. coli,* and *Proteus, Providencia, Klebsiella, Enterobacter,* and *Serratia* species resistant to gentamicin and/or tobramycin. Amikacin is also active against *S. aureus* and *S. epidermidis.* Because of potential toxicity amikacin should not be used for minor infections or against bacteria susceptible to less toxic drugs. Use should be restricted to 2 weeks.

Characteristics

Peak levels: 60 min (IM). Duration: to 12 hr. Protein binding: less than 11%. Half-life: 2 to 3 hr. Excretion: unchanged in urine. Dialysis: yes, H; poor, P.

Administration and dosage
Adult

IM or IV 1. Normal renal function: 15 mg/kg/day in 2 to 4 equally divided doses. Do not exceed 1.5 g per day. When administered IV dilute the dose with 100 to 200 ml of standard IV solution and infuse over 30 to 60 min.

2. Impaired renal function
   a. Normal dosage at prolonged intervals:

   Serum creatinine (100 mg/100 ml) × 9 =
   Dose interval (hr)

   Example: If the serum creatinine is 3, administer the single recommended dose (7.5 mg/kg) every 27 hr.
   b. Reduced dosage at fixed time intervals:
   Loading dose = 7.5 mg/kg

   Maintenance dose every 12 hours =

   $$\frac{\text{Observed CCR (ml/min)}}{\text{Normal CCR (ml/min)}} \times$$
   Calculated loading dose (mg)

   Example: If a patient weighs 60 kg and has a steady creatinine clearance of 35 ml/min:

   $$\frac{35 \text{ ml/min}}{100 \text{ ml/min}} \times (60 \text{ kg} \times 7.5 \text{ mg/kg}) =$$
   157 mg/12 hr

Pediatric
Neonates

IM or IV—Loading: 10 mg/kg; maintenance: 7.5 mg/kg every 12 hr. Infuse IV over 1 to 2 hr.

Older infants and children

IM or IV—15 mg/kg day in 2 to 4 equally divided doses. Infuse IV over 30 to 60 min.

Nurse and patient considerations

＊ See General information on aminoglycosides (p. 43).

Drug interactions

See General information on aminoglycosides (p. 43).

Gentamicin sulfate
(Garamycin)

AHFS 8:12.28
CATEGORY Aminoglycoside
antibiotic

Action and use

At present gentamicin is the most widely used aminoglycoside. Its mode of action is similar to that of the other members of this class. As a result of potential toxicity and the development of resistant organisms, gentamicin should only be used in severe infections caused by susceptible gram-negative organisms such as *P. aeruginosa* and *E. coli; Proteus, Klebsiella, Enterobacter,* and *Serratia* species; and most *Salmonella* and *Shigella* species.

Characteristics

Peak plasma level: 1 to 1½ hr (IM). Protein binding: 25% to 30%. Half-life: 2 hr. Excretion: unchanged in urine. Toxic level: 10 to 12 µg/ml. Dialysis: yes, H; no, P.

Administration and dosage
Adult

PO—Not available.

IM—As for IV.

IV 1. Normal renal function:
   a. Urinary tract infection: 3 mg/kg/24 hr.
   b. Other infections: 3 to 5 mg/kg/24 hr.
   c. Life threatening infections: at least 5 mg/kg/24 hr reduced to 3 mg/kg/24 hr as soon as clinically indicated.

The usual adult dose is 60 mg 3 times daily for those patients weighing less than 60 kg (132 lb) and 80 mg 3 times daily for those patients weighing more than 60 kg (132 lb).

2. Renal failure (see Table 1-4). Dilute with saline solution or dextrose 5% to a concentration not greater than 1 mg/ml. Administer over 30 to 60 min. Alkalinization of the urine provides greater urinary concentrations for treating urinary tract infections.

Pediatric
Neonates

IV 1. First 7 days after birth (premature or full-term): 2.5 mg/kg/12 hr.
   2. After 7 days: 2.5 mg/kg/8 hr.

Table 1-4. Gentamicin dosage in renal failure

CCR (ml/min)	<2	4	8	10	20	30	40	50	60	70*
mg/kg/8 hr	0.13	0.2	0.26	0.33	0.6	0.8	1.0	1.3	1.5	1.7
	mg/8 hr	mg/8 hr	mg/8 hr	mg/8 hr	mg/8 hr	mg/8 hr	mg/8 hr	mg/8 hr	mg/8 hr	mg/8 hr
50 kg (110 lb) L.D. = 85 mg	6.5	10	13	16.5	30	40	50	65	75	85
60 kg (132 lb) L.D. = 102 mg	7.8	12	15.6	20	36	48	60	78	90	102
70 kg (154 lb) L.D. = 120 mg	9	14	18	23	42	56	70	91	105	120
80 kg (176 lb) L.D. = 136 mg	10	16	21	26	48	64	80	104	120	136
90 kg (198 lb) L.D. = 153 mg	12	18	24	30	54	72	90	117	135	153
100 kg (220 lb) L.D. = 170 mg	13	20	26	33	60	80	100	130	150	170

Modified from Chan, R.A., et al.: Ann. Intern. Med. **76:**773-778, 1972.

*For patients with creatinine clearance greater than 70 ml/min, this dosage provides 5 mg/kg/day. In non-life-threatening infections this dosage should be reduced to 3 mg/kg/day or 1 mg/kg/8 hr.

KEY: CCR—Creatinine clearance rate (ml/min × 1.73 m^2).

L.D.—Loading dose of 1.7 mg/kg followed every 8 hr by the calculated maintenance dose.

Children (normal renal function). Administer 2 to 2.5 mg/
kg/8 hr. Dilute with saline solution or dextrose 5% to a
concentration not greater than 1 mg/ml. Administer over
a 1 to 2 hr period. Do not mix with other drugs.

Nurse and patient considerations

* See General information on aminoglycosides (p.
  43).
* As a result of potentially severe neurotoxicity and
  nephrotoxicity, monitoring of renal and eighth cranial nerve function is recommended.

Drug interactions

See General information on aminoglycosides (p. 43).

As a result of chemical and physical incompatibilities,
carbenicillin slowly inactivates gentamicin. Do not mix
together before infusion.

Gentamicin and heparin are chemically incompatible.
Do not mix together before infusion.

Kanamycin sulfate
(Kantrex)

AHFS 8:12.28
CATEGORY Aminoglycoside
antibiotic

Action and use

Kanamycin is an aminoglycoside used in the short-term
treatment of susceptible strains of *E. coli, Proteus, Enterobacter, Klebsiella pneumoniae,* and *S. marcescens.* Kanamycin is not effective against *P. aeruginosa.* PO administration
has been useful in suppression of normal bacterial flora in
the bowel when treating hepatic coma.

Characteristics

Peak plasma level: 1 hr (IM). Protein binding: 0% to
3%. Half-life: 2.5 hr. Excretion: 40% to 80% unchanged in
urine in 24 hr. Dialysis: yes, H, P.

Administration and dosage
Adult
PO—8 to 12 g/day in divided doses.

IM—7.5 mg/kg/12 hr or 15 mg/kg/24 hr in equally divided
doses 3 to 4 times daily. Rotate sites of injection.

NOTE: IV administration should be used only if clinical conditions prevent IM administration.

iv—15 mg/kg/24 hr. Add the contents of 500 mg vial to 200 ml of saline solution or dextrose 5% (providing a solution of 2.5 mg/ml) and administer at 60 to 80 gtt/min. Dosages must not exceed 1.5 g/day regardless of the patient's weight. In renal failure the dosing interval is determined by the following formula:

Serum creatinine (mg/100 ml) × 9 = Dose interval (hr)

Example: If the serum creatinine is 3, administer the recommended dose (7.5 mg/kg) every 27 hr.

Pediatric
Neonates. Consult the following chart for neonatal dosages.

Birth weight (g)	≤7 days of age	>7 days of age
≤2000	7.5 mg/kg every 12 hr	10 mg/kg every 12 hr
>2000	10 mg/kg every 12 hr	10 mg/kg every 8 hr

Modified from Eichenwald, H., and McCracken, G. H., Jr.: J. Pediatr. **93**:339, 1978.

Children. As for adult dosages.

Nurse and patient considerations

* See General information on aminoglycosides (p. 43).

Drug interactions

See General information on aminoglycosides (p. 43).

Neomycin sulfate
(Mycifradin, Neobiotic)

AHFS 8:12.28
CATEGORY Aminoglycoside antibiotic

Action and use

Neomycin has the same actions as the other aminoglycosides but is potentially more toxic, especially when administered parenterally. When no other therapy is effective, intramuscular neomycin may be used in the treatment of urinary tract infections caused by susceptible strains of *P.*

aeruginosa, K. pneumoniae, P. vulgaris, E. coli, Aerobacter aerogenes, and *Salmonella* and *Shigella* species.

Neomycin is poorly absorbed (only 3%) from the gastro-intestinal tract. It is effective in suppressing normal gastro-intestinal bacterial flora when treating hepatic coma, diarrhea caused by enteropathogenic *E. coli,* and in preoperative preparation for abdominal surgery.

Characteristics

Half-life: 2 hr. Excretion: 97% unchanged in feces after PO administration, 30% to 50% unchanged in urine after parenteral administration. Dialysis: yes, H; no, P.

Administration and dosage
Adult and pediatric

PO 1. Hepatic coma: 4 to 12 g/day.
2. Infectious diarrhea: 50 mg/kg/day in divided doses.
3. Preoperative bowel sterilization: low-residue diet and 40 mg of neomycin sulfate per *pound* (90 mg/kg) in 6 equally divided doses (1 dose every 4 hr) for 2 to 3 days after the use of a cathartic and if there is no bowel obstruction.

IM—15 mg/kg day in 4 divided doses. The total daily dose should not exceed 1 g of neomycin sulfate. Therapy should not be continued beyond 10 days. Reconstitute by adding 2 ml of normal saline solution (0.9%) to a 0.5 g vial of neomycin sulfate powder, making a solution of 250 mg/ml.

NOTE: IM use is not recommended in pediatric patients.

Nurse and patient considerations

* Neomycin is commonly used in many topical and irrigant preparations. Long-term or high-dose irrigant solutions other than in the bladder or frequent topical administration on large body surface areas may result in systemic adverse effects of neomycin.
* See General information on aminoglycosides (p. 43).

Drug interactions

Neomycin may inhibit the production and/or absorption of vitamin K from the gut. This may be significant in patients receiving oral anticoagulants (warfarin), resulting in increased bleeding tendency and elevated prothrombin time levels.

See General information on aminoglycosides (p. 43).

Paromomycin sulfate
(Humatin)

AHFS 8:04
CATEGORY Aminoglycoside antibiotic

Action and use

Paromomycin is an aminoglycoside antibiotic structurally related to kanamycin, neomycin, gentamicin, and amikacin. It is used in the treatment of intestinal amebiasis (especially *Entamoeba histolytica*). It may be used alone in mild cases or with asymptomatic carriers but should be used in conjunction with metronidazole, chloroquine, or emetine in treating acute or severe forms of the disease. It is effective against both the trophozoite and the encysted forms. Although not approved for use, paromomycin is also used as alternative therapy to treat intestinal infestations of giardiasis, *Taenia saginata* (beef tapeworm), *Hymenolepis nana* (dwarf tapeworm), *Diphyllobothrium latum* (fish tapeworm), and *Taenia solium* (pork tapeworm).

Characteristics

Absorption (PO): poorly absorbed, but impaired gastrointestinal motility or lesions or ulcerations may enhance absorption. Excretion: fecal—the unabsorbed fraction; renal—the absorbed fraction. Accumulation may occur in patients with renal dysfunction.

Administration and dosage

For amebiasis:

Adult

PO—25 to 35 mg/kg, in 3 divided doses after meals for 5 to 10 days.

Pediatric

PO—As for adults, or 750 mg/m^2 in 3 divided doses after meals for 5 days.

For tapeworms:

Adult

PO—1 g every 15 min for 4 doses.

Pediatric

PO—11 mg/kg every 4 hr for 4 doses.

For *Hymenolepis nana:*

Adult and pediatric

PO—45 mg/kg once daily for 5 to 7 days.

Nurse and patient considerations

* Common side effects associated with oral paromomycin include anorexia, nausea, vomiting, abdominal cramps, epigastric pain and burning, and diarrhea.
* Overgrowth on nonsusceptible organisms, especially *Candida,* may occur.
* See General information on aminoglycosides (p. 43).

Drug interactions

See General information on aminoglycosides (p. 43).

Tobramycin sulfate
(Nebcin)

AHFS 8:12.28
CATEGORY Aminoglycoside antibiotic

Action and use

Tobramycin is a bactericidal agent with a mechanism of action similar to the other aminoglycosides. The spectrum of tobramycin activity is quite similar to gentamicin; however, tobramycin appears to be 2 to 4 times more active against *P. aeruginosa,* on a weight basis.

Characteristics

Peak plasma levels: 30 to 90 min (IM). Half-life: 1½ to 3 hr. Metabolism: insignificant. Excretion: 60% to 90% unchanged in urine in 24 hr. Dialysis: yes, H; no, P.

Administration and dosage
Adult

IM 1. Normal renal function (see Table 1-5):
    a. Serious infection: 1 mg/kg/8 hr (3 mg/kg/day).
    b. Life-threatening infection: 1.66 mg/kg/8 hr (5 mg/kg/day).
  2. Impaired renal function: see Table 1-5.

IV—As for IM administration, dilute the recommended dosage in 50 to 100 ml of dextrose 5% saline solution and infuse over 20 to 60 min. Administration in less than 20 min may result in toxic serum levels. Tobramycin should not be physically premixed with other medications.

Pediatric
Neonates (under 1 week)

IM—Up to 2 mg/kg/12 hr (4 mg/kg/day).
IV—As for children and older infants.

Children and older infants (normal renal function)

IM 1. Serious infection: 1 mg/kg/8 hr (3 mg/kg/day).
2. Life-threatening infection: to 1.66 mg/kg/8 hr (5 mg/kg/day).
IV—Dilute with saline solution or dextrose 5% to a concentration of about 1 mg/ml and administer over 20 to 60 min. Do not mix with other medications.

Nurse and patient considerations

* See General information on aminoglycosides (p. 43).

Drug interactions

See General information on aminoglycosides (p. 43).

Sulfonamides
GENERAL INFORMATION

Sulfonamides are bacteriostatic agents that competitively inhibit bacterial synthesis of folic acid from para-aminobenzoic acid (PABA). Only organisms that synthesize folic acid are inhibited by sulfonamides.

Nurse and patient considerations

As a result of the increasing frequency of organisms resistant to sulfonamides and the relative unreliability of in vitro sulfonamide sensitivity tests, clinical response must be carefully monitored, especially in the treatment of chronic and recurrent urinary tract infections.

Sulfonamides are a class of drugs with many side effects that may occur in nearly all organs.

Table 1-5. Tobramycin administration

CR$_s$ (mg/100 ml)	10	7.6	5.3	3.3	2.4	1.9	1.6	1.4	1.3		
CCR (ml/min)	0	2	5	10	20	30	40	50	60	70	>70
mg/kg/8 hr	0.06 / 0.10	0.08 / 0.13	0.10 / 0.16	0.18 / 0.3	0.28 / 0.46	0.36 / 0.6	0.45 / 0.74	0.55 / 0.9	0.65 / 1	0.75 / 1.2	1 / 1.66
	mg/8 hr	mg/8 hr	mg/8 hr	mg/8 hr	mg/8 hr	mg/8 hr	mg/8 hr	mg/8 hr	mg/8 hr	mg/8 hr	mg/8 hr
40 kg (88 lb) L.D. = 40 mg	2.4 / 4	3 / 5	4 / 7	7.2 / 12	11 / 18	15 / 24	18 / 30	22 / 36	26 / 43	30 / 50	40 / 66
50 kg (110 lb) L.D. = 50 mg	3 / 5	5 / 7	5 / 8	9 / 15	14 / 23	18 / 30	23 / 37	28 / 45	33 / 54	38 / 62	50 / 83
60 kg (132 lb) L.D. = 60 mg	3.5 / 6	5 / 8	6 / 10	11 / 18	17 / 28	22 / 36	27 / 45	33 / 55	39 / 65	45 / 75	60 / 100

Each cell below shows two values: **A** (upper-left of the diagonal) / **B** (lower-right of the diagonal).

Weight											
70 kg (154 lb) L.D. = 70 mg	4 / 7	5.4 / 9	7 / 12	13 / 21	20 / 33	25 / 42	32 / 52	38 / 64	46 / 75	53 / 88	70 / 116
80 kg (176 lb) L.D. = 80 mg	5 / 8	6.4 / 10	8 / 13	14 / 24	22 / 37	29 / 48	36 / 60	44 / 73	52 / 87	60 / 100	80 / 133
90 kg (198 lb) L.D. = 90 mg	5.5 / 9	7 / 12	9 / 15	16 / 27	25 / 42	32 / 54	40 / 68	50 / 83	59 / 98	68 / 113	90 / 150
100 kg (220 lb) L.D. = 100 mg	6 / 10	8 / 13	10 / 17	18 / 30	28 / 47	36 / 60	45 / 75	55 / 91	65 / 108	75 / 125	100 / 166

Modified from Nebcin–Tobramycin sulfate product information, Eli Lilly Co.

KEY: A / B

A — Dosage adjustment for serious infections with renal dysfunction.

B — Adjustment of maximum dosage for life-threatening infections with renal dysfunction. REDUCE AS SOON AS POSSIBLE.

c_{RS} — Serum creatinine level (mg/100 ml).

c_{CR} — Creatinine clearance rate (ml/min).

L.D. — Loading dose followed at 8 hr by the appropriate maintenance dose.

1. Gastrointestinal:
   a. Nausea, vomiting, anorexia, and diarrhea are among the more common side effects.
   b. Stomatitis, pancreatis, hepatitis, and abdominal pains have been reported.
2. Hematologic:
   a. Agranulocytosis may occur 10 to 14 days after therapy is initiated.
   b. Acute hemolytic anemia may occur in the first week of therapy as a result of hypersensitivity or glucose-6-phosphate dehydrogenase deficiency.
   c. Other blood dyscrasias include thrombocytopenia, aplastic anemia, and leukopenia. Signs of blood dyscrasias include sore throat, pallor, fever, purpura, jaundice, and weakness. Routine blood studies should be performed in patients receiving sulfonamides longer than 14 days.
3. Dermatologic:
   a. Patients should be cautioned to avoid unnecessary exposure to sunlight or ultraviolet light, since photosensitivity may occur.
   b. Rash, prúritus, and exfoliative dermatitis may also occur. Since many serious adverse effects of sulfonamide therapy may be heralded by a rash, sulfonamide therapy should be discontinued at once if a rash does develop.
4. Renal: crystalluria caused by precipitation of a sulfonamide in the urinary tract may result in urolithiasis, oliguria, hematuria, proteinuria, and obstruction anuria. Input and output should be monitored, and collected urine should be observed for changes in coloration and sediment. Fluid intake should be encouraged to at least 1.5 L/day.
5. Neurologic: dizziness, headache, mental depression, confusion, acute psychosis, drowsiness, tinnitus, and restlessness occur occasionally.

Sulfonamides may cause hypothyroidism and will suppress ^{131}I uptake for about 7 days after sulfonamide therapy is discontinued.

Drug interactions

Although apparently infrequent, local anesthetics that are derivatives of PABA (benzocaine, procaine, tetracaine) may antagonize the antibacterial activity of sulfonamides. Local infections have occurred in areas of procaine infiltration while patients were receiving sulfonamide therapy.

Sulfonylurea oral hypoglycemics (tolbutamide, aceto-hexamide, tolazamide, chlorpropamide) may be displaced from protein-binding sites, resulting in hypoglycemia.

Sulfonamides may displace warfarin from protein-binding sites, enhancing anticoagulation and prolonging the pro-thrombin time.

Sulfonamides may displace methotrexate from protein-binding sites, resulting in enhanced methotrexate toxicity.

Sulfamethoxazole
(Gantanol)

AHFS 8:24
CATEGORY Sulfonamide antibiotic

Action and use

Similar to sulfisoxazole (p. 59).

Characteristics

Peak levels: 3 to 4 hr. Duration: about 12 hr. Protein binding: about 50% to 70%. Half-life: 10 to 11 hr. Metabolism: hepatic acetylation and glucuronidation. Excretion: 10% to 30% unchanged in urine. Dialysis: yes, H.

Administration and dosage
Adult

PO 1. Mild to moderate infections: 2 g initially, followed by 1 g 2 times daily.
2. Severe infections: 2 g initially, followed by 1 g 3 times daily.
IM—Not available.
IV—Not available

Pediatric (over 2 months of age)

NOTE: Sulfamethoxazole must not be administered to infants under 2 months of age.
PO—50 to 60 mg/kg (23 to 27 mg/lb) initially, followed by 25 to 30 mg/kg/24 hr in 2 divided doses. Do not exceed 75 mg/kg/24 hr.

Nurse and patient considerations

✳ See General information on sulfonamides (p. 53).

Drug interactions

See General information on sulfonamides (p. 53).

Sulfasalazine
(Azulfidine)

AHFS 8:24
CATEGORY Sulfonamide

Action and use

Sulfasalazine is a sulfonamide derivative poorly absorbed from the gastrointestinal tract. It does not have antibacterial properties although the intestinal flora may split the drug into sulfapyridine and a salicylate. Its exact mechanism of action is unknown. It is indicated in the treatment of ulcerative colitis, especially with prolonged administration when it may be effective in reducing the number of relapses in patients receiving maintenance therapy.

Administration and dosage
Adult

PO—Initially, 4 to 12 g daily in 4 to 8 divided doses. The usual adult maintenance dosage is 500 mg 4 times daily.

IM—Not available.

IV—Not available.

Pediatric (over 2 months of age)

PO—Initial, 40 to 60 mg/kg/24 hr in 3 to 6 doses; maintenance, 30 mg/kg/24 hr divided into 4 doses.

Nurse and patient considerations

* Common side effects include nausea, vomiting, anorexia, and gastric distress.
* Sulfasalazine is partially absorbed from the gastrointestinal tract. Its metabolites may impart an orange-yellow color to an alkaline urine.
* Patients who are sensitive to either salicylates or sulfonamides must use caution with this drug.
* This drug has been reported to cause pancreatitis, with marked elevations in serum amylase.
* See General information on sulfonamides (p. 53).

Drug interactions

See General information on sulfonamides (p. 53).

Sulfisoxazole
(Gantrisin)

AHFS 8:24
CATEGORY Sulfonamide antibiotic

Action and use

Sulfisoxazole is a short-acting sulfonamide that differs from other agents in this class because it is distributed only in extracellular body fluid. It is used in acute urinary tract infections caused by susceptible *E. coli, Klebsiella, S. aureus, P. mirabilis,* and *Proteus vulgaris.*

Characteristics

Protein binding: 80% to 90%. Half-life: 3 to 4 hr. Metabolism: hepatic acetylation 30%. Excretion: 95% in urine, 30% in acetylated form, in 24 hr. Therapeutic level: 9 to 10 mg/100 ml. Dialysis: yes, H, P.

Administration and dosage
Adult

PO—2 to 4 g initially, followed by 1 to 2 g every 4 to 6 hr.

IM—4 to 5 g every 12 hr. Injectable Gantrisin may be given without dilution.

IV—4 to 5 g every 12 hr. The 40% (2 g) injectable Gantrisin solution must be diluted to 5% concentration. Dilute one 5 ml ampule with 35 ml of sterile distilled water. This provides a solution containing 50 mg/ml. Diluents other than sterile water may cause precipitation. Administration with other parenteral fluids is not recommended. Maximal urinary concentrations may be attained by alkalinizing the urine with sodium bicarbonate.

Pediatric (over 2 months of age)

NOTE: Sulfisoxazole must not be administered to infants under 2 months of age.

PO—75 mg/kg initially, followed by 150 mg/kg/24 hr in 4 to 6 divided doses. Total daily dose should not exceed 6 g.

IM—50 mg/kg initially, followed by 100 mg/kg/24 hr in 2 to 3 divided doses. Not more than 2 ml of the injection should be given IM in any one site.

IV—As for IM but divided in 4 equal doses.

Nurse and patient considerations

✳ See General information on sulfonamides (p. 53)
✳ Sulfisoxazole may cause a hypersensitivity reaction, resulting in hepatitis with jaundice.
✳ Sulfisoxazole may interfere with Urobilistix, resulting in a false-positive urine urobilinogen test.

Drug interactions

Sulfisoxazole may displace thiopental from protein-binding sites, potentiating the effects of thiopental anesthesia.

Sulfisoxazole has been shown to displace phenytoin (Dilantin) from protein-binding sites, resulting in higher active serum levels of the anticonvulsant.

Methotrexate may be displaced from protein-binding sites to the extent of increasing active methotrexate levels as much as 25%, thus enhancing the potential for methotrexate toxicity.

Co-trimoxazole
(Bactrim, Septra)

AHFS 8:24
CATEGORY Combination sulfonamide-pyrimidine

Action and use

Co-trimoxazole is one of the few antibacterial combination products available. It contains sulfamethoxazole (p. 57) and trimethoprim in a 5:1 ratio. Trimethoprim and sulfamethoxazole act synergistically by blocking the formation of folic acid and the utilization of folic acid already formed by bacteria. This does not affect human use of folic acid, since mammalian cells do not synthesize folic acid and are not as susceptible to trimethoprim, but utilize what is provided by the diet. Co-trimoxazole is used for acute and chronic urinary tract infections caused by susceptible *E. coli, Klebsiella* and Enterobacter species, *P. mirabilis, P. vulgaris,* and *P. morgani.* Co-trimoxazole is also approved for use in treating pneumonia caused by *Pneumocystis carinii,* otitis media caused by *H. influenzae* and *S. pneumoniae,* and enteritis caused by *Shigella flexneri* and *Shigella sonnei.* Investigations are currently under way for its use against other pathogenic organisms.

Characteristics

Sulfamethoxazole—see p. 57.

Trimethoprim—peak plasma levels: 1½ to 3 hr. Protein binding: 30% to 70%. Half-life: 6 to 17 hr. Metabolism: hepatic. Excretion: 50% to 75%, unchanged in urine, 20% to 30% as metabolites in urine. Dialysis: yes, H; no, P.

Administration and dosage

Co-trimoxazole is available in the following dosage forms:

1. Tablets:
   a. 400 mg of sulfamethoxazole and 80 mg of trimethoprim.
   b. 800 mg of sulfamethoxayole and 160 mg of trimethoprim.
2. PO suspension: 200 mg of sulfamethoxazole and 40 mg of trimethoprim in flavored syrup/5 ml.
3. IV solution: 400 mg sulfamethoxazole (80 mg/ml) and 80 mg trimethoprim (16 mg/ml) for infusion with dextrose 5% in water.
   a. This solution must be diluted only in dextrose 5% in water. Add each 5 ml ampule to 125 ml of dextrose 5% in water.
   b. Do not refrigerate the diluted solution, and use within 6 hr. If cloudiness or precipitation occurs, discard and prepare a fresh solution.
   c. Administer by intravenous drip over 60 to 90 min. Avoid rapid infusion or bolus injection.
   d. If fluid restriction is necessary, dilute the ampule with 75 ml of dextrose 5% in water. Mix solution just before use, and administer within 2 hr.

For urinary tract infections and shigellosis:

Adult

PO—800 mg of sulfamethoxazole and 160 mg of trimethoprim every 12 hr (see Nurse and patient considerations).

IV—8 to 10 mg/kg (based on trimethoprim component) given in 2 to 4 equally divided doses every 6, 8, or 12 hr for up to 14 days for severe urinary tract infections and 5 days for shigellosis (see below for renal impairment).

Pediatric

Infants. Not recommended for use in infants under 2 months of age. See dosages for children.

Children

PO—40 mg/kg/24 hr of sulfamethoxazole and 8 mg/kg/24 hr of trimethoprim given in 2 divided doses (see Special remarks and cautions).

For *P. Carinii* pneumonitis:

Adult and pediatric

PO—100 mg/kg/24 hr of sulfamethoxazole and 20 mg/kg/24 hr of trimethoprim given in equally divided doses every 6 hr.

IV—15 to 20 mg/kg (based on trimethoprim component) given in 3 or 4 equally divided doses every 6 to 8 hr for up to 14 days.

With renal impairment:

For patients with a creatinine clearance above 30 ml/min, use the above recommendations. For patients with a creatinine clearance between 15 and 30 ml/min give half (½) the total daily recommended dose once every 24 hr. Do not use in patients with a creatinine clearance below 15 ml/min.

Nurse and patient considerations

* Patients must maintain adequate fluid intake to prevent crystalluria.
* This combination of drugs may produce megaloblastic anemia caused by interference with folic acid and vitamin B_{12} metabolism. Patients especially susceptible are those with low folic acid and vitamin B_{12} levels or those receiving pyrimethamine (Daraprim), a folic acid antagonist.
* Teratogenic effects such as cleft palate have been reported in laboratory animals. Cotrimoxazole should not be used by pregnant or nursing women.
* See General information on sulfonamides (p. 53).

Drug interactions

Leucovorin (folinic acid) may interfere with the antibacterial activity of co-trimoxazole but may also be used to treat hematologic toxicities induced by co-trimoxazole.

See General information on sulfonamides (p. 53).

Trisulfapyrimidines
(Terfonyl)

AHFS 8:24
CATEGORY Sulfonamide antibiotics

Action and use

Trisulfapyrimidines is a combination of 3 sulfonamide antibiotics—sulfadiazine, sulfamerazine, and sulfamethazine. The 3 sulfonamides are bacteriostatic agents, each with a similar spectrum of activity. The rationale for the combination stems from the toxicity of each of the components. Each sulfonamide, when used in full therapeutic doses, has a history of precipitating crystals in the renal tubules, resulting in severe renal damage. Using the 3 agents together provides full therapeutic activity while significantly reducing the frequency of renal complications.

Trisulfapyrimidines is used to treat acute, recurrent and chronic urinary tract infections caused by susceptible *E. coli, Klebsiella,* and *P. mirabilis.* It is also used in pediatric patients to treat acute otitis media caused by *H. influenzae* in combination with other antibiotics.

Administration and dosage
Adult

PO—2 to 4 g initially, followed by maintenance doses of 2 to 4 g every 24 hr divided into 3 to 6 equal doses.

Pediatric (over 2 months of age)

NOTE: Trisulfapyrimidines must not be administered to infants under 2 months of age.

PO—Initial dose: 75 mg/kg. Maintenance dose: 150 mg/kg/24 hrs divided into 4 to 6 equal doses. Maximum dose: 6 g/24 hr.

Nurse and patient considerations

* See General information on sulfonamides (p. 53).
* Trisulfapyrimidines may cause a hypersensitivity reaction, resulting in hepatitis with jaundice.

Drug interactions

See General information on sulfonamides (p. 53).

OTHER ANTIBIOTICS

Chloramphenicol
(Chloromycetin, Amphicol, Mychel)

AHFS 8:12.08
CATEGORY Antibiotic

Action and use

Chloramphenicol is a bacteriostatic antibiotic that inhibits protein synthesis in susceptible organisms by binding to 50 S subunits of ribosomes, thus interfering with the formation of the peptide bond. Chloramphenicol may be the drug of choice in treatment of *Salmonella typhi* and *H. influenzae* meningitis. It may also be quite effective in rickettsial infections and in gram-negative bacteria causing bacteremia or meningitis. *It must not be used in the treatment of trivial infections or when it is not indicated, as in colds, influenza, throat infections, or as a prophylactic agent to prevent bacterial infection.*

Characteristics

Onset: 30 min. Peak plasma level: 2 hr (PO). Duration: 12 to 18 hr. Protein binding: 60%. Half-life: 3 to 4 hr. Metabolism: hepatic. Excretion: 80% to 90% in urine in 24 hours, 5% to 10% active. Dialysis: No, H, P.

Administration and dosage
Adult

PO 1. Normal renal and hepatic function: 50 mg/kg/day in 4 equally divided doses at 6 hr intervals. Moderately resistant organisms may require 100 mg/kg/day in divided doses. Reduce to 50 mg/kg/day as soon as clinically possible.

2. Impaired renal and/or hepatic function: 25 mg/kg/day in 4 equally divided doses.

IM—Not recommended because of maintenance of inadequate blood levels and poor clinical response.

IV—As recommended for PO administration for normal or impaired renal and hepatic function. Reconstitute by adding 11 ml of sterile water for injection and dextrose 5% to 1 g of chloramphenicol to make a solution containing 100 mg/ml. Administer the calculated dose intravenously over a 1 min period. PO therapy should replace parenteral therapy as soon as possible.

Pediatric

PO 1. Newborn infants and children in whom immature hepatic and/or renal function is suspected: 25 mg/kg/24 hr in 4 equally divided doses.
     2. Infants over 2 weeks of age: to 50 mg/kg/24 hr in 4 equally divided doses.

IM—Not recommended.

IV—As for PO dosages. Administer IV over 1 min. Use only chloramphenicol sodium succinate IV in children. Do not use chloramphenicol in 50% *N,N*-dimethylacetamide (Chloromycetin solution). PO therapy should replace parenteral therapy as soon as possible.

Nurse and patient considerations

* Serious and fatal blood dyscrasias (aplastic anemia, hypoplastic anemia, thrombocytopenia, and agranulocytosis) are known to occur after administration of chloramphenicol. Two types of bone marrow suppression occur, one dose-related and reversible, the other non-dose-related and irreversible. Various studies indicated an occurrence of this second type as 1 in 20 to 40 thousand; it may occur weeks to months after the discontinuance of the drug. It is recommended that baseline blood studies should be followed by periodic blood studies every 2 days and that the drug be discontinued as soon as clinically feasible. Early signs of blood dyscrasias include sore throat, malaise, elevated temperature, and petechiae.

* Neurologic toxicities include headache, mental depression, confusion, and delirium.

* Gastrointestinal side effects include nausea, vomiting, diarrhea, glossitis, stomatitis, and unpleasant taste in mouth.

* Allergic manifestations to chloramphenicol include several types of rashes, hemorrhages, urticaria, and anaphylaxis.

* Chloramphenicol produces "gray syndrome" in the fetus and neonatal infants. The syndrome results from immature metabolic enzyme systems. Chloramphenicol readily crosses the placental barrier and is secreted in breast milk and so must be used with extreme caution during pregnancy and in nursing women.

> * Chloramphenicol may cause a false-positive reaction when determining glucose content in the urine by the Clinitest method.

Drug interactions

Chloramphenicol markedly inhibits the metabolism of oral anticoagulants (warfarin). The prothrombin time must be monitored closely and the patient advised to watch for signs of overanticoagulation (easy bruisability, melena, or any episode of bleeding).

Chloramphenicol prolongs the half-life of oral hypoglycemic agents (tolbutamide, chlorpropamide). Reduction of the dosage of the oral hypoglycemic may be required, and the patient advised of signs of hypoglycemia (faintness, pallor, diaphoresis, increased irritability, seizures, or coma).

Chloramphenicol reduces the metabolism of phenytoin (Dilantin), doubling the half-life. Patients may develop manifestations of phenytoin toxicity such as nystagmus, ataxia, malaise, and lethargy. Reduction in the phenytoin dosage may be required.

Chloramphenicol may interfere with oral contraceptive therapy. See General information on oral contraceptives (p. 499).

Clindamycin
(Cleocin)

AHFS 8:12.28
CATEGORY Antibiotic

Action and use

Clindamycin is a bacteriostatic antibiotic that exerts its action by inhibiting protein formation. This agent's spectrum of activity includes gram-positive aerobic staphylococci, pneumococci, and streptococci and a variety of gram-positive and gram-negative anaerobes.

Characteristics

Peak plasma level: 1 hr (PO). Protein binding: 94%. Half-life: 2 to 2½ hr. Metabolism: hepatic. Excretion: 10% unchanged in urine. Dialysis: no, H, P.

Administration and dosage
Adult

PO—150 to 300 mg every 6 hr in mild to moderate infections; 300 to 450 mg every 6 hr in severe infections. To avoid thickening of the PO suspension, do not refrigerate. The solution is stable for 2 weeks at room temperature.

IM—600 to 2700 mg/24 hr. Do not exceed 600 mg/injection. Pain, induration, and sterile abscesses have been reported. Deep IM injection is recommended to help minimize this reaction.

IV—600 to 2700 mg/24 hr. Dilute to less than 6 mg/ml. Administer at a rate less than 30 mg/min. Administration by IV push is not recommended.

Pediatric (over 1 month of age)

PO 1. Suspension:
    a. Mild infections: 8 to 12 mg/kg/24 hr in divided doses.
    b. Moderate infections: 13 to 16 mg/kg/24 hr in divided doses.
    c. Severe infections: 17 to 25 mg/kg/24 hr in divided doses. In patients weighing 10 kg or less the minimum PO dose recommended is 37.5 mg (½ teaspoon) 3 times daily.
  2. Capsules:
    a. Mild to moderate infections: 8 to 16 mg/kg/24 hr in divided doses.
    b. Severe infections: 16 to 20 mg/kg/24 hr in divided doses. Capsules should be taken with a full glass of water to prevent esophageal irritation.

IM 1. Mild to moderate infections: 15 to 25 mg/kg/24 hrs in 3 to 4 divided doses.
  2. Severe infections: 25 to 40 mg/kg/24 hr in 3 or 4 divided doses. It is recommended that children be given no less than 300 mg/day regardless of body weight.

IV—As for IM use. Dilute to less than 6 mg/ml and administer at a rate less than 30 mg/min.

Nurse and patient considerations

∗ Severe and persistent diarrhea may develop from the use of this drug. If significant diarrhea results (more than 5 bowel movements per day), the drug should be discontinued. The use of opiates, meperidine, and diphenoxylate with atropine (Lomotil) may prolong and/or worsen the condition. Large doses of kaolin-pectin (Kaopectate) may be effective in diminishing the diarrhea.

* Hypersensitivity reactions often manifested by rashes, jaundice, abnormal liver function tests, and bone marrow suppression have been reported in patients being treated with this agent.
* Bitter taste caused by possible secretion of clindamycin in saliva has been reported with both oral and parenteral administration.

Drug interactions

Kaolin-pectin may physically absorb clindamycin and impair absorption from the gastrointestinal tract.

Antagonism has been reported between clindamycin and erythromycin when administered concomitantly.

Clindamycin may potentiate neuromuscular blockade in patients recovering from the effects of surgical muscle relaxants (tubocurarine, succinylcholine, gallamine triethiodide [Flaxedil]) and antibiotics (gentamicin, streptomycin, kanamycin, amikacin, and tobramycin).

Clindamycin significantly reduces the metabolism of theophylline. See General information on theophylline derivatives (p. 271).

Erythromycin
(Ilosone, Erythrocin, E-Mycin, Ilotycin)

AHFS 8:12.12
CATEGORY Macrolide antibiotic

Action and use

The mechanism of action of erythromycin is inhibition of protein synthesis in susceptible microorganisms. This bacteriostatic agent is indicated as an alternate drug of choice in the treatment of mild to moderate infections produced by group A beta-hemolytic streptococcus, alpha-hemolytic streptococcus (viridans group), *S. aureus, S. pneumoniae, T. pallidum,* and *Corynebacterium diphtheriae.* Erythromycin may also be used as an alternate antibiotic against susceptible organisms in patients allergic to penicillin.

Characteristics

Peak plasma level: 1 to 4 hr (PO). Protein binding: 73%. Half-life: 1⅕ hr. Excretion: primarily fecal, 2% to 5% unchanged in urine (PO), 12% to 15% unchanged in urine (IV). Dialysis: no, H, P.

Administration and dosage
Adult

PO—250 mg 4 times a day for 10 to 14 days. Administer at least 1 hr before or 2 hr after meals.

IM—100 mg every 4 to 6 hr. As a result of pain on injection, adequate dosages for the treatment of serious or severe infections with IM erythromycin are difficult to achieve. IM injection of erythromycin may also result in sterile abscess formation and necrosis.

IV—15 to 20 mg/kg/day. If erythromycin is to be given IV, the medication should be given by intermittent rapid infusion. One fourth of the total daily dose can be given in 20 to 60 min by infusion of 250 to 500 mg as an initial solution added to 100 to 250 ml of saline solution or dextrose 5%. Thrombophlebitis after IV infusion is a relatively common side effect.

Pediatric

PO—30 to 50 mg/kg/24 hr in 4 divided doses. For severe infections this dose may be doubled.

IM—Not recommended in infants or children.

IV—15 to 20 mg/kg/24 hr in 3 divided doses

Nurse and patient considerations

* The most common side effects of oral erythromycin products are epigastric distress with possible nausea and vomiting.

* The administration of erythromycin estolate (Ilosone) has been associated with an allergic type of cholestatic hepatitis. Some patients receiving Ilosone for more than 2 weeks or in repeated courses have developed jaundice accompanied by right upper quandrant pain, fever, nausea, vomiting, eosinophilia, and leukocytosis.

* Since erythromycin is principally excreted via the liver, caution should be exercised in administering the antibiotic to patients with impaired hepatic function.

Drug interactions

The use of bacteriostatic erythromycin is not recommended in patients receiving bactericidal antibiotics, such as penicillin. If used concomitantly, start the penicillin several hours before the erythromycin and use adequate doses of each antibiotic.

Erythromycin significantly reduces the metabolism of theophylline. See General information on theophylline derivatives (p. 271).

Metronidazole
(Flagyl, Flagyl
IV RTU)

AHFS 8:32
CATEGORY Anaerobic antibiotic,
trichomonacide

Action and use

Metronidazole is a synthetic compound that has antibacterial, trichamonicidal, and protozoacidal activity. Its mechanisms of activity are not fully defined.

Metronidazole has a fairly narrow spectrum of activity as an antibacterial agent. A metabolite of metronidazole is the antibacterial compound, acting by altering DNA, disrupting transcription and replication. Only obligate anaerobic organisms such as *Bacteroides, Clostridium, Fusobacterium, Eubacterium, Peptococcus,* and *Peptostreptococcus* species are capable of producing the reaction that produces the active metabolite. Metronidazole may be used to treat skin and skin structure, gynecologic, bone and joint, and lower respiratory infections, as well as septicemia, meningitis, and endocarditis caused by susceptible anaerobic organisms.

Metronidazole is also active against *Trichomonas vaginalis, Haemophilus vaginalis, Campylobacter fetus, E. histolytica,* and *Giardia lamblia.* The mechanisms of action are yet unknown. It is used to treat trichomoniasis of the urogenital tract, giardiasis, amebic dysentery, and amebic liver abscess.

Characteristics

Protein binding: less than 20%. Half-life: 7.3 to 8.3 hr. Metabolism: hepatic. Excretion: 60% to 80% in urine, less than 10% as unchanged drug; 6 to 15% in feces. Dialysis: yes, H. Breast milk: yes.

Administration and dosage
Adult

PO

TRICHOMONIASIS
1. Males and females: 250 mg 3 times daily for 7 days. Sexual partners must be treated concurrently to prevent reinfection.

2. Single doses of 2 g, or 2 doses of 1 g each administered the same day appears to provide adequate treatment for trichomoniasis in both sexes. Single-dose therapy is used for patients where follow-up or compliance is less than optimal.

AMEBIC DYSENTERY—750 mg 3 times daily for 5 to 10 days.

AMEBIC LIVER ABSCESS—500 to 750 mg 3 times daily for 5 to 10 days.

GIARDIASIS—250 mg 2 to 3 times daily for 5 to 10 days.

ANAEROBIC BACTERIAL INFECTIONS

1. Start with parenteral therapy initially.
2. The usual *oral* dosage is 7.5 mg/kg every 6 hr. Do not exceed 4 g/24 hr.
3. The usual duration is 7 to 10 days; infections of the bone and joint, lower respiratory tract, and endocardium may require longer treatment.

IV

ANAEROBIC BACTERIAL INFECTIONS

1. Loading dose: 15 mg/kg infused over 1 hr.
2. Maintenance dose: 7.5 mg/kg infused over 1 hr every 6 hr. Do not exceed 4 g/24 hr. Convert to oral dosages when clinical condition warrants.
3. Dosage reduction is necessary in patients with hepatic impairment, but not renal impairment.

Pediatric

PO

TRICHOMONIASIS—35 to 50 mg/kg/24 hr in 3 divided doses for 7 days.

AMEBIASIS—35 to 50 mg/kg/24 hr in 3 divided doses for 10 days.

GIARDIASIS—35 to 50 mg/kg/24 hr in 3 divided doses for 7 days.

Nurse and patient considerations

* The most common side effects for both oral and parenteral therapy are nausea, headache, anorexia, and occasionally vomiting, diarrhea, and abdominal cramping. An unpleasant metallic taste is also common by both routes of administration. Thrombophlebitis occurs in about 6% of patients receiving parenteral therapy.

* The most serious reactions are seizures and peripheral neuropathy. Tonic-clonic seizures have been reported in patients receiving higher dosages than recommended. Patients with a history of seizure activity and those with significant hepatic impairment may be at greater risk. Peripheral neuropathy, manifesting as numbness or paresthesias of an extremity, has been reported after prolonged therapy. Resolution of the neuropathy is reported to be slow.

* Metronidazole is carcinogenic in animals and mutagenic *in vitro* but has not increased the incidence of cancer in humans followed for relatively short periods of time.

* Mild, reversible leukopenia is occasionally observed, and follow-up white cell counts with differential are recommended after therapy.

* Overgrowth of oral and vaginal monilia may result in furry tongue, glossitis, stomatitis, vaginal itching and burning, and urethral irritation.

* Metronidazole therapy may impart a reddish brown discoloration to the urine, especially when higher doses are used.

* Metronidazole interferes with serum glutamic oxaloacetic transaminase determinations by spectrophotometric assay, resulting in false-negative values.

* Metronidazole crosses the placental barrier and passes rapidly into fetal circulation. The drug is also excreted in breast milk. Metronidazole should generally not be used in pregnant women. If treating during the second or third trimester, do not use the 1-day course of therapy, because of high serum levels achieved.

Drug interactions

Consumption of alcoholic beverages during metronidazole therapy may result in abdominal cramping, vomiting, and flushing (disulfiram-like reaction).

When metronidazole and disulfiram (Antabuse) are taken concurrently, psychotic episodes and confusional states have been reported.

Metronidazole will increase warfarin (Coumadin) serum levels and enhance anticoagulation by inhibition of warfarin metabolism. Monitor the prothrombin time and reduce the dose of warfarin as necessary.

Spectinomycin hydrochloride
(Trobicin)

AHFS 8:12.28
CATEGORY Antibiotic

Action and use

Spectinomycin binds to and inhibits the 30 S ribosomal unit required for protein synthesis of the bacterial cell.

The drug is a bacteriostatic agent used specifically for the treatment of acute gonorrheal urethritis and proctitis in the male and acute gonorrheal cervicitis and proctitis in the female when caused by susceptible strains of *N. gonorrhoeae*. A particular advantage is that most strains of the organism respond to one administration of the recommended dosage.

Characteristics

Peak serum level: 1 hr (IM). Protein binding: insignificant. Metabolism: insignificant. Excretion: active form in urine.

Administration and dosage

IM—A 20-gauge needle is recommended. IM injections should be made deep into the upper outer quandrant of the gluteal muscle. Male: 2 g (5 ml); female: 2 to 4 g (5 to 10 ml) divided in 2 sites.

NOTE: Safety for use in infants and children has not been established.

Nurse and patient considerations

* Spectinomycin provides an alternative to penicillin in the treatment of acute, susceptible gonococcal infections. It is not effective in the treatment of syphilis.

* Pain at the site of injection is a common side effect.

* Urticaria, nausea, chills, and fever are other possible side effects of single-dose therapy.

* Safe use in pregnancy has not been established.

Drug interactions

None have specifically been reported.

Vancomycin hydrochloride
(Vancocin)

AHFS 8:12.28
CATEGORY antibiotic

Action and use

Vancomycin is a bactericidal antibiotic that exerts its action by binding to precursors necessary for bacterial cell wall synthesis. Its spectrum of activity is primarily against gram-positive bacteria including S. *epidermidis*, S. *pneumoniae*, *Streptococcus viridans*, penicillinase-producing S. *aureus* resistant to methicillin, and some strains of S. *faecalis*. It is indicated for the treatment of endocarditis, osteomyelitis, pneumonia, septicemia, and soft tissue infections caused by the above organisms when other effective, less toxic antibiotics such as the penicillins and cephalosporins cannot be used. It is also effective against antibiotic-associated pseudomembranous colitis caused by C. *difficile*.

Characteristics

Absorption: poor (PO). Protein binding: 10%. Half-life: 6 hrs; 6 to 10 days in renal failure. Metabolism: negligible. Excretion: 90% unchanged in urine in 24 hrs (IV). Dialysis: no, H. Breast milk: unknown.

Administration and dosage
Adult

PO—NOTE: Use oral form only for staphylococcal enterocolitis and antibiotic-associated pseudomembranous colitis. It is *not* effective by the oral route for other types of infection.

STAPHYLOCOCCAL ENTEROCOLITIS—500 mg every 6 hr or 1 g every 12 hrs.

PSEUDOMEMBRANOUS COLITIS—500 mg every 6 hr for 7 to 10 days.

IM—Do not administer intramuscularly. It is very irritating to tissue and may cause necrosis.

IV—The parenteral form may be administered orally for treatment of staphylococcal entercolitis or antibiotic-associated pseudomembranous colitis produced by *C. difficile*.

Dilute the IV dosage in at least 100 to 200 ml of glucose or saline solution and infuse over at least 20 to 30 min to reduce the frequency of thrombophlebitis.

Dose—500 mg every 6 hr or 1 g every 12 hr.

Pediatric

PO—See above **NOTE**.

Neonates. Administer 12 to 15 mg/kg/day in 2 divided doses.

Children. Administer 40 mg/kg/day in 2 to 4 divided doses.

IV—As for PO. Take into consideration the large dilution necessary when calculating the child's 24 hr fluid requirement.

NOTE: Dosages must be empirically adjusted for patients with renal dysfunction.

Nurse and patient considerations

* Vancomycin is both nephrotoxic and ototoxic. Vancomycin should be avoided, if possible, in patients with prior hearing loss or renal impairment. Deafness may be preceded by tinnitus and may be progressive despite cessation of therapy. Patients with reduced renal function and those over 60 years of age should be given serial tests of renal and auditory function during therapy. (See also Drug interactions.)

* Other adverse effects associated with vancomycin therapy include nausea, chills, fever, and hypersensitivity reactions manifested by maculopapular rashes, urticaria, eosinophilia, and anaphylaxis.

* As with other antibiotics, vancomycin therapy may cause an overgrowth of nonsusceptible organisms. If secondary infections develop, initiate treatment as early as possible.

Drug interactions

Concurrent and sequential use of other ototoxic and/or nephrotoxic agents such as neomycin, streptomycin, kanamycin, gentamicin, viomycin, paromomycin, polymyxin B, colistin, tobramycin, amikacin, cephaloridine, and furosemide requires careful monitoring.

Tetracycline

(Panmycin, Sumycin, Mysteclin, Achromycin V, Tetracyn)

AHFS 8:24.24
CATEGORY Tetracycline antibiotic

Action and use

Tetracycline is a bacteriostatic agent that attaches to ribosomes, preventing the binding of transfer-RNA and thus inhibiting protein synthesis in susceptible organisms. Tetracycline is recommended as an alternative for patients hypersensitive to other antibiotics. It is used primarily for the treatment of gram-positive organisms resistant to penicillin, gram-negative bacillary infections, and rickettsial diseases. Because many strains of organisms are becoming resistant to tetracyclines, culture and sensitivity tests are recommended.

Characteristics

Protein binding: 25% to 30%. Half-life: 7 to 11 hr. Metabolism: hepatic. Excretion: 20% to 55% unchanged in urine. Dialysis: no, H, P. See Table 1-6 for a comparison of the tetracyclines.

Administration and dosage
Adult

PO—250 to 500 mg every 6 hr. Administer 1 hr before or 2 hr after the intake of food, milk, or antacids.

IM—250 to 300 mg every 8 to 12 hr. IM injections may cause pain and induration, which may be minimized by deep injections. Patients placed on IM tetracycline should be switched to the PO form as soon as possible.

IV—250 to 500 mg every 6 to 12 hr by infusion over 30 min to 1 hr. Rapid infusions or prolonged therapy may result in a relatively high incidence of thrombophlebitis. Nausea, vomiting, fever, chills, and hypotension may result from rapid infusion and dosages greater than 750 mg.

NOTE: Patients who are pregnant or who have impaired hepatic or renal dysfunction may accumulate toxic serum levels of tetracycline. These patients may also develop further azotemia, hyperphosphatemia, and acidosis caused by enhanced catabolism. Dosages should be reduced to one-third to one-half the normal dose, or the dosage interval extended 2 to 3 times the normal interval. Administration is not recommended if the creatinine clearance is less than 10 ml/min.

Nurse and patient considerations

* Anorexia, nausea, vomiting, and diarrhea are common side effects.
* Photosensitivity manifested by an exaggerated sunburn reaction has been observed. Patients should be cautioned to avoid unnecessary direct sunlight or ultraviolet light and to watch for early erythema when exposed.
* The use of tetracycline during tooth development (the last half of pregnancy, infancy, and childhood to 8 years of age) may cause enamel hypoplasia and permanent staining of the teeth (yellow, gray, or brown). Tetracycline therefore should not be used in this age group unless other drugs are not likely to be effective or are contraindicated.
* Tetracyclines are present in the milk of lactating women; therefore infant nourishment by formula is recommended during the mother's tetracycline therapy.
* In long-term therapy routine evaluation of the hematopoietic, hepatic, and renal organs should be performed. Leukocytosis, neutropenia, hemolytic anemia, elevated transaminases, bilirubin, alkaline phosphatase, and blood urea nitrogen have been reported. All may be caused by toxicity from tetracycline, so plans for clinical therapy must be reevaluated.
* Tetracycline may produce a false-positive urine glucose using Clinitest and a false-negative value when using Clinistix or Tes-Tape. These results may actually be caused by ascorbic acid that is used as a stabilizer in parenteral formulations of tetracycline.

AHFS 8:12.24

Table 1-6. Comparison of the tetracyclines*

Tetracycline	Peak levels	Duration (hr)	Protein binding (%)	Half-life (hr)	Exretion	Dialysis H	P	Neonate	Child	Adult
Chlortetracycline (Aureomycin)	2-4 hr (PO)	—	43-70	9	10%-15% excreted unchanged in urine	No	No	PO: 100 mg/kg/day in 2 divided doses IV: 10-15 mg/kg/day in 2 divided doses	PO: 25-50 mg/kg/day in 4 divided doses IV: 10-20 mg/kg/day in 2 divided doses	PO: 250 mg every 6 hr IV: 250-500 mg every 6-12 hr Do not exceed 2 g daily
Demeclocycline (Declomycin)	—	24-48	36-91	10-17	10%-25% excreted unchanged in urine	No	No	—	PO: 6-12 mg/kg/day in 2-4 divided doses	PO: 600 mg daily in 2-4 divided doses
Methacycline (Rondomycin)	—	24-48	75-90	11-14	50% excreted unchanged in urine	No	No	—	PO: 6-12 mg/kg/day in 2-4 divided doses	PO: 600 mg daily in 2-4 divided doses

Drug									
Minocycline (Minocin, Vectrin)	2 hr (PO)	12	70-75	11-18	12% excreted unchanged in urine	?	?	—	PO or IV: 4 mg/kg initially; 2 mg/kg every 12 hr	PO or IV: 200 mg initially; 100 mg every 12 hr
Oxytetracycline (Terramycin)	2-4 hr (PO)	—	20-35	5	10%-35% excreted unchanged in urine	No	No	PO: 100 mg/kg/day in 2 divided doses; IV: 10-15 mg/kg/day in 2 divided doses	PO: 25-50 mg/kg/day in 2-4 divided doses; IM: 15-25 mg/kg/day in 2-4 divided doses; IV: 10-20 mg/kg/day in 2 divided doses	PO: 250 mg every 6 hr; IM: 100-250 mg every 12 hr; IV: 250-500 mg every 6-12 hr; Do not exceed 2 g daily

*For Nurse and patient considerations see p. 77; for Drug interactions see p. 80; for discussion on doxycycline see p. 80; for discussion on tetracycline see p. 76.

†Food interferes with absorption of PO dosage forms. Administer at least 1 hr before or 2 hr after meals.

Drug interactions

Iron, milk, food, and antacids containing magnesium, calcium, or aluminum inhibit the absorption of tetracycline. PO tetracycline should be administered 1 hr before or 2 hr after these products.

Tetracycline has been shown to decrease plasma pro-thrombin activity through several postulated mechanisms. Patients receiving tetracycline and anticoagulants (warfarin) should have frequent evaluation of the prothrombin time and may require a reduction in the dosage of the oral anticoagulant.

Nephrotoxicity and fatalities have resulted from concomitant use of methoxyflurane (Penthrane) and tetracycline.

The use of bactericidal antibiotics (cephalosporins, penicillins) with bacteriostatic antibiotics such as tetracycline is not recommended except in special situations.

Doxycycline
(Vibramycin)

AHFS 8:12.24
CATEGORY Tetracycline antibiotic

Action and use

Doxycycline has a mechanism of action and spectrum of antibacterial activity against both gram-positive and gram-negative organisms similar to tetracycline. A particular advantage of doxycycline is its use in patients with renal insufficiency. Serum levels do not accumulate and there is no significant rise in the BUN level as often occurs with other tetracyclines in patients with renal dysfunction.

Characteristics

Protein binding: 25% to 93%. Half-life: 14 to 22 hr. Metabolism: hepatic. Excretion: 90% fecal, inactive. Dialysis: no, H, P.

Administration and dosage
Adult

PO—First 24 hr: 100 mg every 12 hr; maintenance: 100 to 200 mg/day.

IM—Not available.

IV—First 24 hr: 200 mg; maintenance: 100 to 200 mg/day.

NOTE: PO therapy should be instituted as soon as possible. The duration of infusion may vary with the dose, but is usually 1 to 4 hr. A recommended minimum infusion time for 100 mg of a 0.5 mg/ml solution is 1 hr. Rapid infusions or prolonged therapy may result in a relatively high incidence of thrombophlebitis. Nausea, vomiting, fever, chills, and hypotension may result from rapid infusion.

Nurse and patient considerations

* * See Nurse and patient considerations for tetracycline (p. 77).
* * If gastric irritation occurs, doxycycline may be given with food or milk. Absorption is not significantly influenced by food or milk as with other tetracyclines.

Drug interactions

See the Drug interactions of tetracycline (p. 77).

Phenytoin (Dilantin) and carbamazepine (Tegretol) may significantly shorten the serum half-life of doxycycline, reducing its therapeutic efficacy.

URINARY ANTIMICROBIAL AGENTS

Cinoxacin
(Cinobac)

AHFS 8:36
CATEGORY Urinary antibacterial agent

Action and use

Cinoxacin is a synthetic organic acid structurally related to nalidixic acid. Its mechanism of action is not fully understood, but it is thought to inhibit DNA polymerization, similar to nalidixic acid. Cinoxacin may be used to treat initial and recurrent urinary tract infections caused by *E. coli, P. mirabilis,* most indole-positive *Proteus, Klebsiella, Citrobacter* and *Enterobacter* organisms, and some *Serratia, Shigella,* and *Salmonella* organisms. This spectrum of activity is similar to that of nalidixic acid, and cross-resistance is seen between cinoxacin and nalidixic acid. Clinical use indicates that cinoxacin, when compared with nalidixic acid, may have advantages of a simpler dosage regimen and milder adverse effects.

Characteristics

Peak urine levels: 3 to 4 hr (PO). Protein binding: 60% to 80%. Half-life: normal renal function—1 to 4.2 hr; renal failure—4 to 16 hr. Metabolism: hepatic, inactive. Excretion: 65% unchanged in urine within 12 to 24 hr, 92% as active drug and inactive metabolites within 24 hr. Dialysis: yes, H. Breast milk: unknown.

Administration and dosage
Adult

Normal renal function: PO—1 g daily in 2 to 4 divided doses for 7 to 14 days.

Impaired renal function: see chart below. Do not administer to anuric patients.

Creatinine clearance (ml/min)	Dosage
>80	500 mg every 12 hr
50-80	250 mg every 8 hr
20-40	250 mg every 12 hr
<20	250 mg daily

Pediatric

Not recommended in children under 12 years of age.

Nurse and patient considerations

* Side effects occur in about 10% of patients and are reversible on discontinuation of therapy. Most frequently occurring are gastrointestinal complaints manifested by nausea (3%) and vomiting, anorexia, diarrhea, and abdominal cramps (1%). Up to 3% of patients develop rash, perineal burning, urticaria, pruritus, or hives. CNS effects are noted in less than 2% of patients reporting headache and dizziness and less than 1% reporting insomnia, photophobia, tingling sensations, and tinnitus.

* Use is not recommended in pregnancy, because of the development of malformations in fetuses of laboratory animals.

* Although it has not been reported, structural similarities with nalidixic acid indicate that hemolysis may occur in patients with glucose-6-phosphate dehydrogenase deficiency. Use cinoxacin with caution in these patients.

> * Although it has not yet been reported, structural similarities with nalidixic acid indicate that cinoxacin may produce false-positive results with urinary glucose tests that utilize the cupric sulfate method (Clinitest). Glucose oxidase tests (Clinistix, Tes-Tape) may be used instead.

Drug interactions

Administration of cinoxacin with probenecid significantly reduces renal excretion of cinoxacin. This may result in inadequate treatment of urinary tract infections with the possible development of organisms resistant to cinoxacin therapy.

Methenamine mandelate
(Mandelamine)

AHFS 8:36
CATEGORY Urinary
antibacterial agent

Action and use

Methenamine mandelate is essentially inactive until it is concentrated and excreted in an acidic urine. Methenamine, in an acidic environment such as an acid urine, produces ammonia and formaldehyde. Formaldehyde is a nonspecific antibacterial agent effective against both gram-positive and gram-negative organisms. The acid portion of the methenamine salt (mandelic acid) provides antiseptic properties while aiding in urinary acidification.

Methenamine mandelate is used in the antibacterial treatment of pyelonephritis, cystitis, pyelitis, and other chronic urinary tract infections. It should not be used alone in the control of acute infections. If urinary acidification is unattainable because of ammonia-producing bacteria such as *P. aeruginosa* or *A. aerogenes,* methenamine therapy is not recommended.

Administration and dosage
Adult

PO—1 g 4 times daily, after meals and at bedtime.

Pediatric
Under 6 years of age

PO—250 mg/13.5 kg 4 times daily. Do not crush the tablets prior to administration.

Six to 12 years of age

PO—50 mg 4 times daily.

Nurse and patient considerations

* The optimal effect of methenamine occurs in urine with a pH of 5.5 or less. Test the urine with pH paper to determine whether a urinary acidifier, such as ascorbic acid 500 mg 4 times daily, may be required.
* Side effects include nausea, vomiting, skin rash, and pruritus.

Drug interactions

Acetazolamide (Diamox) and sodium bicarbonate tend to render the urine more alkaline, preventing proper conversion of methenamine to free formaldehyde in the urine.

Sulfamethizole (Thiosulfil) may form an unsoluble precipitate in acidic urine. Therefore concomitant use of methenamine salts and sulfamethizole should be avoided.

Nalidixic acid
(NegGram)

AHFS 8:36
CATEGORY Urinary
antibacterial agent

Action and use

Although the exact mechanism of action is unknown, nalidixic acid has marked antibacterial activity against gram-negative bacteria. The agent is bactericidal and is effective over a wide urinary pH range.

Nalidixic acid is indicated for the treatment of urinary tract infections caused by susceptible gram-negative microorganisms.

Characteristics

Protein binding: 93% to 97%. Half-life: 8 hr. Metabolism: hepatic, inactive. Excretion: urinary. Dialysis: unknown.

Administration and dosage
Adult

PO—1 g 4 times daily for 1 to 2 weeks. For prolonged therapy administer 2 g daily after the initial treatment period.

Pediatric (3 months to 12 years of age)

NOTE: Do not administer to infants under 3 months of age.

PO—55 mg/kg/24 hr initially in 4 divided doses. For prolonged therapy the total daily dosage should be reduced to 33 mg/kg/24 hr.

Nurse and patient considerations

* The more common side effects of nalidixic acid include nausea and vomiting. Other side effects include drowsiness, headache, dizziness, and weakness.

* Visual disturbances such as overbrightness of lights, change in color perception, difficulty in focusing, and double vision may occur with each dose during the first few days of therapy.

* Toxic psychosis or convulsions have been reported. Predisposing factors include excessive dosage and patients with epilepsy or cerebral arteriosclerosis.

* Patients receiving nalidixic acid therapy should avoid undue exposure to sunlight, since photosensitivity may occur.

* Nalidixic acid may induce a hemolytic anemia in those patients with glucose-6-phosphate dehydrogenase deficiency. This deficiency is found in 10% of blacks and in a small percentage of ethnic groups of Mediterranean and Near Eastern origin.

Drug interactions

The dosage of oral anticoagulants (warfarin) may need to be reduced. Nalidixic acid may displace significant amounts of warfarin from serum protein-binding sites, resulting in hemorrhage.

Nitrofurantoin
(Furadantin, Macrodantin)

AHFS 8:36
CATEGORY Urinary
antibacterial agent

Action and use

Nitrofurantoin is an antibacterial agent for specific urinary tract infections. It is bacteriostatic in low concentrations and possibly bactericidal in higher concentrations. Its mechanism of action is thought to be based on its interference with several bacterial enzyme systems.

Nitrofurantoin is indicated for the treatment of urinary tract infections when caused by susceptible strains of *E. coli*, *Klebsiella*, *Proteus*, and *S. faecalis*. It may be used to treat an *S. aureus* cystitis but should not be used to treat renal cortical or perinephric abscesses caused by this organism. Nitrofurantoin is not effective against *Serratia* or *Pseudomonas* species. The drug does not appear to be effective against bacteria in the blood or tissue outside the urinary tract.

Characteristics

Half-life: 20 min to 1 hr. Excretion: 40% unchanged in urine. Therapeutic level: 0.18 mg/100 ml. Dialysis: yes, H.

Administration and dosage
Adult

PO—50 to 100 mg 4 times daily for 10 to 14 days.

IV 1. Dissolve just before use. Add 20 ml of dextrose 5% or sterile water to a vial containing 180 mg of nitrofurantoin and shake well. Each milliliter of this initial solution should be further diluted with an additional 25 ml of fluid. Therefore 180 mg in 20 ml must be diluted to at least 500 ml of parenteral fluid for infusion.
   2. Do not dilute with solutions containing methylparabens, propylparabens, phenol, or cresol as preservatives. These may cause nitrofurantoin to precipitate out of solution. Therefore do not administer if a precipitate develops.

DOSAGE SCHEDULE

Over 54 kg (120 lb): 180 mg every 12 hr, at a rate of 2 to 3 ml/min. Replace IV therapy with oral administration as soon as possible.

Pediatric (over 1 month of age)

NOTE: Do *not* use in infants under 1 month of age.
PO—5 to 7 mg/kg/24 hr in 4 divided doses.
IV—See instructions for adult IV administration.

DOSAGE SCHEDULE

Under 54 kg (120 lb): 3 mg/kg every 12 hr at a rate of 2 to 3 ml/min. Replace intravenous therapy with oral administration as soon as possible.

Nurse and patient considerations

* Anorexia, nausea, and vomiting are the most frequent side effects of nitrofurantoin. Reduction of dosage and administration with food or milk may minimize gastric upset.
* The clinically effective use of nitrofurantoin is dependent on adequate concentration of the drug in the urine. The agent is not recommended for use in patients with a creatinine clearance of less than 40 ml/min.
* Severe peripheral neuropathies may result from use of nitrofurantoin. Predisposing conditions such as renal impairment, anemia, diabetes, electrolyte imbalance, vitamin B deficiency, and debilitating disease may enhance the risk of this side effect. The drug should be discontinued at the first sign of numbness or tingling in the extremities.
* Metabolites of this agent may change the color of the urine to rust, yellow, or brown.
* Allergic reactions manifested by dyspnea, chills, fever, erythematous rash, and pruritus have been reported. Acute reactions usually develop within 8 hr in previously sensitized patients and within 7 to 10 days in patients who develop sensitivity during the course of therapy.
* Pulmonary reactions, categorized as acute, subacute, or chronic, are thought to be hypersensitivity reactions. These reactions are fairly infrequent and generally quite mild. Women between 40 and 50 are more frequently affected. The danger of the reaction is that it goes undiagnosed long enough for irreversible pulmonary damage to develop. The acute reactions usually occur within the first week of therapy and are manifested by symptoms of dyspnea at rest, nonproductive cough, fever, and rales. Less common symptoms include eosinophilia, nausea, headache, muscle aches, joint tenderness, and chest pain. Chest x-ray films show pleural infiltration with consolidation. Symptoms resolve within 24 to 48 hr after discontinuation of therapy. In subacute reactions, fever and eosinophilia are seen less often. Symptoms may become more severe as nitrofurantoin therapy continues, and full recovery may take several months. Chronic pulmonary reactions

may develop in patients on therapy for 6 months or longer. Common manifestations are the insidious onset of malaise, dyspnea on exertion, cough, and altered pulmonary function. Fever is rarely evident, and x-ray and histologic examination shows interstitial pneumonitis and/or fibrosis. Reversibility of symptoms depends on duration of therapy.

* Nitrofurantoin may induce a hemolytic anemia in those patients with glucose-6-phosphate dehydrogenase deficiency. This deficiency is found in 10% of blacks and in a small percentage of ethnic groups of Mediterranean and Near Eastern origin.

* Nitrofurantoin may induce hemolytic anemia caused by immature enzyme systems in infants younger than 3 months of age. This caution includes mothers nursing these infants since the drug is excreted in breast milk.

Drug interactions

Nitrofurantoin may interfere with oral contraceptive therapy. See General information on oral contraceptives (p. 499).

Phenazopyridine hydrochloride
(Pyridium)

AHFS 8:36
CATEGORY Urinary analgesic

Action and use

Phenazopyridine exerts an anesthetic effect on the mucosa of the urinary tract as it is excreted in the urine. It is used for symptomatic relief of pain, burning, urgency, and frequency arising from irritation of the lower urinary tract.

Administration and dosage
Adult

PO—200 mg 3 times daily.

Pediatric (6 to 12 years of age)

PO—100 mg 3 times daily.

Nurse and patient considerations

* Phenazopyridine produces a reddish orange discoloration of the urine.
* A yellowish tinge to the sclera or the skin may indicate accumulation caused by diminished renal function. The drug should be discontinued if this manifestation results.
* This agent is frequently used in combination with sulfonamides (Azo Gantanol and Azo Gantrisin). The same side effects apply, as well as those of the sulfonamides.

Drug interactions

No clinically significant adverse reactions have been reported.

ANTIFUNGAL AGENTS

Amphotericin B
(Fungizone)

AHFS 8:12.04
CATEGORY Antifungal agent

Action and use

Amphotericin B is a fungistatic agent that binds to sterols in the fungal cell membrane. Alterations in permeability result in the loss of cellular contents. Amphotericin B is primarily used in the treatment of systemic fungal infections and meningitis.

Characteristics

Protein binding: 90%. Half-life: 18 to 24 hr. Metabolism: unknown. Excretion: urine (inactive). Dialysis: No.

Administration and dosage
Adult

NOTE: 1. Amphotericin B must be reconstituted with sterile water for injection without bacteriostatic agent.
2. An in-line membrane filter must *not* be used during infusion.
3. The infusion must be protected from light during administration.
4. The recommended infusion concentration is 1 mg/10 ml of dextrose 5% in water.

IV—Initially 250 µg/kg over a 6 hr period. The daily dose is gradually increased as patient tolerance develops. Dosage may range up to 1 mg/kg daily or up to 1.5 mg/kg on alternate days. Under no circumstances should a single administration dosage exceed 1.5 mg/kg. Venous irritation may be diminished by the addition of 1200 to 1600 units of heparin and/or 10 to 15 mg of hydrocortisone or methylprednisolone to the infusion solution.

INTRATHECAL—25 to 50 µg diluted with 10 to 20 ml of cerebrospinal fluid. The drug is administered 2 or 3 times per week. This dosage is gradually increased to 500 µg to 1 mg, depending on tolerance.

TOPICAL—Amphotericin B is applied liberally to candidal lesions 2 to 4 times daily. Any staining from cream or lotion preparations may be removed by soap and warm water, and any staining from amphotericin ointment may be removed by standard cleaning fluids.

Nurse and patient considerations

* Side effects of this drug are usually dose related and may be minimized by slow infusion, reduction of dosage, and alternate-day administration. They include headache, chills, fever, malaise, muscle and joint pain, cramping, nausea, and vomiting. Antipyretics, antihistamines, and antiemetics may provide some symptomatic relief.

* Amphotericin B is nephrotoxic. The BUN and serum creatinine levels elevate in nearly all patients and should be monitored routinely. Urinary excretion of uric acid, potassium, and magnesium increases, and proteinuria may occur. Other potentially nephrotoxic agents, such as aminoglycoside antibiotics, should be given with caution.

* A reversible normochromic normocytic anemia is common.

Drug interactions

Corticosteroids may enhance the potassium excretion caused by amphotericin B. The patient's electrolyte status should be watched closely.

Candicidin
(Vanobid)

AHFS 84:04.08
CATEGORY Antifungal agent

Action and use

Candicidin is a conjugated heptane antibiotic complex produced by soil actinomycete bacteria. It is both fungistatic and fungicidal and is clinically effective only for the treatment of vaginal infections due to *Candida albicans* and other *Candida* species. It has an advantage in being safe and approved for use during pregnancy.

Administration and dosage

INTRAVAGINAL—1 vaginal applicatorful of ointment or 1 vaginal tablet inserted high in the vagina 2 times daily, morning and at bedtime, for 14 days. During pregnancy, use the applicator only on recommendation from the physician. Digital insertion of tablets may be preferred.

Nurse and patient considerations

* Adverse effects are quite infrequent with this antibiotic. Temporary irritation and sensitization have been reported.
* Patients should be informed (1) to wash the applicator in warm soapy water after each use so that it does not become a vehicle for reinfection, (2) that a pad may be used to protect clothing, (3) to refrain from sexual intercourse during therapy or that the male wear a condom to avoid reinfection, and (4) that contraception other than a diaphragm should be used when the patient is being treated with the vaginal ointment. Prolonged contact with petrolatum-based products may cause deterioration of the diaphragm.

Drug interactions

No specific drug interactions have been reported.

Clotrimazole

AHFS 84:04.08
CATEGORY Antifungal agent

(Lotrimin,
Gyne-Lotrimin)

Action and use

Clotrimazole is a synthetic topical fungicidal agent that apparently acts by altering cell membrane permeability, resulting in loss of intracellular electrolytes. It has been shown to be effective against tinea pedis (athlete's foot), tinea cruris (jock itch), and tinea corporis caused by *Tricophyton rubrum, T. mentagrophytes,* and *Epiderophyton floccosum.* It is also effective in the treatment of vulvovaginitis (candidiasis) caused by *C. albicans.*

Administration and dosage

TOPICAL—Clotrimazole is commercially available as a 1% cream and lotion (Lotrimin). The cream or lotion should be gently rubbed on the affected areas and surrounding skin morning and evening. Clinical improvement should be evident (relief of pruritus) within a week. If there is no improvement within 4 weeks, rediagnosis should be considered. Both the cream and solution should be stored between 2° and 30° C.

INTRAVAGINAL—For the treatment of candidiasis insert 1 clotrimazole 100 mg tablet (Gyne-Lotrimin) into the vagina at bedtime for 7 consecutive days.

Nurse and patient considerations

* The only adverse reactions reported with clotrimazole are in those patients who have developed hypersensitivity reactions to any of the ingredients. Adverse effects are manifested by pruritus, urticaria, blistering, and erythema. Discontinue treatment if any adverse effects develop.
* Therapy with clotrimazole during the first 3 months of pregnancy is not recommended. No adverse effects have been reported when used during the second and third trimesters of pregnancy.

Drug interactions

No specific drug interactions have been reported.

Flucytosine
(Ancobon)

AHFS 8:12.04
CATEGORY Antifungal agent

Action and use

Flucytosine is a nonantibiotic antifungal agent. Mechanism of action is unknown. It is effective against susceptible candidal septicemia, endocarditis, urinary tract infections, cryptococcal meningitis, and pulmonary infections.

Characteristics

Peak plasma levels: 2 hr. Protein binding: 50%. Half-life: 3 to 4 hr. Excretion: 90% unchanged in urine. Dialysis: yes, H, P.

Administration and dosage
Adult

NOTE: Close monitoring of hematologic, renal, and hepatic status is essential.

PO—50 to 150 mg/kg/day given at 6 hr intervals. Doses up to 250 mg/kg/day may be required in cryptococcal meningitis. Nausea may be reduced if capsules are given a few at a time over 20 to 30 min. Dosage adjustment is required in patients with impaired renal function due to the high urinary content of unmetabolized drug.

Nurse and patient considerations

* Many of the potentially serious adverse effects of flucytosine are related to affects on rapidly proliferating tissues, especially in the bone marrow and mucosa of the gastrointestinal tract. Indications of this are leukopenia, pancytopenia, anemia, thrombocytopenia, nausea, vomiting, and diarrhea.
* Decrease in hemoglobin levels and elevation of alkaline phosphatase, SGOT, SGPT, BUN, and serum creatinine levels are common. Elevations of liver function tests generally appear to be dose related and reversible.
* Other side effects include confusion, hallucinations, headache, sedation, and vertigo.
* Caution must be used prenatally and postnatally since flucytosine has produced birth defects in laboratory animals.
* Use with caution in patients with impaired renal function.

Drug interactions

Flucytosine and amphotericin B display synergistic activity when used concomitantly. It is proposed that amphotericin B affects the fungal cell membrane, allowing greater penetration of flucytosine.

Griseofulvin

AHFS 8:12.04

(Grisactin, Grifulvin V, Fulvicin-U/F, Gris-PEG, Fulvicin P/G)

CATEGORY Antifungal agent

Action and use

Griseofulvin is a fungistatic agent used to treat ringworm infections of skin, hair, and nails. Its proposed mechanism of action is destruction of the fungal cell's mitotic spindle structure, preventing cell division and multiplication. Since griseofulvin is only active against certain species of fungi and not against bacterial or yeast infection, the infecting organism should be identified as a dermatophyte before initiating therapy.

Characteristics

Half-life: 9 to 24 hr. Metabolism: minimal. Excretion: less than 1% in urine, primarily unchanged in feces.

Administration and dosage
Adult

PO—Depending on the specific organism and the location of the infection, 500 mg to 4 g in single or divided doses daily. Absorption from the gastrointestinal tract may be increased by giving the drug with a meal high in fat content.

Nurse and patient considerations

∗ The length of treatment depends on the time required for the replacement of infected skin, hair, or nails. Treatment of skin infections may require only a few weeks of therapy, while infections of toenails may require at least 6 months of continuous treatment.

* Hypersensitivity reactions manifesting as skin rashes and urticaria are relatively common adverse effects of griseofulvin. Others include headaches especially in oral therapy, oral thrush, nausea, vomiting, diarrhea, dizziness, and confusion.
* The patient should be advised concerning possible photosensitivity reaction to sunlight. Proper hygiene and continuation of therapy beyond remission of symptoms is essential.
* During prolonged therapy, periodic laboratory tests should be completed to warn of changes in renal, hepatic, and hematopoietic function. Leukopenia and proteinuria have been reported. Acute attacks of intermittent porphyria have been related to the use of griseofulvin.
* Use with caution in pregnancy. Embryogenic and teratogenic effects have been observed in laboratory animals.

Drug interactions

Griseofulvin may induce hepatic enzymes to increase metabolism of warfarin. Griseofulvin therapy must not be started or stopped while patients are taking oral anticoagulants without monitoring the prothrombin time.

Phenobarbital impairs the absorption of griseofulvin. If concomitant therapy is required, divided doses 3 times daily may be absorbed better than large doses taken less often.

Ketoconazole
(Nizoral)

AHFS 8:12.04
CATEGORY Antifungal agent

Action and use

Ketoconazole is an antifungal agent closely related in chemical structure and activity to clotrimazole and miconazole. It too acts by impairing the synthesis of ergosterol, a chemical needed by fungi to maintain cell wall integrity. Inhibition of ergosterol synthesis results in increased permeability and leakage of intracellular potassium and phosphorus. It has been shown to be effective against candidiasis, chronic mucocutaneous candidiasis, oral thrush, canduria, coccidioidomycosis, histoplasmosis, chromomycosis, and paracoccidioidomycosis.

Characteristics

Peak plasma levels: 1 to 2 hr (PO). protein binding: 99%. Half-life: biphasic—2 hr during the first 10 hr, then 8 hr thereafter. Metabolism: extensive. Excretion: biliary—85% to 90% as metabolites; 9% to 11% in urine as metabolites; 2% to 4% in urine as active drug. Breast milk: yes.

Administration and dosage
Adult

PO—200 to 400 mg once daily. Absorption from the gastrointestinal tract is improved when administered with a meal. Patients with achlorhydria should dissolve each tablet in 4 ml of 0.2N hydrochloric acid, ingest through a straw to minimize contact with the teeth, and follow with a glass of water.

Pediatric
Under 20 kg (44 lb)

PO—50 mg once daily.

Between 20 to 40 kg (44 to 88 lb)

PO—100 mg once daily.

Over 40 kg (88 lb)
PO—200 mg once daily.

Duration of treatment depends on the infecting microorganism.

Nurse and patient considerations

* Side effects are usually quite mild and resolve with continued therapy. Nausea and vomiting (3%) are usually controlled by administration just before or with a meal. Other side effects reported are pruritus (1.5%), abdominal pain (1.2%), rash, dizziness, constipation, diarrhea, fever, chills, and headache.
* Gynecomastia (breast pain and fullness) has been reported in men. Symptoms resolve with continued therapy in most cases.
* Transient elevations of liver enzymes have been recorded in several patients, and one case of probable drug-induced hepatitis has been reported.
* Teratogenic and embryotoxic effects have been reported in laboratory animals. Ketoconazole should not be prescribed for pregnant women unless alternative therapy is unsuccessful and benefits significantly outweigh the risks associated with therapy.

Drug interactions

The bioavailability of ketoconazole is significantly increased in an acid media. Antacids, cimetidine, and anticholinergic agents (Bentyl, Donnatal) decrease stomach acidity, decreasing peak ketoconazole levels. Administer these agents at least 2 hr after ketoconazole administration.

Miconazole nitrate
(Monistat, Micatin)

AHFS 84:04.08
CATEGORY Antifungal agent

Action and use

Miconazole nitrate is a topical antifungal agent that has been shown to be effective against tinea pedis (athlete's foot), tinea cruris (jock itch), and tinea corporis caused by *T. rubrum, T. mentagrophytes,* and *E. floccosum.* It is also effective in the treatment of vulvovaginitis (candidiasis) caused by *C. albicans.* Although the exact mechanism of action is unknown, miconazole alters cell membrane permeability, resulting in the loss of intracellular constituents.

Parenteral miconazole may be used to treat the following severe systemic fungal infections: coccidioidomycosis, candidiasis, cryptococcosis, paracoccidioidomycosis, and for the treatment of chronic mucocutaneous candidiasis. Bladder irrigations must be used for fungal cystitis, and intrathecal injections must be used to treat fungal meningitis.

Characteristics

Half-life: first phase—0.4 hr; second phase—2.1 hr; third phase—24.1 hr (IV). Metabolism: liver. Excretion: 14% to 22% excreted in urine, primarily as inactive metabolites. Dialysis: no, H.

Administration and dosage

TOPICAL—Miconazole nitrate is available as a 2% cream or lotion (Micatin). The cream should be gently rubbed on the affected areas and surrounding skin morning and evening. The lotion is recommended for use in intertriginous areas and is applied in the same manner. Clinical improvement should be evident (relief of pruritus) within 1 week. If no improvement is noted within 4 weeks, reexamination and diagnosis should be considered.

INTRAVAGINAL—For treatment of candidiasis insert 1 applicatorful (Monistat-7 vaginal cream) intravaginally once daily at bedtime for 7 days.

NOTE: Miconazole nitrate is not effective in treating vulvovaginitis caused by *Trichomonas* species or *Haemophilus vaginalis*.

INTRAVENOUS

NOTE: Do not use the parenteral form to treat trivial infections. Dilute all infusion solutions with at least 200 ml of 0.9% sodium chloride or dextrose 5% and administer over a period of 30 to 60 min.

Adult

COCCIDIOIDOMYCOSIS—1800 to 3600 mg divided into 3 doses daily.

CRYPTOCOCCOSIS—1200 to 2400 mg divided into 3 doses daily.

CANDIDIASIS—600 to 1800 mg divided into 3 doses daily.

PARACOCCIDIOIDOMYCOSIS—200 to 1200 mg divided into 3 doses daily.

INTRATHECAL—20 mg every 3 to 7 days as an adjunct to IV treatment of fungal meningitis. Administer undiluted by alternating lumbar, cervical, and cisternal punctures.

BLADDER INSTILLATION—200 mg of diluted solution to treat mycoses of the bladder.

Pediatric

A total daily dose of 20 to 40 mg/kg divided into 3 or more equal doses. Do not exceed 15 mg/kg/infusion.

Nurse and patient considerations

* Miconazole nitrate may cause irritation, burning, and erythema in a few patients. If a hypersensitivity reaction or chemical irritation occurs, discontinue use.
* Avoid eye contact with any of the miconazole products. Wash eyes immediately if contact should occur.
* Miconazole is effective in pregnant and nonpregnant women; however, intravaginal use of Monistat-7 is not recommended during the first trimester of pregnancy.

* Adverse effects associated with parenteral therapy include phlebitis (29%), pruritus (21%), nausea (18%), fever and chills (10%), rash (9%), and emesis (7%). Thrombocytopenia and transient drops in hematocrit and serum sodium values have also been reported. The frequency and severity of nausea and vomiting can be reduced with the use of antihistaminic or antiemetic drugs given before infusion or by reducing the dose, slowing the rate of infusion, and by avoiding administration after mealtime.

Drug interactions

No specific drug interactions have been reported with topical miconazole.

Parenteral miconazole may enhance the anticoagulant effects of warfarin (Coumadin). Reduction of warfarin doses may be necessary if the prolongation of the prothrombin time becomes excessive.

Nystatin
(Mycostatin, Nilstat)

AHFS 8:12.04
CATEGORY Antifungal agent

Action and use

Nystatin is an antifungal antibiotic used in the treatment of monilial infections of the skin, oral cavity, vulvovaginal mucosa, and intestinal tract. It is not effective in the treatment of systemic monilial infections. Antifungal activity is derived from nystatin binding to sterols within the fungal cell membrane, resulting in the loss of selective permeability.

Administration and dosage

PO 1. Gastrointestinal tract: 500,000 to 1 million units 3 times daily.
2. Oral cavity: 400,000 to 600,000 units of suspension 4 times daily. The suspension should be retained in the mouth for several minutes before swallowing if possible.

Treatment of the oral cavity and gastrointestinal tract should be continued for at least 48 hr after remission of symptoms and after cultures have returned to normal flora.

Pediatric

Infants. Administer 200,000 units (2 ml) 4 times daily (1 ml in each side of the mouth). For premature and low birth weight infants administer 100,000 units (1 ml) 4 times daily.

Children. As for adult dosages.

Nurse and patient considerations

∗ Side effects are uncommon with nystatin, although administration of the tablets and suspension may produce transient nausea, vomiting, and diarrhea. Hypersensitivity to nystatin is quite rare; however, patients more commonly develop a contact dermatitis to the preservatives in the topical preparations.

∗ When treating topical candidal infection the powder is recommended where the lesions are moist, such as in skin folds or on feet. The affected areas should be kept dry and exposed to air if possible. Concomitant therapy must include proper hygiene to prevent reinfection.

Drug interactions

No specific interactions have been reported.

Tolnaftate
(Tinactin)

AHFS 84:04.08
CATEGORY Antifungal agent

Action and use

Tolnaftate is a fungistatic and fungicidal agent effective against *T. rubrum, T. mentagrophytes, T. tonsurans,* and various *Microsporum* and *Aspergillus* species. Tolnaftate is commonly used to treat tinea pedis (athlete's foot), tinea cruris (jock itch), tinea corporis, and tinea manuum when caused by the above fungal pathogens. The mechanism of action is unknown. Tolnaftate is not effective against the yeastlike *C. albicans.*

Administration and dosage

TOPICAL—Tolnaftate is available in cream, solution, powder, and spray powder, all in 1% concentrations. All the products may be used interchangeably; however, the powder is most effective in intertriginous areas and in cases when a dry environment may enhance the therapeutic response. Only small amounts of the cream or solution are necessary for therapy. Dry the affected areas, apply, and gently massage in until the medication disappears. Apply the medication 2 times daily for 2 to 3 weeks. Clinical improvement should be observed within 2 to 3 days. Treatments may be required for 6 weeks or more with long-standing infections and in areas with thickened skin. If no improvement is evident after 4 weeks, the diagnosis should be reviewed.

Nurse and patient considerations

* Adverse effects with tolnaftate are quite infrequent. Local irritation and burning have been reported when the medication has been applied to excoriated skin or to lesions caused by multiple pathogens. Discontinue therapy if the lesions get worse or if there is evidence of hypersensitivity (pruritus, urticaria, erythema).
* Avoid contact with the eyes. Wash the eyes immediately if contact occurs.

Drug interactions

No specific drug interactions have been reported.

ANTITUBERCULAR AGENTS

Ethambutol hydrochloride   AHFS 8:16
(Myambutol)   CATEGORY Antitubercular agent

Action and use

Ethambutol is a bacteriostatic agent used in combination with other chemotherapy in the treatment of pulmonary tuberculosis. Its mode of action is inhibition of RNA synthesis and phosphate metabolism, resulting in inhibition of cellular multiplication.

Characteristics

Peak plasma level: 2 to 4 hr (PO). Half-life: 8 hr. Excretion: 50% unchanged and 15% as metabolites in urine in 24 hr. Dialysis: yes, H, P.

Administration and dosage

NOTE: Ethambutol should not be used alone, but in combination with other antitubercular agents. Ethambutol is not recommended for use in patients under 13 years of age.

PO   1. Patients who have received no previous antitubercular therapy: 15 mg/kg as a single dose every 24 hr.
   2. Retreatment: 25 mg/kg as a single daily dose. After 60 days reduce the dose to 15 mg/kg and administer as a single dose every 24 hr.
   3. Patients with renal insufficiency should be observed for cumulative effects of the drug. The dosage for those patients with a creatinine clearance of less than 10 ml/min should be 6 to 10 mg/kg.

Nurse and patient considerations

* Approximately 6% of patients receiving therapy exhibit decreased visual acuity and reduction of green color vision. These effects usually appear within 7 months after starting therapy and generally disappear within several weeks after therapy is discontinued.
* Other side effects include dermatitis, pruritus, anorexia, nausea, vomiting, headache, dizziness, mental confusion, disorientation, and hallucinations.
* Elevated serum uric acid levels occur, and precipitation of acute gout has been reported.
* Transient elevations of liver function tests are a common observation.
* Patients should be warned that omission or interrupted intake may result in drug resistance, reversal of clinical improvement, and increased susceptibility of family members to tuberculosis.
* Ethambutol is not recommended in pregnant women.

Drug interactions

No specific interactions have been reported.

Isoniazid
(Hyzyd, Nydrazid)

AHFS 8:16
CATEGORY Antitubercular agent

Action and use

Isoniazid is both a tuberculostatic and tuberculocidal agent effective against *Mycobacterium tuberculosis* as well as other organisms of this genus. The bactericidal effects are exerted only against actively growing tubercle bacilli and do not affect those cells in a resting state. Although the mechanism of action is unknown, isoniazid penetrates sensitive cells well and is effective against intracellularly located bacilli as well as those growing in vitro.

Characteristics

Peak plasma levels: 1 to 2 hr (PO). Half-life: 50 to 110 min in "rapid inactivators," 140 to 250 minutes in "slow inactivators." Metabolism: acetylation in liver. Excretion: 75% to 95% in urine as metabolites. Dialysis: yes, H, P.

Administration and dosage
Adult

PO 1. For treatment of active tuberculosis isoniazid should be used in conjunction with other effective antitubercular agents, 5 mg/kg to a maximum of 300 mg daily.
   2. Prophylactic therapy: 300 mg daily in single or divided doses.
   3. Concurrent administration of pyridoxine, 25 to 50 mg daily, is recommended for prevention of peripheral neurophathies.
   4. Administer on an empty stomach for maximal absorption.

IM—As for PO administration.

Pediatric

Infants and children tolerate larger doses than adults and may be given 10 to 30 mg/kg 24 hr PO in single or divided doses. Maximum dose is 500 mg daily.

Nurse and patient considerations

* Approximately 50% of blacks and whites are slow inactivators, while the majority of Eskimos, American Indians, and Orientals are rapid inactivators. This does not significantly alter the effectiveness of the medication; however, slow inactivators may have higher blood levels and may manifest more toxic symptoms.

* Peripheral neuropathy, often preceded by numbness and tingling of the hands or feet, nausea, vomiting, dizziness, and ataxia are relatively common side effects of isoniazid and are dose related.

* The incidence of hepatotoxicity increases with age to about 2.3% of those patients over 50 years of age. This reaction often occurs within the first 3 months of therapy and is suspected of being an allergic manifestation. Early symptoms include fatigue, weakness, anorexia, and malaise. Serum transaminase levels are not a good indicator of this toxic reaction, since they may already be elevated.

* Hematologic reactions include agranulocytosis, eosinophilia, thrombocytopenia, hemolytic anemia, and methemoglobinemia.

* Patient counseling must emphasize that omission or interrupted intake may result in drug resistance, reversal of clinical improvement, and increased susceptibility of family members to tuberculosis.

Drug interactions

Combined therapy with disulfiram (Antabuse) and isoniazid may result in changes in affect and behavior as well as incoordination.

Concomitant use of meperidine (Demerol) and isoniazid is not recommended, because of the interaction of meperidine and MAO inhibitors. Isoniazid does display some MAO inhibition.

Clinical evidence indicates that concomitant use of isoniazid and rifampin may result in hepatotoxicity, especially in patients with previous liver impairment and/or those patients who are slow acetylators. Either agent when used alone may result in abnormal liver function tests.

Isoniazid inhibits the metabolism of phenytoin (Dilantin), resulting in elevated phenytoin levels. The reaction is usually significant only in slow acetylators, but may result in excessive sedation and incoordination.

Isoniazid inhibits the metabolism of carbamazepine, resulting in signs of carbamazepine toxicity (disorientation, ataxia, lethargy, headache, drowsiness, nausea, vomiting). The reaction may develop within 1 to 2 days of combined therapy and is more likely to occur in patients taking greater than 200 mg of isoniazid daily.

Antacids (aluminum hydroxide, magaldrate) have been shown to reduce the amount of isoniazid absorbed. Administer the isoniazid at least 1 hr before ingestion of antacids to prevent malabsorption.

Isoniazid may inhibit the metabolism of diazepam (Valium), causing moderately prolonged activity. Observe patients for altered response to diazepam when isoniazid therapy is started or stopped.

Rifampin
(Rifadin)

AHFS 8:16
CATEGORY Antitubercular agent

Action and use

Rifampin is a bacteriostatic and bactericidal antibiotic used with other chemotherapy in the treatment of pulmonary tuberculosis. Rifampin exerts its therapeutic effect by interacting with DNA-dependent RNA polymerase.

Characteristics

Peak plasma levels: 2 to 4 hr. Protein binding: 75% to 90%. Half-life: 1½ to 5 hr; the half-life diminishes by up to 40% during the first 14 days of treatment as a result of increased biliary excretion. Excretion: up to 30% in urine, unchanged and as metabolites. Dialysis: unknown.

Administration and dosage

NOTE: Rifampin should not be used alone, but in combination with other antitubercular agents. Administer 1 hr before or 2 hr after meals.

Adult

PO—600 mg once daily.

Pediatric

PO—10 to 20 mg/kg/24 hr with a maximum daily dose of 600 mg.

Nurse and patient considerations

* Gastrointestinal disturbances such as heartburn, anorexia, nausea, vomiting, cramps, gas, and diarrhea are some of the more common side effects. Other adverse reactions include headache, dizziness, mental confusion, visual disturbances, and generalized numbness.

* Transient elevations in serum bilirubin, alkaline phosphatase, SGOT, SGPT, BUN, and uric acid levels have been noted. Rifampin may produce liver dysfunction and should be used with caution in patients with liver disease.

* Rare hematologic side effects include thrombocytopenia, leukopenia, hemolytic anemia, hemoglobinuria, and hematuria.

* The patient should be informed of the possibility of red-orange urine, feces, saliva, sputum, sweat, and tears.

* Patient counseling must emphasize that omission or interrupted intake may result in drug resistance, reversal of clinical improvement, and increased susceptibility of family members to tuberculosis.

* Although birth defects have not been reported, caution must be used prenatally and postnatally, since rifampin diffuses across the placental barrier and is secreted in breast milk.

Drug interactions

Rifampin may decrease the prothrombin time and increase the dosage of warfarin.

Increased liver dysfunction may result from the combined use of isoniazid and rifampin, especially in patients with previous liver impairment and/or in those who are slow isoniazid inactivators.

The contraceptive efficacy of oral contraceptives when taken with rifampin may be impaired. Alternative contraceptive methods should be considered. See General information on oral contraceptives (p. 499).

Rifampin stimulates the metabolism of diazepam. Patients receiving long-term diazepam therapy may require an increase in dosage to maintain therapeutic activity.

Rifampin enhances quinidine metabolism. Patients receiving long-term quinidine and rifampin therapy may require an increase in quinidine dosage to maintain therapeutic activity.

ANTHELMINTIC AGENTS

Mebendazole
(Vermox)

AHFS 8:08
CATEGORY Anthelmintic agent

Action and use

Mebendazole is an oral anthelmintic agent that apparently works by inhibiting carbohydrate transport and metabolism of the intestinal cells of worms. The intestinal cells die, resulting in the death of the parasite. There does not appear to be any alteration of carbohydrate metabolism in humans. Mebendazole is used in the treatment of *Trichuris trichiura* (whipworm), *Enterobius vermicularis* (pinworm), *Ascaris lumbricoides* (roundworm), *Ancylostoma duodenale* (common hookworm), and *Necator americanus,* (American hookworm).

Administration and dosage
Adult and pediatric (over 2 years of age)

PO   1. Pinworm: 1 tablet (100 mg) 1 time, well mixed with food and chewed.
2. Roundworm, whipworm, and hookworm: 1 tablet (100 mg) morning and evening on 3 consecutive days. If evidence of infestation persists beyond 3 to 4 weeks, another course of therapy may be administered.

Special diets, fasting, enemas, or laxatives are not necessary prior to therapy.

The safe use of mebendazole in children under 2 years of age has not been established. The risk versus the benefit of therapy must be considered in these patients.

Nurse and patient considerations

* Side effects are usually minimal; however, patients may experience nausea, diarrhea, and abdominal pain.
* Hygienic procedures should be explained to patients to help prevent reinfection. Precautions should include wearing shoes, washing hands with soap and cleaning under fingernails, especially before eating and after defecation, and washing all fruits and vegetables thoroughly before eating them.

* Mebendazole is *contraindicated* in pregnant women. Teratogenic effects have been reported in pregnant rats after a single dose of this agent.

Drug interactions

No specific drug interactions have been reported.

Piperazine citrate
(Antepar, Multifuge, Vermizine)

AHFS 8:08
CATEGORY Anthelmintic agent

Action and use

Piperazine is an oral anthelmintic agent that acts by blocking the effects of acetylcholine at the neuromuscular junctions of worms, resulting in paralysis. The paralyzed parasites are then expelled from the gastrointestinal tract by normal peristalsis. Piperazine is effective against *E. vermicularis* (pinworm) and *A. lumbricoides* (roundworm).

Administration and dosage
Adult

PO 1. Roundworm: a single daily dose of 3.5 g PO for 2 consecutive days.
    2. Pinworm: a single daily dose of 65 mg/kg (maximum daily dose: 2.5 g) for 7 consecutive days.

Pediatric

PO 1. Roundworm: a single daily dose of 75 mg/kg (maximum daily dose: 3.5 g) for 2 consecutive days.
    2. Pinworm: as for adult dosages.
    Special diets, fasting, enemas, or laxatives are not necessary prior to therapy.

Nurse and patient considerations

* Hygienic procedures should be explained to patients to help prevent reinfection. Precautions should include wearing shoes, washing hands with soap and cleaning under fingernails especially before eating and after defecation, and washing all fruits and vegetables thoroughly before eating them.

* Side effects are usually minimal and transient. Complaints of nausea, vomiting, diarrhea, cramps, dizziness, and headache occur occasionally.
* Hypersensitivity reactions consisting of skin rashes, pruritus, fever, joint pain, purpura, fever, and chills have been reported. Discontinue therapy immediately if these symptoms develop.
* Piperazine may cause central nervous system effects in some patients (especially children). If ataxia, muscle spasticity, nystagmus, muscle weakness, or numbness develops, discontinue therapy immediately. Patients with a history of neurologic disorders such as epilepsy should not be given piperazine.
* Safe use of piperazine in pregnant or lactating patients has not been established.

Drug interactions

Pyrantel pamoate (Antiminth) and piperazine have antagonistic mechanisms of action. Courses of therapy should not be administered concurrently.

Pyrantel pamoate
(Antiminth)

AHFS 8:08
CATEGORY Anthelmintic agent

Action and use

Pyrantel is also a neuromuscular blocking agent, but in contrast to piperazine citrate, pyrantel acts by stimulating acetylcholine release at the neuromuscular junction. It also inhibits acetylcholinesterase, the enzyme necessary for metabolism of acetycholine. The paralyzed worms are then expelled from the gastrointestinal tract by normal peristalsis. Pyrantel may be used to treat *E. vermicularis* (pinworm) and *A. lumbricoides* (roundworm).

Administration and dosage
Adult and pediatric

PO—Administer 11 mg/kg (maximum dose: 1 g) once only. The suspension may be given with food or milk at any time of the day.

Special diets, fasting, enemas, or laxatives are not necessary prior to therapy.

The safe use of pyrantel pamoate in children under 2 years of age has not been established. The risk versus the benefit of therapy must be considered in these patients.

Nurse and patient considerations

* Hygienic procedures should be explained to patients to help prevent reinfection. Precautions should include wearing shoes, washing hands with soap and cleaning under fingernails, especially before eating and after defecation, and washing all fruits and vegetables thoroughly before eating.
* Side effects are usually minimal and transient. Complaints of nausea, vomiting, diarrhea, and headache occur most frequently.
* Pyrantel pamoate should be used with caution in patients with liver disease.
* Safe use of pyrantel pamoate in pregnant or lactating patients has not been established.

Drug interactions

Piperazine Citrate (Antepar, Multifunge, Vermizine) and pyrantel pamoate have antagonistic mechanisms of action. Courses of therapy should not be administered concurrently.

Pyrvinium pamoate
(Povan)

AHFS 8:08
CATEGORY Anthelmintic agent

Action and use

Pyrvinium pamoate is an organic dye that exerts its anthelmintic effects in worms by altering carbohydrate absorption and by inhibiting respiration. Pyrvinium pamoate is used to treat *E. vermicularis* (pinworm).

Administration and dosage
Adult and pediatric

PO—Administer a single dose of 5 mg/kg (maximum dose: 350 mg). Tablets should be swallowed without chewing to prevent staining of teeth.

Special diets, fasting, enemas, or laxatives are not necessary before therapy.

If the infestation persists after 2 to 3 weeks the treatment may be repeated.

Nurse and patient considerations

* Pyrvinium pamoate is a bright red dye that will stain clothing, stools, and vomitus. The staining is harmless to patients but may be unremovable if spilled on most materials.
* Hygienic procedures should be explained to patients to help prevent reinfection. Precautions should include wearing shoes, washing hands with soap and cleaning under fingernails, especially before eating and after defecation, and washing all fruits and vegetables thoroughly before eating them.
* Nausea, vomiting, cramping, and diarrhea are the most frequently reported side effects. Vomiting occurs more commonly in adults who receive large doses; it is also more common with the suspension than with the tablets.
* Do not use in patients with conditions such as inflammatory bowel disease. Gastrointestinal absorption is enhanced, and toxic effects may result.
* Safe use in pregnant and lactating patients has not been established.

Drug interactions

No specific drug interactions have been reported.

Quinacrine hydrochloride
(Atabrine hydrochloride)

AHFS 8:08
CATEGORY Anthelmintic agent

Action and use

The mechanism of action of quinacrine hydrochloride is unknown except that it causes detachment of the parasite from the intestinal wall, allowing it to be removed by purging. Quinacrine may be effective against *Taenia saginata* (beef tapeworm), *T. solium* (pork tapeworm), *Diphyllobothrium latum* (fish tapeworm), and *Hymenolepis nana* (dwarf tapeworm). Quinacrine may also be used to treat malaria and giardiasis.

Administration and dosage

For tapeworm:
Restrict the patient to a bland, nonfat, liquid, or semisolid diet for 24 to 48 hr.

The patient should not eat or drink anything after the last evening meal.

A saline cathartic and/or cleansing enema may be given before treatment.

Adult

PO—Administer 4 doses of 200 mg, 10 min apart (total dose: 800 mg) accompanied by 600 mg of sodium bicarbonate with each dose to reduce vomiting.

Pediatric

Ages 5 to 10 years. Administer 2 doses of 200 mg 10 min apart (total dose: 400 mg) followed by 300 mg of sodium bicarbonate with each dose.

Ages 11 to 14 years. Administer 3 doses of 200 mg 10 min apart (total dose: 600 mg) followed by 300 mg of sodium bicarbonate after each dose.

Over 14 years of age. As for adult dosages.

A saline cathartic should be administered 1 to 2 hr after administration of quinacrine to expel the tapeworm.

The worm will be stained yellow and should be examined carefully for the presence of the scolex (head). If the scolex is not found, the patient may be considered cured only if segments do not reappear in the stool over the next 3 to 6 months.

Episodes of nausea and vomiting are frequent, especially when large doses are administered in the treatment of tapeworm. Use of a duodenal tube may reduce emesis. If a tube is used, administer the saline cathartic about 30 min after quinacrine.

For giardiasis:

Adult

PO—100 mg 3 times daily for 5 to 7 days.

Pediatric

PO—7 mg/kg daily in 3 divided doses (maximum dose: 300 mg/day) for 5 days. Repeat in 2 weeks if stool specimens still indicate the presence of giardia.

Nurse and patient considerations

* Other side effects noted with chronic administration for malaria include headaches, anorexia, and diarrhea. CNS stimulation manifested by restlessness, nightmares, anxiety, emotional changes, aggressive behavior, and acute psychoses have been reported.

✳ Patients should be informed that the drug imparts a yellowish color to skin and urine. This color change is reversible on discontinuation of therapy.

✳ The drug should be used with great caution in patients with liver disease, alcoholism, renal disease, and glucose-6-phosphate dehydrogenase deficiency. Patients receiving prolonged therapy should periodically have an ophthalmologic examination and a complete blood count.

✳ Use with caution in patients with psoriasis. Quinacrine may seriously exacerbate the disease.

✳ Because of possible teratogenic effects, quinacrine must not be administered to pregnant women.

Drug interactions

Toxic levels of primaquine may result if quinacrine and primaquine are administered concurrently.

Thiabendazole
(Mintezol)

AHFS 8:08
CATEGORY Anthelmintic agent

Action and use

Thiabendazole has a spectrum of activity against a large variety of helminths, making it quite useful as in the treatment of mixed helminthic infestations. The exact mechanism of action of thiabendazole has not been determined; however, it is an enzyme inhibitor in the parasitic worm. Thiabendazole is effective in the treatment of *E. vermicularis* (pinworm), *A. lumbricoides* (roundworm), strongyloidiasis (threadworm), cutaneous larva migrans (creeping eruption), *A. duodenale* (common hookworm), and *N. americanus* (American hookworm).

Characteristics

Onset: rapid. Peak levels: 1 to 2 hr. Duration: 7 to 8 hr. Metabolism: hepatic to glucuronide and sulfate conjugates. Excretion: 90% in urine as inactive metabolites. Dialysis: unknown.

Administration and dosage
Adult

PO—25 mg/kg for patients under 70 kg; 1.5 g for patients over 70 kg. Maximum daily dose: 3g.

Pediatric

PO—22 mg/kg.

Administer preferably after meals.

For pinworms, the dose is given once in the morning and once in the evening on 1 day only. Repeat regimen in 7 days.

For roundworm, hookworm, threadworm, and creeping eruption, the dosage is given once in the morning and once in the evening on 2 successive days. Special diets, fasting, enemas, or laxatives are not necessary before therapy.

The safe use of thiabendazole in children under 2 years of age has not been established. The risk versus the benefit of therapy must be considered in these patients.

Nurse and patient considerations

* Hygienic procedures should be explained to patients to help prevent reinfection. Precautions should include wearing shoes, washing hands with soap and cleaning under fingernails, especially before eating and after defecation, and washing all fruits and vegetables thoroughly before eating them.
* About one third of patients treated with thiabendazole complain of some side effects from therapy. Most are mild and transient, occurring 3 to 4 hr after administration and lasting for 2 to 8 hr. The most frequent adverse effects are nausea and dizziness. Diarrhea, lethargy, drowsiness, and headache are less common. Patients should be warned not to attempt tasks requiring mental alertness.
* Hypersensitivity reactions consisting of skin rashes, fever, chills, and facial flushing have been reported. Discontinue therapy immediately if these symptoms develop.
* Because of significant hepatic metabolism and renal excretion, thiabendazole should be used with caution in patients with hepatic or renal impairment.
* Safe use in pregnancy and lactation has not been established.

Drug interactions

No specific drug interactions have been reported.

ANTIPARASITIC AGENTS

Benzyl benzoate
AHFS 84:04.12
CATEGORY Antiparasitic agent

Action and use

Benzyl benzoate is an organic compound toxic to arthropods such as *Sarcoptes scabiei* (scabies), *Pediculus humanis* var. *capitis* (head lice), and *Phthirus pubis* (crab lice). The mechanism of action is not known. Although gamma benzene hexachloride 1% (p. 116) is considered the drug of choice for the treatment of scabies in adults, benzyl benzoate is most frequently used in infants and young children because of its lower potential for toxicity.

Administration and dosage

NOTE: For external use only. Do not administer orally; do not apply to inflamed or raw, weeping skin. Benzyl benzoate lotion is available as a 28% and a 50% solution. Dilute the 50% solution with an equal volume of water before using.

For scabies:

1. Have the patient bathe with soap and water to scrub and remove scaly skin. Towel dry.
2. While skin is still slightly damp, apply a thin layer of 28% lotion over the entire body from neck to toes (cover all extremities, including soles of feet). Gently rub into all skin surfaces, especially between fingers, toes, and skin folds. Avoid contact with the face, eyes, mucous membranes, and urethral meatus.
3. Apply a second coat after the first layer has dried. Some clinicians recommend that 2 more coats be applied the next day.
4. The drug should be removed by bathing 24 to 48 hr after the last application.
5. Repeat treatment in 7 to 10 days if mites appear or new lesions develop.

For head or pubic (crab) lice:

1. Bathe as above.
2. Rub 28% benzyl benzoate lotion into the affected hairy areas. Avoid exposure to eyes.

3. Remove with soap and water after 12 to 24 hr.
4. Comb air with a fine-toothed comb to remove nit shells.
5. Repeat in 1 week if the first application was not adequate.

Nurse and patient considerations

∗ The first manifestations of scabies infestation may not occur until 2 to 6 weeks after contact. During this period scabies is highly contagious. All family members and close social contacts should be carefully examined and treated if necessary. Pruritus from scabies and their by-products may last for several weeks after treatment. Unless new lesions develop or the patient is recontaminated, there is no indication for further treatment.

∗ All clothing and bedding should be machine-washed or dry-cleaned to prevent reinfestation. Combs and brushes should be washed with gamma benzene hexachloride shampoo and then rinsed thoroughly to remove the drug.

∗ Even when applied in appropriate quantities, topical benzyl benzoate may cause minor local irritation with itching and burning. If major irritation or a rash develops, discontinue therapy.

Drug interactions

No specific drug interactions have been reported.

Gamma benzene hexachloride (lindane)

(Kwell)   AHFS 84:04.12
                                  CATEGORY Antiparasitic agent

Action and use

Gamma benzene hexachloride is a synthetic, chlorinated hydrocarbon insecticide. It is particularly effective topically against *S. scabiei* (scabies), *P. humanis* var. *capitis* (head lice), *P. corporis* (body lice), and *P. pubis* (crab lice). Gamma benzene hexachloride acts as a CNS stimulant to arthropods, resulting in convulsions and death.

Administration and dose

NOTE: For external use only. Do not administer orally. Do not apply to inflamed or raw, weeping skin. Gamma benzene hexachloride is available as a 1% cream, lotion, or shampoo. Shake well before use.

For scabies:
1. Have the patient bathe with soap and water to scrub and remove scaly skin. Towel dry.
2. Apply a thin layer of cream or lotion uniformly over the body from neck to toes (cover all extremities, including soles of feet). Gently rub into all skin surfaces, especially between fingers, toes, and skin folds. Avoid contact with face, eyes, mucous membranes, and urethral meatus.
3. After 12 to 24 hr bathe and remove the drug.
4. Dress with freshly laundered clothing.
5. One application is usually adequate; however, 1 or 2 more applications may be required at weekly intervals.

For body lice:
1. Bathe as above.
2. Apply a thin layer of cream or lotion to hairy infested areas and adjacent skin (avoid contact with the face, mucous membranes, and urethral meatus).
3. Bathe thoroughly after 12 to 24 hr to remove all medication. Dress in freshly laundered clothing.
4. Repeat in 4 days if necessary.

For head or pubic (crab) lice:
1. Bathe as above.
2. Apply 15 to 30 ml of shampoo (long hair may require 60 ml) to head or pubic hair and lather well for 5 min.
3. Rinse the hair thoroughly and rub with a dry towel.
4. Comb hair with a fine-toothed comb to remove nit shells.
5. Repeat in 24 hr if needed. Do not apply more than twice in 1 week.
6. Dress in freshly laundered clothing.

Nurse and patient considerations

* The first manifestations of scabies infestation may not occur until 2 to 6 weeks after contact. During this period scabies is highly contagious. All family members and close social contacts should be carefully examined and treated if necessary. Pruritus from scabies and their by-products may last for several weeks after treatment. Unless new lesions develop or the patient is recontaminated, there is no indication for further treatment. Repeated application frequently causes contact dermatitis.

* All clothing and bedding should be machine-washed or dry-cleaned to prevent reinfestation. Combs and brushes should be washed with gamma benzene hexachloride shampoo and then rinsed thoroughly to remove the drug.

* This product is not effective as a prophylactic agent against scabies or lice. Do not use the shampoo routinely.

* Avoid contact with the eyes. If accidently contaminated, wash eyes immediately with water.

* Use cautiously and sparingly in infants and small children. Avoid ingestion via hand-to-mouth (thumbsucking) or hand-to-eye contact.

* Oral ingestion or chronic exposure may result in serious CNS, renal, and hepatic toxicities. If ingested orally, treat immediately with gastric lavage and follow with saline cathartics. Do not use oil laxatives such as castor or mineral oil since absorption may be enhanced.

Drug interactions

No specific drug interactions have been reported.

ANTIVIRAL AGENTS

Acyclovir
(Zovirax)

AHFS 8:18
CATEGORY Antiviral agent

Action and use

Acyclovir is an antiviral agent that acts by accumulating in virus-infected cells, where it competitively inhibits viral DNA polymerase, resulting in inhibition of viral cell replication. It is used topically to treat initial infections of herpes genitalis and non-life-threatening cases of mucocutaneous herpes simplex virus infections in immunocompromised patients. The intravenous form is used to treat initial and recurrent mucosal and cutaneous herpes simplex type 1 and 2 infections in immunosuppressed adults and children and for treatment of severe initial clinical episodes of herpes genitalis in patients who are not immunocompromised.

Characteristics

Absorption: topical—minimal. Onset: immediate (IV). Duration of action: 8 hr (IV). Half-life: normal renal function—2.1 to 3.8 hrs (IV); Ccr < 10 ml/min—20 hr. Protein binding: 9% to 33%. Metabolism: liver—8.5% to 14.1%. Excretion: renal—62% to 91% within 72 hr. Breast milk: unknown.

Administration and dosage

TOPICAL

NOTE: Acyclovir will not prevent transmission of herpes genitalis and will not prevent recurrent infections when applied in the absence of signs and symptoms of the disease.

Acyclovir ointment 5% should be applied to each lesion every 3 hr, 6 times daily for 7 days. A finger cot or rubber gloves should be used to avoid the spread of virus to other tissues and persons. (This is not an ophthalmic ointment; do *not* apply to the eye.)

NOTE: Bolus or rapid IV infusions may result in renal tubular damage. Reconstitute and administer only as directed.

Adult

1. Normal renal function: 5 mg/kg every 8 hr for 5 to 7 days.
2. Impaired renal function: based on estimated creatinine clearance (see chart below).

Creatin clearance rate (ml/min)	Dosage
> 50	5 mg/kg every 8 hr
25 = 50	5 mg/kg every 12 hr
10 = 25	5 mg/kg every 24 hr
< 10	2.5 mg/kg every 24 hr

Pediatric (under 12 years of age)

Administer 250 mg/m^2 every 8 hr for 7 days at a constant infusion rate over 1 hr.

PREPARATION—Acyclovir powder (500 mg vial) is reconstituted with 10 ml of preservative-free sterile water for injection to provide a solution concentration of 50 mg/ml (stable for 12 hr). This solution should be further diluted by any glucose and electrolyte IV fluid to a concentration of 1 to 7 mg/ml before administration (stable for 24 hr). Infuse over at least 1 hr to well-hydrated patients. Observe for phlebitis at the infusion site.

Nurse and patient considerations

* Common complaints associated with topical application include transient burning and stinging, pruritus, and rash. Symptoms are mild and do not cause discontinuation of therapy.

* Side effects that developed after IV administration included phlebitis (14%), transient elevation in serum creatinine (4.7%), and rash or hives (4.7%). Other adverse effects reported included diaphoresis, hematuria, hypotension, headache, and nausea. Approximately 1% of patients receiving parenteral acyclovir manifested neurologic changes characterized by varying degrees of lethargy, obtundation, tremors, confusion, hallucinations, agitation, seizures, or coma.

* Patients who are not well hydrated, do not have the dosage adjusted to account for reduced renal function, and receive bolus administration are quite susceptible to renal tubular damage by precipitation of crystals in the tubules. This complication is characterized by a rise in serum creatinine and blood urea nitrogen (BUN), hematuria, and a decrease in renal creatinine clearance. Renal tubular damage may result in acute renal failure.

* Safe use in pregnancy has not been established. Use only if the benefits significantly outweigh the risks of therapy.

Drug interactions

Concomitant therapy with probenecid and acyclovir will prolong serum concentrations of acyclovir because probenecid blocks renal tubular secretion of acyclovir.

Idoxuridine
(Dendrid, Herplex
Liquifilm, Stoxil)

AHFS 52:04.06
CATEGORY Antiviral
agent

Action and use

Idoxuridine is chemically related to trifluridine and acts by the same mechanisms of incorporation into viral DNA during replication producing abnormal protein formation. Idoxuridine inhibits the growth of herpes simplex virus types 1 and 2, varicella zoster, vaccinia, and cytomegalovirus but is used primarily against initial ophthalmic epithelial infections of herpes simplex when the dendritic figure is present. Deep infections involving the stromal layers or chronic or recurrent infections do not respond well to idoxuridine therapy.

Characteristics

After ophthalmic instillation, idoxuridine is poorly absorbed into systemic circulation.

Administration and dosage

NOTE: Success of therapy is highly dependent on adherence to the dosage schedule. Idoxuridine is optimally effective when consistently high concentrations of the drug are in contact with the lesion.

OPHTHALMIC SOLUTION—Initially, 1 drop in each infected eye every hour during the day and every 2 hr after bedtime. After significant improvement as shown by loss of staining with fluorescein, reduce the dose to 1 drop every 2 hr during the day and every 4 hr at night. Continue therapy for 3 to 5 days after healing appears to be complete to minimize recurrences.

OPHTHALMIC OINTMENT—Place a ribbon of ointment in the conjunctival sac of the infected eye 5 times daily, approximately every 4 hr, with the last dose at bedtime. Continue therapy for 3 to 5 days after healing appears to be complete to minimize recurrences.

NOTE: If significant improvement is not seen within 7 to 8 days, consider other forms of therapy. If the patient shows improvement, therapy is continued up to 21 days.

Make sure that the patient understands how to instill the eye drops or ointment and realizes the importance of aseptic technique in the instillation procedure.

Nurse and patient considerations

* Side effects are usually quite mild and include irritation, pain, pruritus, inflammation, or edema of the conjunctiva and eyelids. Allergic reactions have rarely occurred.
* Photophobia, manifested by sensitivity to bright light, occasionally occurs but can be minimized by wearing sunglasses. Use of the ointment may produce a temporary visual haze.
* Idoxuridine has produced fetal malformations in certain species of pregnant laboratory animals. Idoxuridine therapy in pregnant women should be avoided unless the benefits significantly outweigh the risks of therapy. Secretion in breast milk is unknown.

Drug interactions

No significant drug interactions have been reported.

Trifluridine
(Viroptic)

AHFS 52:04.06
CATEGORY Opthalmic antiviral agent

Action and use

Trifluridine is an antiviral agent that appears to act by alteration and inhibition of viral replication. Since trifluridine is a pyrimidine nucleoside, it is incorporated into viral DNA during replication, resulting in the formation of defective proteins and mutated viruses. Trifluridine is effective against herpes simplex virus, types 1 and 2, and vaccinia virus. It is not active against bacteria, fungi, and *Chlamydia* organisms.

Trifluridine is used topically to treat recurrent epithelial keratitis and primary keratoconjunctivitus caused by herpes simplex virus, types 1 and 2. It is particularly effective in those patients who are intolerant of or resistant to idoxuridine or vidarabine therapy, since cross-sensitivity with these other agents has not been reported.

Characteristics

Absorption: when instilled into the eye, trifluridine penetrates the cornea and may be found in the aqueous humor; systemic absorption appears to be negligible.

Administration and dosage
Adult

Trifluridine, 1% solution—1 drop onto cornea of affected eye every 2 hr (maximum of 9 drops daily) until reepithelialization occurs. Continue for 7 more days to prevent reoccurrence, using 1 drop every 4 hr (at least 5 drops daily). If reepithelialization has not occurred in 14 days, other therapy should be considered. Do not exceed 21 days of continuous therapy due to potential ocular toxicity.

NOTE: Make sure that the patient understands how to instill the eye drops and realizes the importance of aseptic technique in the installation procedure.

Nurse and patient considerations

∗ Side effects are quite mild, since essentially no systemic absorption takes place. Patients may notice a mild, transient stinging, burning, and redness to the conjunctiva and sclera and palpebral edema on instillation. Other adverse effects that have rarely been reported include epithelial keratopathy, stromal edema, hypersensitivity reactions, and increased intraocular pressure.

∗ Although there is minimal apparent systemic absorption and no evidence of teratogenicity has been reported, it is recommended that trifluridine therapy in pregnant or nursing women be avoided unless the benefits significantly outweigh the risks of therapy. Secretion in breast milk is unknown.

Drug interactions

No significant drug reactions have been reported.

Vidarabine
(Vira-A)

AHFS 52:04.06; 8:18
CATEGORY antiviral agent

Action and use

Vidarabine is an antiviral agent derived from the bacteria *Streptomyces antibioticus*. Its mechanism of activity is not fully known, but it does inhibit viral replication and inhibits viral DNA synthesis by inhibiting viral DNA polymerase. It has shown antiviral activity against several viruses, but is used intravenously in the treatment of encephalitis caused by herpes simplex virus and topically as an opthalmic ointment to treat keratitis and keratoconjunctivitis caused by herpes simplex virus types 1 and 2. Vidarabine does not show cross-sensitivity to idoxuridine and may be effective in treating recurrent keratitis that is resistant to idoxuridine.

Characteristics

Absorption: very minimal from ophthalmic, subcutaneous, or intramuscular routes. Metabolism: cornea and blood to ara-hypoxanthine (ara-Hx), which has some antiviral activity. Plasma half-life: normal renal function, vidarabine—1.5 hr; ara-Hx—3.3 hr. Protein binding: vidarabine—20% to 30%; ara-Hx—0% to 3%. Excretion: renal—1% to 3% as vidarabine, 41% to 53% as ara-Hx within 24 hr. Fecal excretion: none. Breast milk: unknown.

Administration and dosage

For encephalitis:

SC, or IM—Do not administer.

IV—15 mg/kg daily for 10 days. Administer over 12 to 24 hr using an in-line filter (0.45 μm or smaller). Make sure vidarabine is completely dissolved. It requires 2.2 ml of fluid to dissolve 1 mg of vidarabine (1 L dissolves 450 mg at 25° C). Dissolution may be facilitated by prewarming the IV infusion fluid to 35° to 40° C. Dilution should be made just prior to administration and used within 48 hr. Do *not* refrigerate the solution. Administer with any parenteral fluid except blood, protein, and lipid products. Reduce dosage in renal impairment.

For keratitis:

NOTE: Success of therapy is highly dependent on adherence to the dosage schedule. Vidarabine is optimally effective when consistently high concentrations of the drug are in contact with the lesion.

TOPICAL—Place a 1 cm ribbon of ointment 3% inside the lower conjunctival sac of the infected eye 5 times daily at 3 hr intervals. If there are no signs of improvement after 7 days or if complete reepithelialization has not occurred within 21 days of treatment, other forms of therapy should be considered. Vidarabine therapy should be continued for an additional 5 to 7 days at a dosage of 1 cm twice daily after reepithelialization has occurred to prevent recurrence of the infection.

NOTE: Make sure that the patient understands how to instill the ointment and realizes the importance of aseptic technique in the instillation procedure.

Nurse and patient considerations

* Minor side effects associated with the use of vidarabine ointment include temporary visual haze, burning, itching, redness, and lacrimation. Photophobia, manifested by sensitivity to bright light, occasionally occurs, but can be minimized by wearing sunglasses. Allergic reactions have rarely been reported.
* The most common side effects to IV vidarabine are nausea, vomiting, diarrhea, anorexia, and weight loss. These reactions begin on the second or third day of therapy and resolve in another 1 to 4 days. Hallucinations, psychosis, confusion, tremor, and dizziness may be dose related and reverse following discontinuation of therapy.
* Elevated SGOT and bilirubin levels frequently occur with intravenous vidarabine therapy but are reversible. Decreased levels of leukocytes, platelets, reticulocytes, hemoglobin, and hematocrit have been reported but are reversible 3 to 5 days after discontinuation of therapy. Dosages over 20 mg/kg may cause bone marrow depression. Serum levels should be monitored.
* IV vidarabine should be used with caution in patients with impaired liver or kidney function and in patients susceptible to fluid overload or cerebral edema.
* Vidarabine has produced fetal malformations in certain species of pregnant laboratory animals. Vidarabine therapy in pregnant women should be avoided unless the benefits significantly outweigh the risks of therapy. Secretion in breast milk is unknown.

Drug interactions

No significant drug interactions have been reported.

CHAPTER TWO

Cardiovascular agents

Cardiac glycosides
GENERAL INFORMATION

Digitalis glycosides have played an active role in medicine for more than 200 years. The glycosides are a recurrent topic in the literature and are perhaps the most frequently discussed class of compounds in the armamentarium of therapeutic medication.

Digitalis glycosides have two primary pharmacologic actions on the heart. The exact mechanisms of action have been difficult to determine, partially as a result of differences in compensatory extracardiac activity in patients with a normal heart versus those with impaired cardiac function.

Digitalis provides an increased force of contraction (positive inotropy) by acting on cellular structures of the heart to increase the quantity of intracellular free calcium. Calcium ions potentiate the binding of proteins (actin and myosin) necessary for myocardial contraction, thus increasing the force of contraction and cardiac output in the failing heart.

Digitalis slows the heart rate (negative chronotropy) by directly suppressing the conduction of electric impulses at the atrioventricular (AV) node. As cardiac output increases and peripheral circulation improves, mechanisms needed to compensate for the failing heart are no longer required, further decreasing the heart rate.

The most frequent use of digitalis is in the treatment of congestive heart failure. By improving contractility, digitalis helps restore circulatory function. Another major use of digitalis is slowing the ventricular rate in atrial fibrillation, atrial flutter, supraventricular tachycardia, and premature extrasystoles by increasing block of the AV node, so that fewer atrial beats will be followed by a ventricular beat.

Although it may be used, digitalis is usually less effective in heart failure secondary to respiratory insufficiency, infection, and hyperthyroidism (so-called high-output failures).

Characteristics

Although there are structural similarities between the digitalis glycosides, the small structural dissimilarities make a significant difference in the characteristics of the individual digitalis preparations. Compare the characteristics on the monographs for digoxin and digitoxin (pp. 129 and 131).

Administration and dosage

As a result of a more complete understanding of the pharmacokinetics of the digitalis glycosides, more precise dosage adjustments may be made with a lower incidence of toxicity. It is important to realize that in most patients the optimal dose is considerably below that of digitalis intoxication. Patients do not need to receive large doses to produce toxic nausea and vomiting to determine the maintenance level.

The most appropriate dosage is obviously that which provides the greatest recovery in cardiac efficiency with maximal reduction in initial symptomatology. The most effective way to determine this optimal dosage is by careful and frequent observation of the patient.

See the individual monographs on digoxin and digitoxin for administration and dosage (pp. 129 and 131).

Nurse and patient considerations

Hypokalemia, hypomagnesemia, and hypercalcemia sensitize the heart to digitalis intoxication. Attempts must be made to restore and maintain electrolyte balance prior to initiation of digitalis therapy. Lower doses of digitalis should be used initially, and patients should be placed on ECG monitors if possible (see Table 4-1, p. 237). Monitor serum electrolytes and cardiac rate and rhythm.

Clinical conditions other than electrolyte imbalance that may require lower doses of digitalis glycosides include myxedema (hypothyroidism), acute myocardial infarction, renal disease, severe respiratory disease, and far-advanced heart failure. Those that may require higher than average doses include hyperthyroidism and atrial arrhythmias. Remember, however, that it is essential to treat the patient and the clinical symptomatology and that individual variation is frequently observed with the digitalis glycosides.

The most common toxic manifestations are fatigue, anorexia, nausea, vomiting, blurred vision, mental confusion, and arrhythmias. Many of the arrhythmias for which digitalis is used are also observed in digitalis intoxication. If the arrhythmias occur while a patient is receiving digitalis, it is often difficult to determine whether the arrhythmias are secondary to digitalis treatment or an indication of inadequate treatment. Clinical judgment is certainly required, but if the possibility of intoxication cannot be ruled out, digitalis should be temporarily withheld. Monitoring of both serum electrolyte and specific digitalis (digoxin or digitoxin) levels may be beneficial in formulating a clinical impression.

Drug interactions

Drugs that may alter digitalis response and the incidence of toxicities by alteration of electrolyte imbalance include:

Hypokalemia	*Hyperkalemia*	*Hypomagnesemia*
Amphotericin B (Fungizone)	Potassium chloride	Chlorthalidone (Hygroton)
Chlorthalidone (Hygroton)	Potassium supplements— K-Lyte, Kaon, K-Lor, and others	Ethacrynic acid (Edecrin)
Ethacrynic acid (Edecrin)		Furosemide (Lasix)
Furosemide (Lasix)		Metolazone (Zaroxolyn)
Metolazone (Zaroxolyn)	Spironolactone (Aldactone)	Ethanol
Thiazide diuretics	Triamaterene (Dyrenium)	Thiazide diuretics
Corticosteroids	Amiloride	Neomycin (Mycifradin)
	Beta blockers	
	Succinylcholine	
	Heparin	
	Potassium penicillin G	
	Mannitol infusions	
	Salt substitutes	

Parenteral calcium gluconate and chloride administration may potentiate the therapeutic and arrhythmic effects of any of the digitalis preparations. If used concomitantly, the calcium should be given slowly and in low doses, accompanied by careful electrocardiographic monitoring.

Succinylcholine (Anectine, Quelicin) may enhance arrhythmias in the digitalized myocardium.

Concomitant use of propranolol and digitalis may potentiate the bradycardia associated with either agent.

Cholestyramine (Questran) decreases intestinal absorption of digitalis glycosides, altering expected response.

Digoxin
(Lanoxin)

AHFS 24:04
CATEGORY Cardiac glycoside

Action and use

See General information on cardiac glycosides (pp. 126).

Characteristics

Absorption: 80% to 90% (PO, liquids), 50% to 85% (PO, tablets). Onset: 5 to 30 min (IV), 30 to 60 min (PO). Peak activity: 5 to 6 hr. Protein binding: 23%. Half-life: 36 hr with normal renal function. Metabolism: liver, minimal, inactive; enterohepatic recirculation: 7%. Excretion: 35% of total amount in body in 24 hr, 20% in urine unchanged, 14% primarily fecal. Therapeutic level: 0.7 to 1.6 ng/ml. Toxic level: 2 ng/ml. Fatal level: 4 ng/ml. Dialysis: no, H, P.

Administration and dosage

A baseline ECG is recommended before initiation of therapy.

Assuming the patient has not ingested digoxin for the previous week or other digitalis preparations for the previous 2 weeks:

Adult

PO 1. Digitalizing: 0.50 to 0.75 mg initially, followed by 0.25 mg every 6 hr until adequate digitalization is achieved.
2. Maintenance: 0.125 to 0.25 mg daily for inotropic therapy. Some patients may require 0.375 to 0.5 mg daily for chronotropic effects.

IV 1. Digitalizing: 0.25 to 0.5 mg initially, followed by 0.25 mg every 6 hr until adequate digitalization is achieved. Administer at a rate of 0.5 to 1 ml/min.
2. Maintenance: as for PO administration.

Pediatric
Premature

IM or IV 1. Digitalizing: 0.015 to 0.02 mg/kg initially, followed by 0.01 mg every 6 to 8 hr for 2 doses (total digitalizing dose: 0.03 to 0.05 mg/kg).
2. Maintenance: 0.003 to 0.006 mg/kg every 12 hr.

Ages 2 weeks to 2 years

PO 1. Digitalizing: 0.03 to 0.04 mg/kg initially, followed by 0.02 mg/kg every 6 to 8 hr for 2 doses (total digitalizing dose: 0.06 to 0.08 mg/kg).
2. Maintenance: 0.006 to 0.01 mg/kg every 12 hr.
IM or IV 1. Digitalizing: 0.02 to 0.03 mg/kg initially, followed by 0.01 to 0.015 mg/kg every 6 to 8 hr for 2 doses (total digitalizing dose: 0.04 to 0.06 mg/kg).
2. Maintenance: 0.003 to 0.006 mg/kg every 12 hr.

Over 2 years of age

PO 1. Digitalizing: 0.02 to 0.03 mg/kg initially, followed by 0.01 to 0.015 mg every 6 to 8 hr for 2 doses (total digitalizing dose: 0.04 to 0.06 mg/kg).
2. Maintenance: 0.004 to 0.009 mg/kg every 12 hr.
IM or IV 1. Digitalizing: 0.01 to 0.02 mg/kg initially, followed by 0.005 to 0.01 mg/kg every 6 to 8 hr for 2 doses (total digitalizing dose: 0.02 to 0.04 mg/kg).
2. Maintenance: 0.002 to 0.004 mg/kg every 12 hr.

NOTE: Elderly patients and those with impaired renal function tend to accumulate the drug. These patients often require reduced dosage. Also note the differences in absorption, depending on the route and preparation for administration.

Routine safety precautions require that a patient's pulse be monitored before administration of each dose. Usually the medication administration should be withheld if the patient's heart rate is less than 60 beats/min (less than 90 beats/min for infants) (an early sign of increasing AV block).

Nurse and patient considerations

* See General information on cardiac glycosides (p. 126).

Drug interactions

See General information on cardiac glycosides (p. 126).

Gastrointestinal absorption of digoxin is inhibited by neomycin and antacids. Patients should be observed more closely for clinical effect or the lack of it. Monitoring digoxin serum levels may also be particularly useful.

Quinidine, by unknown mechanisms, may cause an increase in digoxin serum levels, resulting in increased gastrointestinal and cardiac toxicity. Monitor serum digoxin levels, ECG readings, and the clinical course of the patient closely.

The chronic use of the calcium antagonists, nifedipine and verapamil, increase serum digoxin levels by about 50% during the first week of therapy, potentially resulting in digitalis toxicity. Reduce maintenance and digitalization doses when nifedipine or verapamil is initiated, and monitor the patient closely to prevent overdigitalization or underdigitalization.

Verapamil and digitalis may be used concomitantly but may result in additive effects on cardiac conduction. Monitor patients for excessive bradycardia and AV block.

Some patients extensively metabolize digoxin in the gut. This metabolism is dependent on bacterial concentrations of normal gastrointestinal flora. Antibiotic therapy can significantly reduce metabolism of digoxin by destruction of GI flora, causing serum levels of digoxin to accumulate. Patients most susceptible to toxicity are those already on higher dosages of digoxin. This effect on digoxin metabolism may last from several weeks to several months.

Digitoxin
(Crystodigin)

AHFS 24:04
CATEGORY Cardiac glycoside

Action and use

See General information on cardiac glycosides (p. 126).

Characteristics

Absorption: 100% (PO). Onset: 1 to 2 hr. Peak activity: 4 to 12 hr. Protein binding: 90% to 95%. Half-life: 5$\frac{7}{10}$ days with normal renal function. Metabolism: liver—92% inactive, 8% digoxin (active); enterohepatic recirculation: 26%. Excretion: 11% of total amount in body in 24 hr, 4% urinary, 7% nonurinary. Therapeutic level: 20 to 30 ng/ml. Toxic level: 45 ng/ml. Dialysis: no, H, P.

Administration and dosage

A baseline ECG is recommended before initiation of therapy.

Assuming the patient has not ingested a digitalis preparation in the preceding 3 weeks:

Adult

PO 1. Digitalizing: 0.6 mg initially, followed by 0.4 mg and then 0.2 mg at intervals of 4 to 6 hr.
2. Maintenance: 0.05 to 0.3 mg once daily. The average dose is 0.1 to 0.15 mg daily.

IV 1. Digitalizing: 0.6 mg initially followed by 0.4 mg 4 to 6 hr later and by 0.2 mg every 4 to 6 hr thereafter until therapeutic effects are apparent. These effects are usually observed within 8 to 12 hr.
2. Maintenance: As for PO maintenance therapy.

Pediatric

PO 1. Digitalizing
    a. Premature, full-term, and infants with impaired renal function: 0.022 mg/kg.
    b. Ages 2 weeks to 1 year: 0.045 mg/kg.
    c. Over 2 years of age: 0.03 mg/kg.

NOTE: Divide total digitalizing dose into 3 or more doses administered at least 6 hr apart.

2. Maintenance: Give one tenth the total digitalizing dose daily.

IV—As for PO therapy.

NOTE: Elderly patients and those with impaired renal function tend to accumulate digitoxin. These patients often require reduced dosage.

Routine safety precautions require that a patient's pulse be measured before administration of each dose. Usually the medication administration should be withheld if the patient's heart rate is less than 60 beats/min (less than 90 beats/min for infants) (an early sign of increasing AV block).

Drug interactions

See General information on cardiac glycosides (p. 126).

Phenobarbital, phenylbutazone (Butazolidin), and phenytoin (Dilantin) have been reported to enhance the metabolism of digitoxin to digoxin, possibly as a result of enzyme induction. This has resulted in decreased digitoxin serum levels, shortened half-life, and diminished therapeutic effect caused by underdigitalization.

Cholestyramine (Questran) may bind digitoxin in the gastrointestinal tract, preventing reabsorption after enterohepatic recirculation. The half-life of digitoxin will be shortened, possibly leading to a diminished therapeutic effect.

ADRENERGIC AGENTS

Dobutamine
(Dobutrex)

AHFS 12:12
CATEGORY Beta$_1$-Adrenergic stimulant

Action and use

Dobutamine is a synthetic sympathomimetic agent that direcly stimulates beta$_1$-adrenergic receptors. In therapeutic doses, it has essentially no activity on beta$_2$- or alpha-adrenergic receptors and does not stimulate the release of norepinephrine as dopamine does. It does not have dopaminergic receptor activity and causes no renal or mesenteric vasodilation.

The primary therapeutic response to dobutamine is cardiac stimulation. It produces a positive inotropic effect on the myocardium, which results in increased cardiac output in normal patients and patients with congestive heart failure. Total peripheral resistance is reduced only to a minor extent. Dobutamine is used in patients who require short-term inotropic support secondary to organic heart disease or from cardiac surgical procedures.

Characteristics

Onset: less than 2 min (IV). Peak activity: within 10 min. Half-life: 2 min. Metabolism: liver and other tissues to

Table 2-1. Dobutamine administration*

amps/500 ml	1	2	4	8
mg/ml	250/500 ml	500/500 ml	1000/580 ml	2000/660 ml
μg/ml	500	1000	1724	3030
50 kg μgtts/min	μg/kg/min	μg/kg/min	μg/kg/min	μg/kg/min
10	1.6	3.2	5.5	9.7
20	3.3	6.6	11.3	20
30	5	10	17.2	30
40	6.6	13.2	22.7	40
50	8.3	16.6	28.6	50.3
60	10	20	34.5	60.6
60 kg μgtts/min				
10	1.3	2.6	4.6	8.1
20	2.7	5.4	9.5	16.6
30	4.2	8.4	14.4	25.5
40	5.5	11	19	33.3
50	6.9	13.8	23.8	41.9
60	8.3	16.6	28.7	50.5
70 kg μgtts/min				
10	1.1	2.6	3.9	6.9
20	2.3	4.6	8.1	14.3
30	3.5	7	12.3	21.6
40	4.7	9.4	16.2	28.5
50	5.9	11.8	20.4	35.9
60	7.1	14.2	24.6	43.3
80 kg μgtts/min	μg/kg/min	μg/kg/min	μg/kg/min	μg/kg/min
10	1	2	3.5	6.0
20	2	4	7.1	12.5
30	3.1	6.2	10.7	18.9
40	4.1	8.2	14.2	25
50	5.1	10.2	17.9	31.4
60	6.2	12.4	21.5	37.8

*Using a microdrip administration set—60 gtts/ml.

Table 2-1. Dobutamine administration—cont'd

amps/500 ml	1	2	4	8
mg/ml	250/500 ml	500/500 ml	1000/580 ml	2000/660 ml
μg/ml	500	1000	1724	3030
90 kg μgtts/min				
10	.9	1.8	3	5.4
20	1.8	3.6	6.3	11.1
30	2.7	5.4	9.5	16.8
40	3.6	7.2	12.5	22.2
50	4.6	9.2	15.9	27.9
60	5.5	11	19.1	33.6
100 kg μgtts/min				
10	.8	1.6	2.7	4.8
20	1.65	3.3	5.7	9.6
30	2.5	5	8.6	15.1
40	3.3	6.6	11.3	19.9
50	4.1	8.2	14.3	25.1
60	5	10	17.2	30.3

inactive compounds. Excretion: primarily in urine as inactive metabolites. Dialysis: unknown. Breast milk: unknown.

Administration and dosage

NOTE: Dobutamine is contraindicated in patients with idiopathic hypertrophic subaortic stenosis.

Patients must be adequately hydrated before dobutamine therapy. The central venous pressure should be 10 to 15 cm of H_2O, or the pulmonary wedge pressure should be 14 to 18 mm Hg.

Reconstitute by adding 20 ml of dextrose 5% or sodium chloride 0.9% to the 250 mg dobutamine powder. (This reconstituted solution is stable under refrigeration for 48 hr or at room temperature for 6 hr.) This solution must be further diluted before administration. A slight pinkish color may be observed but does not indicate loss of potency (See Table 2-1).

IV   1. Begin administration of the diluted solution at a dose of 2.5 to 3 μg/kg/min. The usual dosage range is 2.5 to 10 μg/kg/min, but doses up to 40 μg/kg/min may occasionally be necessary.

2. The rate of administration and the duration of therapy should be readjusted according to the patient's response as determined by heart rate, presence of ectopic heart beats, blood pressure, urine flow, and, whenever possible, by measurement of central venous or pulmonary wedge pressure and cardiac output.

3. Do not add dobutamine to sodium bicarbonate solutions, since the drug is inactivated in alkaline solution.

Nurse and patient considerations

* The most frequent adverse reactions are ectopic beats, angina, chest pain, and palpitations. Heart rate routinely increases 5 to 15 beats/min but may exceed 30 beats/min. The systolic blood pressure routinely increases by 10 to 20 mm Hg but has been reported to exceed 50 mm Hg. Patients with preexisting hypertension may be predisposed to developing exaggerated responses. All these effects are dose related and can usually be controlled by a reduction in dosage or discontinuations of therapy.

* Since dobutamine enhances atrioventricular (AV) conduction, patients with atrial fibrillation are at risk for developing a rapid ventricular response. These patients should be adequately digitalized before the administration of dobutamine.

Drug interactions

Beta-adrenergic blocking agents (propranolol, nadolol, timolol, and others) will antagonize the cardiac activity of dobutamine and result in greater alpha-adrenergic activity and increased peripheral vascular resistance.

There is an increased incidence of ventricular arrhythmias when dobutamine is used during halothane or cyclopropane anesthesia.

Patients who have been treated with MAO inhibitors (isoniazid [Marplan], pargyline hydrochloride [Eutonyl] tranylcypromine sulfate [Parnate]) require a substantially reduced dosage of dopamine. The starting dose in such patients should be reduced to at least one tenth the usual dose. MAO inhibitors block the metabolism of dopamine.

Dopamine hydrochloride
AHFS 12:12
(Intropin)
CATEGORY Adrenergic stimulant

Action and use

Dopamine is a precursor in the synthesis of norepinephrine in the body and acts on alpha- and beta-adrenergic receptors. It also acts on specific dopamine receptors to cause vasodilatation of the renal and mesenteric vascular beds. It produces an inotropic and chronotropic effect on the myocardium, resulting in an increased cardiac output. It usually produces an increased systolic and pulse pressure with either no effect or a slight increase in diastolic pressure. Dopamine is indicated in shock caused by myocardial infarction, trauma, renal failure, and endotoxic septicemia.

Administration and dosage

The central venous pressure should be 10 to 15 cm of H_2O, or the pulmonary wedge pressure should be 14 to 18 mm Hg (see Table 2-2).

Table 2-2. Dopamine administration*

amps/500 ml	1	2	4	8
mg/ml	200/500 ml	400/500 ml	800/520 ml	1600/540 ml
μg/ml	400	800	1538	2962
50 kg μgtts/min	μg/kg/min	μg/kg/min	μg/kg/min	μg/kg/min
10	1.3	3	5	10
20	2.6	5	10	20
30	4	8	15	30
40	5.3	11	20	39
50	6.6	13	26	49
60	8	16	31	59
60 kg μgtts/min				
10	1.1	2	4	8
20	2.2	4	8	16
30	3.3	7	13	25
40	4.4	8	17	33
50	5.5	11	21	41
60	6.6	13	26	49

*Using a microdrip administration set—60 gtts/ml. *Continued.*

Table 2-2. Dopamine administration—cont'd

amps/500 ml	1	2	4	8
mg/ml	200/500 ml	400/500 ml	800/520 ml	1600/540 ml
μg/ml	400	800	1538	2962
70 kg μgtts/min				
10	0.9	2	3	7
20	1.9	4	7	14
30	2.8	6	11	21
40	3.8	8	15	28
50	4.7	10	18	35
60	5.7	11	22	42
80 kg μgtts/min				
10	0.8	2	3	6
20	1.6	3	6	12
30	2.5	5	10	18
40	3.3	7	13	24
50	4.2	8	16	31
60	5	10	19	37
90 kg μgtts/min				
10	0.7	1	3	5
20	1.4	3	6	11
30	2.2	4	9	16
40	2.9	6	11	22
50	3.7	7	14	27
60	4.4	9	17	33
100 kg μgtts/min				
10	0.6	1	3	5
20	1.3	3	5	10
30	2	4	8	15
40	2.6	5	10	20
50	3.3	7	13	25
60	4	8	15	30

Begin administration of the diluted solution at doses of 2 to 5 μg/kg/min. Increase gradually using 5 to 10 μg/kg/min increments up to 20 to 50 μg/kg/min. Dosage should be adjusted according to the patient's response. Observe particularly for diminished urine output, increasing tachycardia, or the development of arrhythmias.

Do not add dopamine to sodium bicarbonate, since the drug is inactivated in alkaline solution.

NOTE: Safety in children has not been established.

Nurse and patient considerations

* The most frequent adverse reactions are ectopic beats, nausea, vomiting, tachycardia, anginal pain, dyspnea, hypotension, and headache.
* If a disproportionate rise in the diastolic pressure (a marked decrease in pulse pressure) is noted, the infusion rate should be decreased and the patient watched for further evidence of vasoconstrictor activity such as decreased urine output.
* In overdosage, as noted by elevated blood pressure, reduce the administration rate or discontinue infusion. Dopamine's duration of action is quite short (1 to 5 min), and usually no other action is needed. If blood pressure remains elevated, the short-acting alpha-adrenergic blocking agent, phentolamine (Regitine), should be considered.
* Extravasation of large amounts may cause ischemia and tissue necrosis. Gangrene of fingers and toes has been reported after prolonged infusion.

Drug interactions

All beta blockers (propranolol, timolol, nadolol, others) antagonize the cardiac activity of dopamine.

Patients who have been treated with MAO inhibitors (isocarboxazid [Marplan], pargyline hydrochloride [Eutonyl], tranylcypromine sulfate [Parnate]) require a substantially reduced dosage of dopamine. The starting dose in such patients should be reduced to at least one-tenth the usual dose. MAO inhibitors block the metabolism of dopamine.

Epinephrine
(Adrenalin)

AHFS 12:12
CATEGORY Cardiac stimulant

Action and use

Epinephrine is one of the primary catecholamines of the body, stimulating both alpha- and beta-receptor cells. It is a very potent cardiac stimulant, acting directly on the beta receptors of the myocardium, pacemaker cells, and conducting tissue. Stimulation results in increased spontaneous contractions (automaticity), heart rate (positive chronotropic effect), myocardial contraction (positive inotropic effect), cardiac ouput, coronary blood flow, and oxygen consumption.

Administration and dosage
Adult

IV—Cardiac resuscitation: epinephrine 1:1000, 0.2 to 1 ml (0.2 to 1 mg); epinephrine 1:10,000, 2 to 10 ml (0.2 to 1 mg).

INTRACARDIAC—As for IV administration.

ENDOTRACHEAL TUBE—As for IV administration.

Pediatric

IV—Cardiac resuscitation: epinephrine 1:1000, 0.01 ml/kg/dose; epinephrine 1:10,000, 0.1 ml/kg/dose.

NOTE: Dosages are given in milliliters rather than in milligrams.

Epinephrine conversion chart

Epinephrine	1:1000	1:10,000
1 ml	1 mg	0.1 mg
10 ml	10 mg	1.0 mg

NOTE: Do not use if discolored (red to brown) or if sediment is present. Do not mix with solutions containing aminophylline, phenytoin (Dilantin), or sodium bicarbonate.

Nurse and patient considerations

* Be extremely cautious with dosage calculations and administration.
* Isoproterenol and epinephrine should not be administered simultaneously, since both drugs are potent cardiac stimulants. They may be given alternately, however.
* Palpitation, tachycardia, headache, tremor, weakness, and dizziness are common side effects. Serious arrhythmias, ventricular fibrillation, anginal pain, nausea, respiratory difficulty, and cerebral hemorrhage may also occur.
* Dosage should be adjusted carefully in the elderly, in patients with coronary insufficiency, diabetes, hyperthyroidism, hypertension, and in psychoneurotic individuals. These patients are particularly sensitive to sympathomimetic amines.

Drug interactions

Tricyclic antidepressants (doxepin, nortriptyline, amitriptyline, protriptyline, imipramine, desipramine) strongly potentiate the actions of epinephrine. If they must be used concurrently, start with significantly lower doses of epinephrine.

Use epinephrine with caution in patients receiving propranolol. Vagal reflex has resulted in marked bradycardia.

Epinephrine causes hyperglycemia. Diabetics may require increased doses of insulin of oral hypoglycemic agents.

Epinephrine may produce arrhythmias in patients anesthetized with cyclopropane.

Isoproterenol hydrochloride AHFS 12:12
(Isuprel)
CATEGORY Beta-adrenergic stimulant

Action and use

Isoproterenol is a beta-receptor stimulant. Cardiac output is raised by inotropic and chronotropic action combined with an increase in venous return to the heart. Usual doses maintain or raise the systolic pressure, although the mean pressure is reduced. Peripheral vascular resistance is lowered in skeletal muscle and renal and mesenteric vascular beds. Diastolic pressure falls.

Isoproterenol is used primarily in cardiac standstill (arrest), AV block, carotid sinus hypersensitivity, ventricular arrhythmias—especially those occurring during the course of AV block—and bronchospasm. For its use as a bronchodilator see p. 265.

Administration and dosage
Adult and pediatric

Infusion rates of 0.5 to 5 μg/min have been recommended. The rate of infusion should be adjusted on the basis of heart rate, central venous pressure, systemic blood pressure, and urine output. Rates over 30 μg/min have been used in advanced stages of shock (Table 2-3).

Nurse and patient considerations

* Administration of isoproterenol is contraindicated in patients with tachycardia caused by digitalis intoxication.
* Isoproterenol and epinephrine should not be administered simultaneously, since both drugs are direct cardiac stimulants. They may be given alternately, however.
* Dosage should be adjusted carefully in patients with coronary insufficiency, diabetes, and hyperthyroidism, and in patients sensitive to sympathomimetic amines.
* If the cardiac rate increases sharply, patients with angina pectoris may experience anginal pain until the cardiac rate decreases.
* Palpitation, tachycardia, headache, and flushing of the skin are common side effects. Serious arrythmias, anginal pain, nausea, tremor, dizziness, weakness, and sweating occasionally occur.
* Although there have been no teratogenic effects reported, safe use in pregnant or lactating women has not been established.

Drug interactions

The beta-adrenergic stimulant effects of isoproterenol are blocked by propranolol, a beta-adrenergic blocker.

Isoproterenol may produce arrhythmias in patients anesthetized with cyclopropane.

Patients who have been treated with MAO inhibitors (isocarboxazid [Marplan], pargyline hydrochloride [Euto-

Table 2-3. Isoproterenol administration for cardiac standstill and arrhythmias in adults*

1. *Intravenous infusion*

5 ml amps/500 ml		2	4	8	12	16
mg/500 ml		2	4	8	12	16
μg/ml		4	8	16	24	32
μgtts/min	ml/min	μg/min	μg/min	μg/min	μg/min	μg/min
5	0.08	0.3	0.6	1.2	1.9	2.5
10	0.16	0.6	1.2	2.4	3.8	5.3
15	0.25	1	2	4	6	8
20	0.33	1.3	2.6	5.3	8	11
25	0.41	1.6	3.3	6.5	9.8	13.1
30	0.5	2	4	8	12	16
35	0.58	2.3	4.6	9.3	13.9	18.5
40	0.66	2.6	5.3	10.5	15.8	21.1
45	0.75	3	6	12	18	24
50	0.83	3.3	6.6	13.3	20	26.5
55	0.91	3.6	7.3	14.5	21.8	29.1
60	1.0	4	8	16	24	32

	Preparation	*Initial dose*	*Subsequent dosage range*
2. *Intramuscular*	Use solution 1:5000 undiluted	0.2 mg (1 ml)	0.02 to 1 mg (0.1 to 5 ml)
3. *Subcutaneous*	Use solution 1:5000 undiluted	0.2 mg (1 ml)	0.15 to 0.2 mg (0.75 to 1 ml)
4. *Intracardiac*	Use solution 1:5000 undiluted	0.2 mg (1 ml)	

*Using a microdrip administration set—60 gtts/ml. Each milliliter of the sterile 1:5000 solution contains 0.2 mg isoproterenol (Isuprel). The drug is available in 5 ml (1 mg) ampules and should be diluted in dextrose 5% before administration. Normal saline solution is not a recommended diluent.

nyl], tranylcypromine sulfate [Parnate]) require a substantially reduced dosage of isoproterenol. The starting dose in such patients should be reduced to at least one tenth the usual dose. MAO inhibitors block the metabolism of isoproterenol.

Isoxsuprine hydrochloride
(Vasodilan)

AHFS 24:12
CATEGORY Beta-adrenergic stimulant

Action and use

Isoxsuprine has beta-receptor stimulant properties that result in dilatation of blood vessels of skeletal muscle and cardiac stimulation. Increased circulation in skeletal muscle and lowered peripheral vascular resistance is present. As a result of increased cardiac output the mean blood pressure stays about the same, but there appears to be improved circulation to skeletal muscle and cerebral circulation. Isoxsuprine may be effective in relieving symptoms of cerebral vascular insufficiency, Buerger's disease, and Raynaud's disease. Because of its ability to relax uterine musculature, it may also be used in cases of premature labor and threatened abortion.

Administration and dosage

For peripheral vasodilatation:

PO—10 to 20 mg 3 to 4 times daily.

IM—5 to 10 mg (1 to 2 ml) 2 to 3 times daily. IM administration may result in hypotension and tachycardia.

IV—Not recommended because of increased incidence of side effects.

Guidelines for use in premature labor:

1. Initiate a control IV of dextrose 5%, Ringer's lactate, or saline solution and administer 400 to 500 ml in 15 to 20 min before initiation of the medication. Then decrease dosage to 100 to 125 ml/hr.
2. Add 400 mg of isoxsuprine to 1000 ml of dextrose 5% (400 μg/ml).
3. An initial loading dose used in premature labor is 0.5 to 1 mg/min (see Table 2-4). This rate is continued for the first ½ hr to 1 hr of therapy until control of contractions has been established or tachycardia (pulse over 120), hypotension (systolic below 100, diastolic below 60), or vomiting results. The initial uterine response should occur within the first 15 min.
4. A maintenance infusion of 0.25 to 0.75 mg/min can be given for 2 to 12 hr or more.
5. After control of uterine activity is established, the IV dose is tapered while control is maintained by PO isoxsuprine, 20 mg every 4 to 6 hr.
6. The maintenance PO dosage ranges from 10 to 20

**Table 2-4. Isoxsuprine administration
for premature labor***

ml/hr	ml/min	mg/min
15	0.25	0.11
20	0.33	0.13
25	0.42	0.17
50	0.82	0.33
75	1.25	0.5
100	1.67	0.67
125	2.08	0.83
150	2.5	1
175	2.91	1.16
200	3.33	1.33

*Administer 400 mg/1000 ml or 400 μg/ml.

mg 4 to 6 times daily, depending upon clinical response.
7. If labor begins again, restart the IV infusion as above.

Nurse and patient considerations

* When isoxsuprine is used for premature labor, a sometimes significant drop in blood pressure (due to the vasodilatory effect), can be seen in the first 10 to 15 min of the infusion. Blood pressure and pulse monitoring should be done prior to and every 5 min after the infusion has been started until the patient's condition is stable. Use continuous electronic fetal monitoring. If maternal pulse exceeds 120 beats/min and does not decrease with an increase in fluids or if there is any evidence of a decrease in uterine perfusion, discontinue the infusion.
* Other dose-related side effects include tachycardia, dizziness, nausea, and vomiting.
* Long-term PO administration has resulted in severe skin rashes. If a rash should develop, the drug should be discontinued.

Drug interactions

Patients who have been taking antihypertensive agents (hydralazine hydrochloride, diuretics, methyldopa) may be more susceptible to the hypotensive effects of isoxsuprine.

Levarterenol (norepinephrine)

(Levophed) AHFS 12:12

CATEGORY Adrenergic stimulant

Action and use

Levarterenol acts predominantly on alpha receptors and has little action on beta receptors, except in the heart. As a result of general peripheral vasoconstriction (alpha stimulation) and beta stimulation of the heart, systolic, diastolic, and usually, pulse pressure levels are increased. Compensatory vagal reflex activity slows the heart, overcoming the direct cardioaccelerator action, thus increasing the stroke volume. The peripheral vasoconstriction reduces blood flow through the kidney, brain, liver, and usually skeletal muscle. Glomerular filtration rate is maintained unless the decrease in renal blood flow is quite marked. Coronary circulation is increased probably because of both indirect coronary dilatation and elevated blood pressure. Levarterenol is used to restore blood pressure after an acute hypotensive episode such as myocardial infarction, cardiac arrest, drug reaction, septicemia, blood transfusions, and surgical procedures.

Administration and dosage

NOTE: Levarterenol infusions must *never* be left unattended. Monitor blood pressure and infusion rate continuously.

IV—See Table 2-5.

Extravasation ischemia: Care must be taken that necrosis and sloughing do not occur at the site of IV infusion as a result of extravasation of the drug. Blanching along the course of the infused vein may be an early indication of extravasation. The area will later develop a cold, hard, and pallid appearance. Whenever possible, levarterenol should be administered through a large vein. To prevent sloughing and necrosis in areas where extravasation has taken place, the area should be infiltrated as soon as possible with 10 to 15 ml of saline solution containing from 5 to 10 mg of phentolamine (Regitine), an alpha-adrenergic blocking agent. Administration with whole blood or plasma is not recommended. If these fluids are required, use separate infusion sites or Y tubing with the connections as close to the infusion site as possible.

Table 2-5. Levarterenol administration*

amps/500 ml	1	2	4
mg base/500 ml	4	8	16
μg base/ml	8	16	32

μgtts/ml	ml/min	μg base/min	μg base/min	μg base/min
5	0.08	0.64	1.3	2.5
10	0.16	1.3	2.6	5.2
15	0.25	2.0	4	8
20	0.33	2.6	5.3	10.5
25	0.41	3.3	6.6	13.2
30	0.5	4.0	8	16
35	0.58	4.6	9.3	18.5
40	0.66	5.3	10.6	21.2
45	0.75	6	12	24
50	0.83	6.6	13.3	26.5
55	0.91	7.3	14.6	29.2
60	1.0	8.0	16	32

*Using a microdrip administration set—60 gtts/ml.

Each 1 ml of the 0.2% solution contains 2 mg of levarterenol bitartrate or the equivalent of 1 mg levarterenol base (1 ml solution = 1 mg of base). Dilute in dextrose 5%. Saline solution is not recommended. Adding one 4 ml ampule of 0.2% levarterenol to 1000 ml of dextrose 5% gives a concentration of 4 μg levarterenol base/ml of final solution.

Although the clinical condition of the patient must be a major determinant, the recommended initial dosage is 8 to 12 μg of base/min. The average maintenance dose ranges from 2 to 4 μg of base/min. Great individual variation occurs in the dose required to attain and maintain normotension. Dosage must be titrated to the response of the patient. The pressor response can readily be controlled since the drug is rapidly metabolized. Activity-response is insignificant 1 to 2 min after the infusion is stopped.

Overdoses may cause severe hypertension with violent headache, photophobia, stabbing chest and neck pain, pallor, intense sweating, and vomiting.

Levarterenol infusions must never be left unattended. Blood pressure must be monitored at least every 5 min and more frequently when the dosage is being adjusted.

Nurse and patient considerations

* Severe hypotension may result if levarterenol is suddenly discontinued. Plasma volumes must be adequate and the dosage reduced in increments while the blood pressure response is monitored.
* Other side effects include severe hypertension, reflex bradycardia, and hyperglycemia. Violent headache, photophobia, stabbing chest and neck pain, pallor, intense sweating, and vomiting may be indications of overdose.
* A decrease in urinary output should be expected. Monitor fluid intake and output to avoid overhydration.
* Use of levarterenol in pregnant women must be used on a risk versus benefit basis. Levarterenol increases the frequency of contraction of the gravid uterus.

Drug interactions

General anesthetics such as cyclopropane and halothane increase cardiac autonomic irritability. Patients receiving levarterenol during or immediately after anesthesia have an increased risk of ventricular tachycardia or fibrillation. The same type of arrhythmias may result from the use of levarterenol in patients with profound hypoxia or hypercarbia.

Levarterenol should be used with extreme caution in patients receiving MAO inhibitors (pargyline [Eutonyl, Eutron], tranylcypromine sulfate [Parnate]), tricyclic antidepressants (imipramine, amitriptyline, Triavil), and guanethidine (Ismelin) because severe, prolonged hypertension may result.

Metaraminol
(Aramine)

AHFS 12:12
CATEGORY Adrenergic stimulant

Action and use

Metaraminol is a sympathomimetic amine that acts indirectly by stimulating the release of stored norepinephrine from nerve ending storage granules and directly by stimulating the sympathetic receptor. There are both alpha- and beta-receptor effects, causing cardiac stimulation and peripheral arteriolar vasoconstriction in all vascular beds, resulting in a rise in both systolic and diastolic pressure. Metaraminol may be used to treat paroxysmal atrial tachycardia and acute hypotensive states induced by spinal anesthesia, drug reactions, and shock.

Administration and dosage

IM—2 to 10 mg (0.2 to 1 ml).

IV 1. Direct injection: 0.5 to 5 mg (0.05 to 0.5 ml undiluted). Administration by direct injection is recommended only in a life-threatening emergency.
   2. Infusion: Initially, 15 to 100 mg (1.5 to 10 ml) in 500 ml of dextrose 5% or saline solution. Adjust the rate of infusion to maintain the blood pressure at the desired level. More concentrated solutions may be used to restrict fluid intake. Concentrations of 150 to 500 mg/500 ml of dextrose 5% or saline solution may be used. When IV infusions are discontinued the dosage should be gradually tapered with close observation of the blood pressure. Avoid abrupt withdrawal.

Extravasation ischemia: Injections and infusions may occasionally result in abscess formation, tissue necrosis, and sloughing. Administer with caution in patients with peripheral vascular disease or shock. Blanching along the course of the infused vein may be an early indication of extravasation. The area will later develop a cold, hard, and pallid appearance. To prevent sloughing and necrosis in mottled, cold tissue, infiltrate the area as soon as possible with 10 to 15 ml of saline solution containing 5 to 10 mg of phentolamine (Regitine), an alpha-adrenergic blocking agent.

Nurse and patient considerations

* Metaraminol may cause tachycardia or arrhythmias, particularly in patients with previous myocardial injury. Other side effects include severe hypertension, reflex bradycardia, headache, anginal pain, nausea, and vomiting.
* Patients potentially more sensitive to metaraminol are those with impaired hepatic function, thyroid disease, hypertension, heart disease, hyperthyroidism, and diabetes. Therefore use with caution in these patients.

* After discontinuation of therapy, prolonged hypertension may occur due to cumulative effects of metaraminol. However, the converse is more likely to occur. Hypotension, partially due to depletion of norepinephrine stores, may require the administration of levarterenol to replace tissue stores of norepinephrine.
* Use with extreme caution in pregnant patients. Metaraminol may cause uterine contractions and decreased uterine blood flow, resulting in fetal hypoxia and bradycardia.

Drug interactions

Patients who have been treated with MAO inhibitors (isocarboxazid [Marplan], pargyline [Eutonyl], tranylcypromine sulfate [Parnate]) require much smaller doses of metaraminol. MAO inhibitors block the metabolism of norepinephrine, prolonging and intensifying the activity of metaraminol.

Metaraminol may produce arrhythmias in patients anesthetized with halothane or cyclopropane.

Phentolamine (Regitine) decreases but does not completely block the vasoconstriction of metaraminol.

Atropine sulfate blocks the reflex bradycardia caused by metaraminol.

Guanethidine (Ismelin) and tricyclic antidepressants (imipramine, amitriptyline) potentiate the pressor effects of metaraminol.

Phenylephrine hydrochloride AHFS 12:12
(Neo-Synephrine) CATEGORY Alpha-adrenergic stimulant

Action and use

Phenylephrine is a sympathomimetic agent that acts predominantly by direct stimulation of alpha-adrenergic receptors. There is also a minor indirect component of activity due to release of norepinephrine from nerve ending storage granules. Most vascular beds are constricted, and renal, splanchnic, cutaneous, and limb blood flow is reduced. In contrast to levarterenol and metaraminol, there are essentially no direct effects on receptors within the heart. A reflex bradycardia is frequently seen, however, secondary to peripheral vasoconstriction.

Phenylephrine may be used to maintain systolic and diastolic blood pressure during spinal and inhalation anesthesia and shock. It is also used to terminate episodes of paroxysmal superventricular tachycardia by induction of reflex bradycardia.

Administration and dosage

For mild to moderate hypotension:

Adult

sc—Usual dose: 2 to 5 mg (0.2 to 0.5 ml). Range: 1 to 10 mg (0.1 to 1 ml). Initial dose should not exceed 5 mg (0.5 ml).

im—As for SC administration.

iv—Usual dose: 0.2 mg. Range: 0.1 to 0.5 mg. Initial dose should not exceed 0.5 mg. Dilute 1 ml of phenylephrine with 9 ml of saline solution to make a concentration of 0.1 mg phenylephrine/0.1 ml, or 1 mg/ml, for ease of administration.

iv infusion—See Table 2-6.

Pediatric

sc—0.1 mg/kg.

im—As for SC administration.

NOTE: Injections should not be repeated more often than every 10 to 15 min. (A 5 mg dose IM should raise blood pressure for 1 to 2 hr; a 0.5 mg dose IV should raise blood pressure for about 15 min.)

For paroxysmal supraventricular tachycardia:

Adults

iv—0.5 mg over 20 to 30 sec. Further doses may be increased by increments of 0.1 to 0.2 mg depending on blood pressure response. The systolic blood pressure should generally not rise above 160 mm Hg. The maximum single dose should not exceed 1 mg.

Extravasation ischemia: Injections and infusions may occasionally result in abscess formation, tissue necrosis, and sloughing. Administer with caution in patients with peripheral vascular disease or shock. Blanching along the course of the infused vein may be an early indication of extravasation. The area will later develop a cold, hard, and pallid appearance. To prevent sloughing and necrosis in mottled, cold tissue, infiltrate the area as soon as possible with 10 to 15 ml of saline solution containing 5 to 10 mg of phentolamine (Regitine), an alpha-adrenergic blocking agent.

Table 2-6 Phenylephrine administration*

amps/500 ml		1	2	4	6	8	10	12
mg/500 ml		10	20	40	60	80	100	120
	μg/ml	20	40	80	120	160	200	240
μgtts/min	ml/min	μg/min	μg/min	μg/min	μg/min	μg/min	μg/min	μg/min
5	0.08	1.6	3.2	6.4	9.6	12.8	16	19
10	0.16	3.2	6.4	12.8	19.2	25.6	32	38
15	0.25	5	10	20	30	40	50	60
20	0.33	6.6	13.2	26.4	39.6	52.8	66	79
25	0.41	8.2	16.4	32.8	49.2	65.6	82	98
30	0.5	10	20	40	60	80	100	120
35	0.58	11.6	23.2	46.4	69.6	92.8	116	139
40	0.66	13.2	26.4	52.8	79.2	105.6	132	158
45	0.75	15	30	60	90	120	150	180
50	0.83	16.6	33.2	66.4	99.6	132.8	166	200
55	0.91	18.2	36.4	72.8	109.2	145.6	182	218
60	1.0	20	40	80	120	160	200	240

*Using a microdrip administration set—60 gtts/ml. Each 1 ml of the 1% solution contains 10 mg of phenylephrine (1 ml = 10 mg). Dilute in dextrose 5% or saline solution.

Although the clinical condition of the patient must be a primary determinant, the recommended initial dosage is 100 to 180 μg/min. After the blood pressure stabilizes, 40 to 60 μg/min is usually adequate. There is great patient variation in the dosage required to attain and maintain the desired blood pressure. Dosage must be titrated to the response of the patient.

Nurse and patient considerations

* Side effects of phenylephrine include restlessness, anxiety, nervousness, respiratory distress, arrhythmias, anginal pain, and numbness and/or cool sensations of the extremities. Overdosage may result in hypertension, palpitations, cerebral hemorrhage, and convulsions. Headache may be an early indication of hypertension and overdose.
* Phenylephrine should be administered with extreme caution to the elderly and to patients with hyperthyroidism, bradycardia, partial heart block, myocardial disease, or hypertension.
* A decrease in urinary output should be expected. Monitor fluid intake and output to avoid overhydration.
* Use with caution in patients with peripheral circulatory insufficiency. Vasoconstriction produced by phenylephrine may cause further necrosis.
* Use with extreme caution in late pregnancy and during delivery. Phenylephrine increases uterine contractility and reduces uterine blood flow, which may result in fetal hypoxia and bradycardia.

Drug interactions

Phentolamine (Regitine) may be used to reduce vasoconstriction and hypertension induced by phenylephrine.

Atropine sulfate blocks the reflex bradycardia induced by phenylephrine.

Propranolol (Inderal) may be used to treat cardiac arrhythmias arising from phenylephrine therapy.

Arrhythmias may result from concurrent administration of halothane or cyclopropane anesthesia and phenylephrine. This reaction is much less likely to occur with phenylephrine than with levarterenol or metaraminol therapy.

Patients who have been treated with MAO inhibitors (isocarboxazid [Marplan], pargyline [Eutonyl], tranylcypromine sulfate [Parnate]) require much smaller doses of phenylephrine. MAO inhibitors diminish the metabolism of phenylephrine.

Guanethidine (Ismelin) and tricyclic antidepressants (imipramine, amitriptyline) potentiate the vasoconstriction induced by phenylephrine.

ANTIARRHYTHMIC AGENTS

Bretylium tosylate
(Bretylol)

AHFS 24:04
CATEGORY Antiarrhythmic;
adrenergic blocking agent

Action and use

Bretylium tosylate is an antiarrhythmic adrenergic blocking agent indicated for use in patients with life-threatening arrhythmias, ventricular tachycardia, or ventricular fibrillation uncontrollable by other antiarrhythmic agents or electrical cardioversion. The mechanism of action has not been established, but pharmacologic actions observed include inhibition of the release of norepinephrine from adrenergic nerve terminals, positive inotropic and chronotropic effects on the heart, and restoration of the resting membrane potential toward normal in damaged myocardial cells.

Characteristics

Onset: Ventricular fibrillation, 5 to 10 min (IV), 20 to 60 min (IM), ventricular tachycardia, 20 to 120 min (IM and IV). Duration: 6 to 8 hr (IM and IV). Half-life: about 10 hr (range: 4 to 17 hr). Metabolism: no apparent metabolites. Excretion: unchanged in urine, 70% to 80% in 24 hr.

Administration and dosage

For ventricular fibrillation:

After failure of electrical cardioversion, 5 mg/kg IV undiluted. Repeat cardioversion. If fibrillation persists, the dosage may be increased to 10 mg/kg and repeated every 15 to 30 min. Maximum total dosage should not exceed 30 mg/ kg.

For other ventricular arrhythmias:

Administer 5 to 10 mg/kg IV over 8 to 10 min. Dilute the solution at least fivefold (500 mg/10ml diluted in at least 50 ml with dextrose 5% or saline solution). If nausea or vomiting occurs, reduce the rate of infusion. The dose may be repeated in 1 to 2 hr if the arrhythmia persists.

IV—Continuous infusion: recommended dosage is 1 to 2 mg/min (Table 2-7).

IM—5 to 10 mg/kg. Do *not* dilute before IM injection. Dosage may be repeated in 1 to 2 hr if the arrhythmia still persists. Thereafter repeat every 6 to 8 hr.

Table 2-7. Bretylium administration*

Add 2 ampules of 1000 mg/20 ml bretylium to any of the following volumes of dextrose 5%.

Dextrose 5% (ml)		150	250	500	1000
Final volume (ml)		170	270	520	1020
	mg/ml	5.88	3.70	1.92	1
μgtts/min	ml/min	mg/min	mg/min	mg/min	mg/min
5	0.08	0.47	0.3	0.15	0.08
10	0.16	0.94	0.6	0.30	0.16
15	0.25	1.47	0.92	0.48	0.25
20	0.33	1.94	1.22	0.63	0.33
25	0.41	2.4	1.51	0.78	0.41
30	0.5	2.94	1.85	0.96	0.5
35	0.58	3.41	2.14	1.11	0.58
40	0.66	3.88	2.44	1.26	0.66
45	0.75	4.41	2.77	1.44	0.75
50	0.83	4.88	3.07	1.6	0.83
55	0.91	5.35	3.36	1.75	0.91
60	1.0	5.88	3.70	1.92	1.0

*Using a microdrip administration set—60 gtts/ml. The drug is available in 10 ml ampules containing 500 mg of bretylium.

For routine bretylium administration add 2 ampules (1000 mg/20 ml) of bretylium to dextrose 5% as shown in Table 2-7.

For bretylium administration in patients with restricted fluid intake add bretylium to 500 mg of dextrose 5% as shown in Table 2-8.

NOTE: The dosage of bretylium should be tapered and discontinued within 3 to 5 days under electrocardiographic monitoring.

Table 2-8. Bretylium administration: patients with restricted fluid intake*

amp/500ml		1	2	4	6
	mg/ml	500/ 500 ml	1000/ 520 ml	2000/ 540 ml	2500/ 560 ml
	mg/ml	1	1.92	3.7	4.46
μgtts/min	ml/min	mg/min	mg/min	mg/min	mg/min
5	0.08	0.08	0.15	0.3	0.35
10	0.16	0.16	0.3	0.6	0.71
15	0.25	0.25	0.48	0.9	1.11
20	0.33	0.33	0.63	1.2	1.47
25	0.41	0.41	0.78	1.5	1.82
30	0.5	0.5	0.96	1.85	2.23
35	0.58	0.58	1.11	2.14	2.60
40	0.66	0.66	1.26	2.44	2.94
45	0.75	0.75	1.44	2.77	3.34
50	0.83	0.83	1.6	3.07	3.70
55	0.91	0.91	1.75	3.36	4.05
60	1.0	1.0	1.92	3.7	4.46

*Using a microdrip administration set—60 gtts/ml. The drug is available as 10 ml ampules containing 500 mg of bretylium.

Nurse and patient considerations

* When bretylium therapy is initiated, transient hypertension followed by postural hypotension may be observed. Patients may complain of dizziness, light-headedness, vertigo, or syncope. Symptoms may be reduced by keeping the patient in a supine position. Avoid the use of subtherapeutic dosages (that is, less than 5 mg/kg), since hypotension may occur at dosages lower than those needed to suppress arrhythmias. Hypotension with systolic blood

may be treated with infusions of dopamine or levarterenol. Initiate catecholamine therapy at low dosages, since the pharmacologic effects of bretylium may enhance the pressor activity of these agents. Transient tachycardia, increased frequency of arrhythmias, bradycardia, and precipitation of anginal attacks have been reported in a few patients.

Drug interactions

Bretylium therapy may aggravate digitalis glycoside toxicity. Use only in digitalized patients if the arrhythmia does not appear to be induced by digitalis and if other antiarrhythmic agents are not effective.

Disopyramide phosphate
(Norpace)

AHFS 24:04
CATEGORY Antiarrhythmic agent

Action and use

Disopyramide is an antiarrhythmic agent with properties similar to those of quinidine and procainamide. It is indicated for the suppression and treatment of ventricular arrhythmias, especially in patients refractory to procainamide or quinidine therapy or in patients in whom the side effects of other antiarrhythmic therapy are unacceptable.

Characteristics

Peak plasma levels: less than 2 hr. Protein binding: 50%. Half-life: 5 to 10 hr. Excretion: 50% unchanged, 30% as metabolites, in urine, 10% in feces. Therapeutic level: 2 to 4 μg/ml. Toxic level: more than 9 μg/ml. Dialysis: unknown.

Administration and dosage

PO 1. Normal renal function:
   a. Initial: 300 mg.
   b. Maintenance: Initially, 150 mg every 6 hr. Individual dosage adjustments must be made; some patients may require as much as 400 mg every 6 hr.
2. Moderately impaired renal function (creatinine clearance greater than 40 ml/min), hepatic insufficiency, or severe cardiac disease:
   a. Initial: 200 mg.
   b. Maintenance: Initially, 100 mg every 6 hr.

3. Severe renal impairment (creatinine clearance less than 40 ml/min):
   a. Initial: 200 mg.
   b. Maintenance: 100 mg according to the following chart:

Creatinine clearance (ml/min)	40-15	15-5	5-1
Dosage interval (hr)	10	20	30

Nurse and patient considerations

* Disopyramide is a myocardial depressant. Myocardial toxicity may be manifested by premature ventricular contractions (PVCs), bradycardia, AV block, ventricular tachycardia, ventricular fibrillation, or an increase in congestive heart failure. Electrocardiographic changes may include prolongation of the PR interval, widened QRS interval (greater than 25%), widened QT interval (greater than 25%), ST segment depression, idioventricular rhythm, SA block, AV block, and asystole.
* More common adverse effects of therapy include dry mouth, nose, and throat, urinary hesitancy and retention, constipation with bloating and gas, and occasional diarrhea.
* Use disopyramide with *extreme* caution in heart block and digitalis intoxication.
* Complete effects of disopyramide therapy during pregnancy and delivery have not been evaluated. It is not known as yet whether disopyramide is excreted in human breast milk. Studies on lactating rats indicate that milk concentrations may be 1 to 3 times greater than maternal plasma concentration. Therefore nursing during disopyramide therapy is not recommended.

Drug interactions

Disopyramide may potentiate the hypotensive effects of the thiazides, other diuretics, and antihypertensive agents.

Disopyramide may be additive with procainamide (Pronestyl), quinidine, digitalis, and propranolol (Inderal), resulting in further myocardial depression.

Phenytoin (Dilantin) may significantly decrease serum levels of disopyramide. Patients should be observed for redevelopment of arrhythmias, which may require an increase in dosage of disopyramide.

Other drug interactions may be observed as more clinical experience is gained. Patients receiving disopyramide with other medications should be monitored closely for potential multiple drug toxicity.

Lidocaine hydrochloride
(Xylocaine hydrochloride)

AHFS 24:04
CATEGORY
Antiarrhythmic agent

Action and use

Lidocaine exerts its antiarrhythmic effect by increasing the electric stimulation threshold of the ventricles without depressing the force of ventricular contractions. Lidocaine is the drug of choice for the treatment of ventricular arrhythmias associated with acute myocardial infarction and ventricular tachycardia.

Characteristics

Onset: 1 to 2 min (IV bolus), 5 to 15 min (IM). Duration of antiarrhythmic affect: 10 to 20 min (IV bolus), 60 to 90 min (IM). Distribution: after bolus administration lidocaine is rapidly distributed to almost all body tissues. The serum half-life of the initial (active) phase of distribution is 8 to 9 min. To maintain serum blood levels initiated by the bolus, a continuous infusion must be started within about 10 min (see p. 160). The half-life of the second phase is 1½ to 2 hr. Metabolism: primarily liver. Excretion: <5% unchanged in urine. Therapeutic level: 1 to 5 μg/ml. Toxic level: 6 to 10 μg/ml. Dialysis: unknown.

Administration and dosage

NOTE: Lidocaine should not be used in patients with complete heart block.

Adult

IM—200 to 300 mg in the deltoid muscle. IM administration is recommended only in emergency conditions when IV facilities are not available and when the potential benefits outweigh the risks.

NOTE: IM injections may result in increased creatine phosphokinase levels, invalidating the use of this

Table 2-9. Routine lidocaine administration*

Add 50 ml of 40 mg/ml (2 g) lidocaine to any of the following volumes of dextrose 5%

Dextrose 5% (ml)	100	250	450	500	1000
Final volume (ml)	150	300	500	550	1050
mg/ml	13.3	6.6	4	3.6	2
μgtts/min	mg/min	mg/min	mg/min	mg/min	mg/min
10	2.2	1.1	0.66	0.6	0.33
20	4.4	2.1	1.3	1.2	0.66
30	6.6	3.3	2	1.8	1.0
40	8.8	4.4	2.6	2.4	1.3
50	11.0	5.5	3.3	3	1.6
60	13.3	6.6	4	3.6	2

*Using a microdrip administration set—60 gtts/ml.

NOTE: If the infusion rate is to be increased, a loading bolus of 25 to 50 mg of lidocaine should also be administered. Toxicity is usually seen at administration rates greater than 5 mg/min or with prolonged administration rates greater than 4 mg/min. There will be variation, especially in patients with shock, hypovolemia, congestive heart failure, and hepatic insufficiency. Serum levels accumulate, since the volume of distribution and/or metabolism is diminished.

enzyme determination, without isoenzyme separation, in diagnosing acute myocardial infarction.

IV—The initial dose (bolus) is 50 to 100 mg (1 mg/kg) at a rate of 25 to 50 mg/min. Boluses of 50 to 100 mg may be given every 3 to 5 min until the desired effect is achieved or side effects appear. Do not exceed 300 mg by intermittent bolus. To maintain the antiarrhythmic effect an IV infusion must be initiated. The usual rate of administration is 1 to 4 mg/min (see Table 2-9).

Pediatric

IV 1. Initial (bolus): 1 mg/kg up to 15 mg if under 25 kg (55 lb); up to 25 mg if over 25 kg (55 lb).
2. Continuous infusion: 20 to 40 μg/kg/min (maximum total dose: 5 mg/kg).

For routine lidocaine administration for cardiac arrhythmias add 50 ml of 40 mg/ml (2 g) of lidocaine hydrochloride to dextrose 5% as shown in Table 2-9.

For lidocaine administration for cardiac arrhythmias in patients with restricted fluid intake add lidocaine hydrochloride to 500 ml of dextrose 5% as shown in Table 2-10.

Table 2-10. Lidocaine administration: patients with restricted fluid intake*

Lido-caine (g)	1	2	3	4	5	6
Final volume (ml)	525	550	575	600	625	650
mg/ml	1.9	3.6	5.2	6.6	8	9.2
μgtts/min	mg/min	mg/min	mg/min	mg/min	mg/min	mg/min
10	0.3	0.6	0.8	1	1.3	1.5
20	0.6	1.2	1.7	2.2	2.6	3
30	0.9	1.8	2.6	3.3	4	4.6
40	1.2	2.4	3.4	4.3	5.3	6
50	1.6	3	4.3	5.5	6.6	7.6
60	1.9	3.6	5.2	6.6	8	9.2

*Using a microdrip administration set—60 gtts/ml.

NOTE: If the infusion rate is to be increased, a loading bolus of 25 to 50 mg of lidocaine should also be administered. Toxicity is usually seen at administration rates greater than 5 mg/min or with prolonged administration rates greater than 4 mg/min. There will be variation, especially in patients with shock, hypovolemia, congestive heart failure, and hepatic insufficiency. Serum levels accumulate, since the volume of distribution and/or metabolism is diminished.

Nurse and patient considerations

* Most side effects are dose related and of short duration when the administration rate is decreased. Minor side effects include light-headedness, tinnitus, muscle twitches, and blurred or double vision. Adverse effects mediated through the CNS are depression, stupor, restlessness, euphoria, hypotension, and convulsions. Infrequently, lidocaine may produce bradycardia and/or aggravate arrhythmias.
* Safe use in pregnancy has not been established. Lidocaine does cross the placental barrier.

Drug interactions

Large IV doses of lidocaine have been shown to enhance the neuromuscular blocking action of succinylcholine. Use the combination with caution particularly if large doses of lidocaine are used.

Phenytoin
(Dilantin)

AHFS 28:12
CATEGORY Antiarrhythmic agent

Action and use

Phenytoin is considered an anticonvulsant, but it may also be effective in treatment of ventricular arrhythmias, particularly those produced by overdoses of digitalis. It depresses automaticity as do quinidine and procainamide, but improves conduction in depressed myocardial tissue. Reduction in automaticity helps control arrhythmias, while enhanced conduction of electric impulses through previously depressed conduction tissue (e.g., that seen in digitalis intoxication) may improve cardiac function.

Characteristics

Onset: Within 1 hr following an IV loading dose of 1 to 1.5 g, 2 to 24 hr following a PO loading dose of 1 g. Protein binding: 95%. Half-life: 18 to 24 hr. Metabolism: liver to inactive metabolites. Excretion: 1% unchanged in urine, 75% in urine as metabolites. Therapeutic level: 7.5 to 20 μg/ml. Toxic level: 10 to 50 μg/ml. Dialysis: yes, H.

Administration and dosage

For treatment of arrhythmias:

Adult

PO—250 mg 4 times during the first day, 500 mg daily on days 2 and 3, and 300 to 400 mg on subsequent days.

IM—Not recommended as a result of erratic absorption and pain on injection.

IV—250 mg initially, at a rate no faster than 50 mg/min until the arrhythmia is abolished, a total of 1000 mg has been given, or side effects appear.

Pediatric

IV—1 to 5 mg/kg slow IV push. Repeat as needed. Maximum total dose: 500 mg in a 4 hr interval.

NOTE: If given too rapidly by the IV route, bradycardia and severe hypotension may result. The diluent, propylene glycol, will also potentiate the hypotensive effect of phenytoin and cause ECG changes. Cardiac and respiratory arrest may occur with excessive dosage and speed of administration. Blood pressure and the ECG should be monitored carefully, especially during administration.

Phenytoin should not be mixed with any drugs or added to any IV infusion solutions. The solubility is very pH dependent, and use with other medications or solutions will result in a white precipitate.

Each IV injection should be followed by an injection of sterile saline through the same needle or IV catheter to avoid local venous irritation.

Nurse and patient considerations

* Frequent side effects include nystagmus, ataxia, slurred speech, and mental confusion. Dizziness and transient nervousness may also occur. These side effects are usually dose related and disappear at reduced administration rates. If these symptoms appear before the arrhythmias are controlled, it is less likely that phenytoin will be effective, and therapy may have to be altered.

* Phenytoin may elevate blood glucose levels, especially if larger doses are used. Patients with diabetes mellitus or renal insufficiency may be more susceptible to hyperglycemia.

* Fatal dermatologic manifestations sometimes accompanied by fever, blood dyscrasias, toxic hepatitis, and liver damage have been attributed to phenytoin.

* Gingival hyperplasia occurs frequently, but the incidence may be reduced by good oral hygiene including gum massage, frequent brushing, and proper dental care.

* Phenytoin will occasionally discolor urine with shades from pink to red to red-brown.

* There have been reports suggesting a correlation between birth defects and the administration of anticonvulsant drugs. Use of phenytoin must be based on risk versus benefit.

Drug interactions

Barbiturates may enhance the rate of metabolism of phenytoin.

Warfarin (Coumadin), disulfiram (Antabuse), phenylbutazone (Butazolidin), chloramphenicol (Chloromycetin), and isoniazid (INH) inhibit the metabolism of phenytoin, resulting in signs of phenytoin toxicity (nystagmus, ataxia, lethargy, and confusion).

Complex relationships exist between folic acid, phenytoin, and anticonvulsant activity. Phenytoin may induce folic acid deficiency, while folic acid replacement may result in partial loss of seizure control.

Phenytoin stimulates microsomal enzyme activity that enhances the metabolism of corticosteroids and theophylline. Serum theophylline levels should be monitored closely when phenytoin is either added or removed from the drug therapy of patients who are also taking theophylline.

Phenytoin may interfere with oral contraceptive therapy. See General information on oral contraceptives (p. 499).

Valproic acid (Depakene) may increase or decrease phenytoin serum levels. Serum phenytoin levels should be determined periodically and dosages adjusted if necessary.

Phenytoin may significantly decrease serum levels of disopyramide. Patients should be observed for redevelopment of arrhythmias, which may require an increase in dosage of disopyramide.

Procainamide hydrochloride AHFS 24:04
(Pronestyl) CATEGORY Antiarrhythmic agent

Action and use

The actions and uses of procainamide are similar to those of quinidine. Procainamide increases the threshold to electric stimulation in both the atria and the ventricles. Conduction in the atria and the ventricles is diminished, while the refractory period of the atria is prolonged.

Procainamide is most commonly used for the treatment of PVCs and ventricular tachycardia. Procainamide is used in atrial arrhythmias, but usually after quinidine has failed.

Characteristics

Peak plasma level: 15 to 60 min (IM), 60 min (PO). Protein binding: 15%. Half-life: 3 to 4 hr. Metabolism: liver to active *N*-acetylprocainamide, other inactive metabolites. Excretion: 2% to 10% unchanged drug, 50% as metabolites, in urine. Therapeutic level: 0.4 mg/100 ml to 0.8 mg/100 ml. Toxic level: 1 mg/100 ml. Dialysis: yes, H.

Administration and dosage

NOTE: Do not use in complete AV block, and use with extreme caution in partial AV block.

Adult

PO 1. Loading: 1 to 1.25 g.
2. Second: 750 mg 1 hr after the loading dose if the arrhythmia is still present.
3. Maintenance: 0.5 to 1 g every 4 to 6 hr. As a result of the short half-life, some patients may require maintenance doses every 3 to 4 hr to maintain adequate control of arrhythmias. Patients should be advised of the importance of adhering to the administration schedule.

IM—0.5 to 1 g every 6 hr until PO therapy is possible.

IV—100 mg every 5 min at 25 to 50 mg/min until arrhythmias are suppressed, a maximum of 1 g has been administered, or side effects develop. Once arrhythmias are suppressed, a continuous infusion may be started at 25 to 30 μg/kg/min. If arrhythmias recur, suppress the arrhythmias with bolus therapy as above and increase the rate of infusion (see Table 2-11).

Pediatric

PO—50 mg/kg divided in 4 to 6 doses for treatment of cardiac arrhythmias.

IV—2 mg/kg diluted in dextrose 5% and given over 5 min. Repeat the dose every 10 to 15 min until arrhythmias are controlled. Maximum total dosage is 1 g. Normal sinus rhythm may then be maintained by an infusion of 20 to 80 μg/kg/min.

NOTE: Cardiovascular toxicities include hypotension, particularly with IV administration. The blood pressure, the apical-radial pulses, and the electrocardiogram must be monitored. If the fall in blood pressure exceeds 15 mm Hg, the infusion should be discontinued. Other manifestations of cardiotoxicity include bradycardia, partial or complete heart-block, extrasystole, asystole, ventricular tachycardia, or fibrillation. If the QRS complex widens beyond 50% or if the PR interval widens, the drug should be discontinued.

Psychoses with hallucinations, giddiness, confusion, CNS stimulation, and convulsions have been reported.

If the infusion is continued for more than 8 to 10 hr, the infusion rate should be reduced as tolerated. Procainamide as well as an active metabolite, *N*-acetylprocainamide, may accumulate, particularly in those patients with congestive heart failure, hepatic insufficiency, or renal impairment. Dosage adjustments are best guided by monitoring of the serum procainamide concentrations.

Text continued on p. 170.

Table 2-11. Procainamide administration*

g/500ml	1.25		1.5		1.75		2.00		2.25		2.50	
mg/ml	2.5		3		3.5		4		4.5		5	
µg/ml	2500		3000		3500		4000		4500		5000	
50 kg µgtts/min	µg/kg/min	mg/min	µg/kg/min	mg/min	µg/kg/min	mg/min	µg/kg/min	mg/min	µg/kg/min	mg/min	µg/kg/min	mg/min
10	8.3	0.4	9.96	0.5	11.6	0.6	13.3	0.66	14.4	0.75	16.6	0.83
20	16.5	0.8	19.8	1.0	23	1.2	26.4	1.3	29.7	1.5	33	1.65
30	25	1.2	30	1.5	35	1.7	40	2.0	45	2.2	50	2.5
40	33	1.65	39.6	2	46.2	2.3	52.8	2.6	59.4	3	66	3.3
50	41.5	2.0	49.8	2.5	58.1	2.9	66.4	3.3	74.7	3.7	83	4.1
60	50	2.5	60	3	70	3.5	80	4.0	90	4.5	100	5
60 kg µgtts/min												
10	6.9		8.3		9.7		11.0		12.5		13.8	
20	13.7		16.5		19.2		21.9		24.7		27.5	
30	20.8		24		29.1		33.3		37.5		41.6	
40	27.5		33		38.5		43.9		49.5		55	
50	34.5		41.5		48.4		55.3		62.2		69.1	
60	41.6		50		58.3		66.6		75		83.3	

70 kg

µgtts/min												
10	5.9	0.4	7.1	0.5	8.3	0.6	9.5	0.66	10.7	0.75	11.8	0.83
20	11.7	0.8	14.14	1.0	16.5	1.2	18.8	1.3	21.2	1.5	23.5	1.65
30	17.8	1.2	21.4	1.5	25	1.7	28.5	2.0	32.1	2.2	35.7	2.5
40	23.5	1.65	28.3	2	33	2.3	37.7	2.6	42.4	3	47.1	3.3
50	29.6	2.0	35.5	2.5	41.5	2.9	47.4	3.3	53.4	3.7	59.3	4.1
60	35.7	2.5	42.8	3	50	3.5	57.1	4.0	64.3	4.5	71.4	5

80 kg

µgtts/min												
10	5.2		6.22	0.5	7.2	0.6	8.3	0.66	9.3	0.75	10.3	0.83
20	10.3		12.3	1.0	14.4	1.2	16.5	1.3	18.5	1.5	20.6	1.65
30	15.6		18.7	1.5	21.8	1.7	25	2.0	28.1	2.2	31.2	2.5
40	20.6		24.7	2	28.8	2.3	33	2.6	37.1	3	41.2	3.3
50	25.9		31.1	2.5	36.3	2.9	41.5	3.3	46.7	3.7	51.8	4.1
60	31.2		37.5	3	43.7	3.5	50	4.0	56.2	4.5	62.5	5

*Using a microdrip administration set—60 gtts/ml.

Continued.

Table 2-11. Procainamide administration—cont'd

g/500ml	1.25		1.5		1.75		2.00		2.25		2.50	
mg/ml	2.5		3		3.5		4		4.5		5	
µg/ml	2500		3000		3500		4000		4500		5000	
90 kg µgtts/min												
10	4.6	0.4	5.53	0.5	6.4	0.6	7.37	0.66	8.3	0.75	9.2	0.83
20	9.14	0.8	11	1.0	12.8	1.2	14.6	1.3	16.5	1.5	18.3	1.65
30	13.85	1.2	16.6	1.5	19.4	1.7	22.2	2.0	25	2.2	27.7	2.5
40	18.28	1.65	22	2	25.6	2.3	29.3	2.6	33	3	36.6	3.3
50	23	2.0	27.6	2.5	32.2	2.9	36.8	3.3	41.5	3.7	46.1	4.1
60	27.7	2.5	33.3	3	38.8	3.5	44.4	4.0	50	4.5	55.5	5

100 kg

μgtts/min						
10	4.15	4.98	5.8	6.64	7.5	8.3
20	8.25	9.9	11.5	13.2	14.9	16.5
30	12.5	15	17.5	20	22.5	25
40	16.5	19.8	23.1	26.4	29.7	33
50	20.75	24.9	29	33.2	37.3	41.5
60	25	30	35	40	45	50

110 kg

μgtts/min												
10	3.77	0.4	4.5	0.5	5.3	0.6	6.0	0.66	6.8	0.75	7.5	0.83
20	7.5	0.8	9	1.0	10.5	1.2	12	1.3	13.5	1.5	15	1.65
30	11.3	1.2	13.6	1.5	15.9	1.7	18.18	2.0	20.5	2.2	22.7	2.5
40	15	1.65	18	2	21	2.3	24	2.6	27	3	30	3.3
50	18.8	2.0	22.6	2.5	26.3	2.9	30.17	3.3	33.9	3.7	37.7	4.1
60	22.72	2.5	27.2	3	31.8	3.5	36.36	4.0	40.9	4.5	45.5	5

Nurse and patient considerations

* When the drug is taken orally, the most common side effects are anorexia, nausea, vomiting, flushing, bitter taste, and diarrhea.
* Hypersensitivity reactions including chills, fever, joint and muscle pain, pruritus, urticarial or maculopapular skin rashes, photosensitivity, and anaphylaxis have been reported.
* Patients on long-term therapy are more susceptible to blood dyscrasias, including agranulocytosis and thrombocytopenia, and clinical manifestations of systemic lupus erythematosus. These conditions are usually reversible, but the symptoms may last for weeks or months.

Drug interactions

Procainamide may potentiate the hypotensive effects of the thiazides, other diuretics, and antihypertensive agents.

Procainamide may be additive with quinidine, digitalis, and propranolol (Inderal), resulting in further myocardial depression.

Procainamide may potentiate neuromuscular blockade in patients recovering from the effects of surgical muscle relaxants (tubocurarine, succinylcholine, gallamine triethiodide [Flaxedil]) and aminoglycoside antibiotics (gentamicin, streptomycin, kanamycin).

Long-term propranolol therapy increases the half-life and decreases the elimination of procainamide. Observe patients for possible toxicity and reduce the procainamide dose if necessary.

Cimetidine (Tagamet) inhibits the metabolism and excretion of procainamide and its metabolite, N-acetylprocainamide. Observe patients closely for an altered procainamide response if cimetidine therapy is started or stopped.

Quinidine

AHFS 24:04

CATEGORY Antiarrhythmic agent

Action and use

Quinidine has been used clinically for its antiarrhythmic effects for several decades. It is a myocardial depressant having both direct and indirect effects on the heart. Directly, quinidine decreases the excitability of the cardiac muscle to electric stimulation, depresses conduction velocity, prolongs the refractory period, and depresses myocardial contractility. The direct depressant actions of quinidine are complicated by a "vagolytic effect" that in some patients may result in a paradoxic increased heart rate. Quinidine also exhibits alpha- and beta-adrenergic blocking activity as well as anticholinergic properties.

Quinidine is used for the prevention and treatment of cardiac arrhythmias. Those arrhythmias most frequently suppressed are atrial fibrillation, atrial flutter, paroxysmal supraventricular and ventricular tachycardia, and PVCs.

Characteristics

Peak activity: 30 to 90 min (IM), 1 to 3 hr (PO). Duration: 6 to 8 hr. Protein binding: 60%. Half-life: 5 hr. Metabolism: liver, active and inactive. Excretion: kidney, 10% to 50% unchanged in urine in 24 hr. Therapeutic level: 0.3 mg/100 ml to 0.6 mg/100 ml. Toxic level: 1 mg/100 ml. Fatal levels: 3 mg/100 ml to 5 mg/100 ml. Dialysis: yes, H, P.

Administration and dosage

NOTE: As a result of the variable effects of quinidine, dosage must be individualized and patients monitored closely, particularly when initiating therapy.

Adult

PO—Quinidine sulfate: 200 to 400 mg 3 to 5 times daily. Higher doses may be used, but the maximum single dose should not exceed 600 to 800 mg.

IM—Quinidine gluconate: 600 mg initially, then 400 mg every 2 hr as needed.

IV—Quinidine gluconate: 800 mg diluted to 40 ml with dextrose 5% and infused at a rate of 1 ml/min. (IV administration is extremely hazardous. Blood pressure and ECG readings should be monitored continuously as hypotension and arrhythmias may occur.)

Pediatric

PO—Quinidine sulfate: 30 mg/kg/24 hr divided into 4 to 6 doses.

IM—Quinidine gluconate: As for PO administration.

Nurse and patient considerations

* Myocardial toxicity may be manifested by PVCs, bradycardia, AV block, ventricular tachycardia, ventricular fibrillation, or an increase in congestive heart failure. Electrocardiographic changes include notched P waves, widened QRS complex interval, (greater than 25%—0.14 sec indicates impending toxicity) widened QT interval, ST segment depression, development of U waves, idioventricular rhythm, SA block, AV block, and cardiac arrest.

* The most common side effects are diarrhea, nausea, and vomiting. Other symptoms of cinchonism (salivation, tinnitus, vertigo, headache, visual disturbances, confusion) may occur but will diminish if the dosage is lowered.

* Hypersensitivity reactions include skin rash, hemolytic anemia, thrombocytopenia, agranulocytosis, or drug fever. Vascular collapse is manifested by severe hypotension, restlessness, cold sweat, pallor, and fainting.

* Use quinidine only with *extreme* caution in heart block and digitalis intoxication.

* Quinidine should be used with caution during pregnancy and in nursing mothers.

Drug interactions

Quinidine may potentiate the hypotensive effects of the thiazides, other diuretics, and antihypertensive agents.

Quinidine may be additive with procainamide (Pronestyl), digitalis, and propranolol (Inderal) resulting in further myocardial depression.

Quinidine may cause an increase in digoxin serum levels, resulting in increased gastrointestinal and cardiac toxicity. Monitor serum digoxin levels, ECG readings, and the clinical course of the patient closely.

Phenothiazines may have an additive effect when administered with quinidine, increasing myocardial depression, ventricular tachycardia, and/or hypotension.

Quinidine may potentiate neuromuscular blockade in patients recovering from the effects of surgical muscle relaxants (tubocurarine, succinylcholine, gallamine triethiodide [Flaxedil]) and aminoglycoside antibiotics (gentamicin, kanamycin).

Patients receiving both quinidine and warfarin derivatives may be more susceptible to increased anticoagulation and bleeding caused by suppression of vitamin K–dependent coagulation factors.

Rifampin enhances quinidine metabolism. Patients on long-term quinidine and rifampin therapy may require an increase in quinidine dosage to maintain therapeutic activity.

Limited evidence indicates that cimetidine may inhibit the metabolism of quinidine. Observe patients for evidence of quinidine toxicity and reduce the dosage if necessary.

CALCIUM ION ANTAGONISTS

Diltiazem hydrochloride
(Cardizem)

AHFS Unlisted
CATEGORY Calcium antagonist

Action and use

Diltiazem is a calcium ion influx inhibitor, or slow channel blocker, structurally unrelated to other calcium antagonists. Its mechanisms of action are not completely known, but its therapeutic activity is thought to be derived from its ability to inhibit the influx of calcium ions across the cell membrane during membrane depolarization of cardiac and vascular smooth muscle. Physiologically, this reduces conduction velocity through the sinoatrial (SA) and atrioventricular (AV) nodes, resulting in a reduced heart rate (negative chronotropic activity), and vasodilation of the coronary and peripheral arteries, resulting in improved myocardial oxygenation and reduced peripheral vascular resistance (afterload). Diltiazem is currently being used to treat angina pectoris caused by coronary artery spasm (Prinzmetal's variant angina) and chronic stable angina (exertional angina) in patients who cannot tolerate or do not receive adequate relief from beta blocker or nitrate therapy.

Characteristics

Bioavailability (PO after first-pass effect): 40%. Onset: 30 to 60 min. Peak plasma levels: 2 to 3 hr. Diltiazem activity is not dose-linear in higher dosages; a 120 mg dose gives blood levels 3 times that of a 60 mg dose. Half-life: 3.5 hr. Protein binding: 70% to 80%. Metabolism: hepatic; desacetyldiltiazem is present at levels of 10% to 20% of diltiazem, with 25% to 50% of the activity of the parent compound. Excretion: 2% to 4% unchanged in urine. Dialysis: unknown. Breast milk: unknown.

Administration and dosage

NOTE: Diltiazem is contraindicated in (1) patients with sick sinus syndrome except in the presence of a functional ventricular pacemaker, (2) patients with second- or third-degree AV block, and (3) patients with a systolic pressure less than 90 mm Hg.

Adult

PO 1. Initially, 30 mg 4 times daily before meals and at bedtime. The dosage is gradually increased to 60 mg 4 times daily at 1- to 2-day intervals.
2. Patients may continue nitroglycerin therapy for acute anginal attacks.

NOTE: To treat overdosage or exaggerated response:

Gastric lavage

Bradycardia: atropine 0.6 to 1 mg IV; isoproterenol cautiously

AV block: atropine, isoproterenol, pacemaker

Cardiac failure: inotropic agents (dopamine, dobutamine) and diuretics

Hypotension: dopamine or levarterenol

Nurse and patient considerations

* Since diltiazem is a fairly new drug available, it is possible that more adverse effects may be reported with greater usage than those that were reported during clinical investigational trials. Two cases of hepatocellular injury after a few days of therapy, manifested by hyperbilirubinemia and elevated transaminase levels, have been reported.
* Other side effects reported are nausea (2.7%), swelling and edema (2.4%), arrhythmias (2%), headache (2%), rash (1.8%), and fatigue (1.1%). The following adverse effects were reported with a frequency of less than 1%: bradycardia, hypotension, congestive heart failure, depression, confusion, hallucinations, pruritus, petechiae, urticaria, photosensitivity, and paresthesias.
* Diltiazem has produced skeletal deformities in laboratory animals. It should be used in pregnancy only when the benefits significantly outweigh the risks of therapy to the fetus.

Drug interactions

Concomitant use of diltiazem with beta blockers (propranolol, nadolol, timolol, others) and digitalis glycosides may result in additive depressant effects on cardiac conduction. Monitor patients for excessive bradycardia and AV block.

Concomitant use with antihypertensive agents should result in additive hypotensive effects.

Nifedipine
(Procardia)

AHFS 24:04
CATEGORY Calcium antagonist

Action and use

Nifedipine is a calcium ion influx inhibitor, or slow channel blocker, structurally unrelated to other calcium antagonists. Its mechanisms of action are not completely known, but its therapeutic activity is thought to be derived from its ability to inhibit the influx of calcium ions across the cell membrane during depolarization of cardiac and vascular smooth muscle. Physiologically, nifedipine is a potent vasodilator of coronary and peripheral arteries. It has essentially no effect on the sinoatrial or atrioventricular nodes and has no antiarrhythmic activity. Nifedipine causes decreased peripheral vascular resistance (reduced afterload) with a fall in systolic and diastolic blood pressure. There is usually a reflex increase in heart rate, secondary to a drop in peripheral resistance. Coronary artery vasodilatation results in improved oxygenation to the myocardium. Nifedipine is currently being used to treat angina pectoris caused by coronary artery vasospasm and chronic stable angina (exertional angina) in patients who cannot tolerate or who do not receive adequate relief from beta blockers or nitrate therapy. Lack of activity at the SA and AV nodes allows nifedipine to be used more effectively in patients with impaired AV conduction or nodal disease and in combination with digitalis and beta blockers.

Characteristics

Onset: 10 min. Peak activity: 30 min. Half-life: 2 hr. Metabolism: extensive, to inactive metabolites. Excretion: 80% of active drug and metabolites in urine.

Administration and dosage
Adult

PO
1. Initially, 10 mg 3 times daily. Adjust dosage upward over the next 7 to 14 days to balance between antianginal and hypotensive activity. Usual effective dose is 10 to 20 mg 3 times daily. Doses above 180 mg are not recommended.
2. Sublingual nitroglycerin therapy may be continued for acute anginal attacks, especially during titration of therapy.

Nurse and patient considerations

* Patients have reported an increased frequency, duration, or severity of angina pectoris when starting nifedipine or at the time of dosage increases. Mechanisms proposed for this phenomenon are decreased diastolic pressure with increased heart rate or increased demand resulting from increased heart rate alone.
* The most common adverse effects include dizziness or lightheadedness, peripheral edema, nausea, weakness, headache, and flushing, each occurring in about 10% of patients. Transient hypotension develops in about 5%, palpitation in about 2%, and syncope in 0.5% of patients. Hypotension and peripheral edema occurred much more frequently in patients receiving higher dosages of nifedipine.
* Other adverse effects that develop in less than 2% of patients include nasal and chest congestion, constipation, cramps, jitteriness, sleep disturbances, nervousness, pruritus, urticaria, sweating, fever, and chills.
* Nifedipine has been shown to be teratogenic and embryotoxic in laboratory animals. It should be used in pregnancy only when the benefits significantly outweigh the risks of therapy to the fetus.

Drug interactions

Concomitant use with antihypertensive agents should result in additive hypotensive effects.

Although concomitant use of nifedipine and beta blocker agents (propranolol, others) is usually well tolerated, cases of severe hypotension, exacerbation of angina, and congestive heart failure have been reported. It is important to taper beta blockers, if possible, rather than stop them abruptly before beginning nifedipine.

Nifedipine treatment increases serum digoxin levels by 45% to 50%, potentially resulting in digitalis toxicity. Reduce maintenance and digitalization doses when nifedipine is initiated, and monitor the patient closely to prevent overdigitalization or underdigitalization.

Nifedipine has complex effects on glucose metabolism. It appears to increase oral hypoglycemic agent dosages in non-insulin-dependent diabetes mellitus. Its effects on insulin-controlled diabetes are unknown, but clinicians should be aware of the possibility of poor control.

Verapamil hydrochloride
(Calan, Isoptin)

AHFS 24:04
CATEGORY Calcium antagonist

Action and use

Verapamil is a calcium ion influx inhibitor, or slow channel blocker, structurally unrelated to other calcium antagonists. Its mechanisms of action are not fully known, but its therapeutic activity is thought to be derived from its ability to inhibit the influx of calcium ions across the cell membrane during membrane depolarization of cardiac and vascular smooth muscle. Physiologically, it slows atrioventricular (AV) conduction and prolongs the effective refractory period within the AV node, thus reducing rapid ventricular rate in supraventricular tachycardia caused by atrial flutter or atrial fibrillation. It also produces coronary and peripheral arterial vasodilatation, resulting in improved mycardial oxygenation and reduced afterload. The negative inotropic action (depressed myocardial contractility) of verapamil is usually counterbalanced by reduction of afterload so that the cardiac index remains essentially unchanged.

Verapamil is currently being used as an antiarrhythmic agent to treat supraventricular arrhythmias and as an antianginal agent. It is effective in treating angina pectoris at rest caused by coronary artery spasm (Prinzmetal's variant angina) and unstable (crescendo, preinfarction) angina as well as chronic stable (exertional) angina.

Characteristics

Bioavailability: 20% to 35% (PO after first-pass effect). Peak therapeutic activity: 3 to 5 minutes (IV); 1 to 2 hr (PO). Protein binding: 90%. Half-life: IV—2 to 5 hr; PO—single dose, 2.8 to 7.4 hr; repetitive dosing, 4.5 to 12 hr; half-life increases due to saturation of hepatic enzyme systems; hepatic impairment—14 to 16 hr. Metabolism: hepatic, to 12 metabolites, levels of activity unknown. Excretion: 3% to 4% unchanged in urine, 70% as metabolites in urine; 16% in feces, all within 5 days. Dialysis: no. Breast milk: unknown.

Administration and dosage

NOTE: Verapamil is contraindicated in (1) patients with sick sinus syndrome except in the presence of a functional ventricular pacemaker, (2) patients with second- or third-degree AV block, and (3) patients with a systolic pressure less than 90 mm Hg.

Dosage adjustments must be made for patients with hepatic or renal failure. These patients should be observed closely for a prolonged duration of activity.

Adult

PO 1. Initially, 80 mg 3 to 4 times daily. Increase daily to keekly until optimal clinical response is achieved. The total daily dose ranges from 240 to 480 mg. Most patients respond in the 320 to 480 mg daily range.
    2. Sublingual nitroglycerin therapy may be continued for acute anginal attacks.

IV 1. Initial dose: 5 to 10 mg administered over 2 to 3 mins with continuous ECG monitoring.
    2. Repeat dose: 10 mg 30 mins after the first dose if therapeutic response was not achieved.
    3. Administer over at least 3 mins in elderly patients.

Pediatric
Birth to 1 year of age

IV—0.1 to 0.2 mg/kg over 2 min. with continuous ECG monitoring.

One to 15 years of age

IV—0.1 to 0.3 mg/kg over 2 min with continuous ECG monitoring. Do not exceed 5 mg.

Repeat above doses 30 min after the first dose if the initial response is inadequate.

NOTE: To treat overdosage or exaggerated response:
Gastric lavage
Bradycardia—atropine 0.6 to 1 mg IV; isoproterenol cautiously.
AV block, asystole—atropine, isoproterenol, pacemaker.
Cardiac failure—inotropic agents (dopamine, dobutamine) and diuretics.

Hypotension—levarterenol, metaraminol, dopamine, dobutamine.

Excessive ventricular rate—DC cardioversion, procainamide, lidocaine.

In patients with idiopathic, hypertrophic, subaortic stenosis, use alpha-adrenergic agents such as phenylephrine or
metaraminol to maintain blood pressure. Avoid isoproterenol
and levarterenol.

Nurse and patient considerations

* The following adverse effects have been reported
  with oral verapamil therapy: hypotension (2.9%);
  peripheral edema (1.7%); third-degree AV block
  (0.8%); bradycardia, less than 50 beats/min (1.1%);
  congestive heart failure or pulmonary edema
  (0.9%); dizziness (3.6%); headache (1.8%); fatigue
  (1.1%); constipation (6.3%); and nausea (1.6%).
* The following adverse effects have been reported
  with IV verapamil therapy: symptomatic hypotension (1.5%), bradycardia (1.2%), severe tachycardia
  (1.0%), dizziness and headache (1.2%), nausea
  (0.9%), and abdominal discomfort (0.6%).
* No teratogenic effects have been identified in off-
  spring of laboratory animals; however, verapamil
  should be used in pregnancy only when the benefits
  significantly outweigh the risks of therapy.

Drug interactions

Concomitant use of verapamil with beta blockers (propranolol, nadolol, timolol, others) may result in additive
depressant effects on cardiac conduction. Monitor patients
for excessive bradycardia and AV block.

It is recommended that disopyramide should *not* be
administered within 48 hr before or 24 hr after verapamil
administration.

Chronic verapamil treatment increases serum digoxin
levels by 50% to 70% during the first week of therapy, potentially resulting in digitalis toxicity. Reduce maintenance and
digitalization doses when verapamil is initiated, and monitor
the patient closely to prevent overdigitalization or underdigitalization. Verapamil and digitalis may be used concomitantly but may result in additive effects on cardiac conduction.
Monitor patients for excessive bradycardia and AV block.

Verapamil has complex effects on glucose metabolism. It appears to decrease oral hypoglycemic agent dosages in non-insulin-dependent diabetes mellitus. Its effects on insulin-controlled diabetics are unknown, but clinicians should be aware of the possibility of poor control.

"Coronary vasodilators"
GENERAL INFORMATION

The nitrites (organic nitrites and nitrates) have long been the treatment of choice for angina pectoris. The primary action of these agents is dilation of vascular smooth muscle, causing decreased peripheral arterial vascular resistance (afterload) and a decrease in venous blood return (preload) to the heart. The net result is a decreased workload on the heart with a reduction in myocardial oxygen consumption. The nitrites may also allow a redistribution of coronary blood flow, improving the supply of oxygen to the hypoxic areas. For various preparations see Table 2-12.

Table 2-12. Preparations of nitrites and organic nitrates

Generic name	Trade name	Doses, routes of adminis- tration	Preparations
SHORT-ACTING			
Amyl nitrite	Vaporole	0.18 ml or 0.3 ml, in- halation	Pearls: 0.18 and 0.3 ml
Nitroglycerin (glyceryl trini- trate)	Nitrostat	0.15 to 0.6 mg, sub- lingual	Tablets: 0.15, 0.3, 0.4, and 0.6 mg
	Nitrobid	2.5 mg PO every 12 hr	Tablets: 2.5 and 6.5 mg
	Nitrol	Topical to skin every 3 to 4 hr and at bedtime	Ointment: 2%
	Tridil	IV infusion	Ampules: 50 mg
	Nitro-BID- IV		Ampules: 5, 25, and 50 mg
	Nitrostat- IV		Ampules: 8 mg

Table 2-12. Preparations of nitrites and organic nitrates—cont'd

Generic name	Trade name	Doses, routes of adminis- tration	Preparations
LONG-ACTING			
Erythrityl tet- ranitrate	Cardilate	5 to 15 mg, sublingual 15 to 60 mg PO	Tablets: 5, 10, 15 mg PO and sublingual
Pentaerythritol tetranitrate	Peritrate	10 to 40 mg PO	Tablets: 10 and 20 mg
	SK-PETN	30 to 80 mg PO every	30 to 80 mg*
	Duotrate*	12 hr*	
Isosorbide din- itrate	Isordil	2.5 to 10 mg, sub- lingual	Tablets: 2.5, 5 mg sublingal
	Sorbitrate	10 to 60 mg PO	5 and 10 mg PO
Mannitol hexanitrate	Nitranitol	32 to 64 mg PO	Tablets: 32 mg
Nitroglycerin	Susadrin*	1 to 2 mg 3 to 6 times daily, transmu- cosal (PO)	1 and 2 mg transmucosal tablets
	Nitrodisk* Nitro-Dur* Transderm- Nitro*	1 disk topical to skin ev- ery 24 hours	Variable, de- pending on surface area covered and permeability of skin and mem- brane

*Sustained-release preparation.

Characteristics

The nitrites (amyl nitrite) and the nitrates (nitroglycerin, pentaerythritol tetranitrate) appear to act through release of the nitrite ion. The parent nitrate compounds appear to be very rapidly metabolized to nitrite ions at specific "nitrate" receptors located in smooth muscle, resulting in relaxation of the smooth muscle.

Amyl nitrite is administered via inhalation while the nitrates are absorbed quite rapidly through the sublingual mucosa and the gastrointestinal tract. The sublingual route is clinically much more preferable, however, because degradation by the liver is so rapid and complete that little of the active drug reaches systemic circulation. Nitroglycerin may also be readily absorbed through the skin (as evidenced by the use of nitroglycerin 2% ointment, transdermal disks, and transmucosal tablets).

Nurse and patient considerations

All nitrites and nitrates may cause cutaneous vasodilation and flushing, along with a severe or persistant headache. Patients may complain of transient episodes of dizziness, weakness, and faintness as well as other signs of cerebral ischemia associated with vasodilatation and postural hypotension that may develop.

An occasional patient may show marked sensitivity to the hypotensive effects of nitrites with normal therapeutic doses. Severe hypotensive episodes may occur, manifested by nausea and vomiting, weakness, restlessness, pallor, cold sweat, and collapse.

Drug rash and/or exfoliative dermatitis is produced by all the organic nitrates, but appears most commonly with pentaerythritol tetranitrate.

Insufficient data has been accumulated to establish the safety of the use of nitrates during the acute phase of a myocardial infarction.

Drug interactions

Ethanol accentuates the vasodilatation and postural hypotension of the nitrites and nitrates. Patients should be cautioned about vasodilatation and hypotension with the ingestion of alcohol while receiving nitrite therapy.

Nitroglycerin (glyceryl trinitrate)

AHFS 24:12

(Numerous brands) CATEGORY Vasodilator

Action and use

See General information on the "coronary vasodilators" (p. 180).

Administration and dosage

SUBLINGUAL
1. Sit or lie down at the first sign of oncoming anginal attack.

2. Place a tablet under the tongue and allow to dissolve; do not swallow saliva.
3. Do not take more than 3 tablets in 15 min.
4. 1 or 2 tablets may be taken prophylactically a few minutes before engaging in activities that may trigger an anginal attack.

PO—Sustained-release tablets or capsules: 1.3, 2.5, or 6.5 mg 2 to 3 times daily at 8 and 12 hr intervals.

TRANSMUCOSAL TABLETS—This dosage form is for prophylactic use against angina pectoris. It contains nitroglycerin in a slow-release tablet. When placed under the upper lip or buccal pouch, it releases nitroglycerin for absorption by the oral mucosa over the next 3 to 5 hr. Patients may eat, drink, and talk while the tablet is in place. The usual initial dose is 1 tablet 3 times daily on arising, after lunch, and after the evening meal. Do not administer more than 1 tablet every 2 hr. Development of headache, dizziness, and hypotension are indications of overdose.

TOPICAL OINTMENT (nitroglycerin 2%)—This dosage form is more for prophylactic use, especially for patients who suffer from the fear of nocturnal attacks of angina pectoris. If the dosage is adjusted properly, the ointment may be used every 3 to 4 hr and at bedtime.
1. Lay the dose-measuring applicator with the printed side down.
2. Squeeze the proper amount of ointment onto the applicator.
3. Place the measuring applicator on the skin, ointment down, spreading in a thin, uniform layer. Do not massage or rub in. The applicator allows measuring of the proper dose and also prevents absorption through the fingertips.
4. Close the tube tightly and store in a cool place.

NOTE: A chronic headache is a sign of overdosage, requiring the dose to be reduced. Sudden dizziness and faintness (postural hypotension) may result from sudden changes in position. Patients should be cautioned to change positions slowly when arising from a recumbent or sitting position. When terminating the use of the topical ointment, gradually reduce the dose and frequency of application over 4 to 6 weeks.

TOPICAL DISKS—This dosage form is for prophylactic use. It provides a controlled release of nitroglycerin through a semipermeable membrane for 24 hr when applied to intact skin. The dosage released is dependent on the surface area of the disk. Therapeutic effect can be observed in about 30 min after attachment and is maintained for about 30 min after removal.

1. The disk should be applied to a hairless/clean shaven area of skin on the upper chest or side, pelvis, or inner upper arm. Avoid scars, skin folds, or wounds. Rotate skin sites daily.
2. Wash hands before you apply and after you remove the product.
3. Transderm-Nitro and Nitro-Dur may be worn while showering. Nitrodisc should be replaced after bathing.
4. If a disk becomes partially dislodged, discard it and replace with a new disk.
5. Sublingual nitroglycerin may be necessary for anginal attacks, especially while the dosage is adjusted.

NOTE: Transient headaches are the most common side effect, especially when higher doses are being used. These headaches should be treated with mild analgesics while therapy is adjusted and continued. If the headache is unresponsive to treatment, it should be considered a sign of overdosage and the dosage dropped or the nitroglycerin disk discontinued. When terminating the use of the topical disk, gradually reduce the dose over a period of 4 to 6 weeks to prevent sudden withdrawal reactions.

iv—Intravenous nitroglycerin is used to control perioperative hypertension, congestive heart failure associated with acute myocardial infarction, and angina pectoris in patients not responsive to other forms of nitrites or beta blockers and to produce controlled hypotension during surgical procedures.

1. It must not be given by direct IV, but diluted in D_5W or normal saline to dilutions of 25 to 400 μg/ml before use.
2. Nitroglycerin binds significantly (40% to 80%) to plastic (PVC) bags and tubing routinely used. Use only glass bottles and IV administration sets provided with each specific brand, thus allowing lower doses to be used. Do not use in-line filters.
3. Initial dosage (administered by infusion pump) is 5 μg/min. Increase by 5 μg every 3 to 5 min until some response is noted. Then increase in smaller increments. There is no optimum or maximum dosage.

4. All patients must be monitored continuously for blood pressure, heart rate, and pulmonary capillary wedge pressure.
5. Overdosage is manifested by severe hypotension and reflex tachycardia. Treat by reduction of dosage and elevation of limbs. Although rarely necessary, an alpha agonist such as phenylephrine or methoxamine may be considered.

Nurse and patient considerations

* Nitroglycerin tablets are inactivated by light, heat, air, and moisture. The tablets should be stored at room temperature in amber glass containers with a tight-fitting screw-on cap. Patients should be warned not to store nitroglycerin tablets within other containers, such as pill boxes, or with other medications, so as to maintain maximum potency.
* It should be explained that even though only a few tablets may have been used from a bottle, the patient should test the tablets once a month, and if found subpotent, to discard the bottle and replace it with a fresh supply. A new, potent nitroglycerin tablet should produce a headache or a burning sensation under the tongue when administered sublingually.
* See General information on "coronary vasodilators" (p. 180).

Drug interactions

See General information on "coronary vasodilators" (p. 180).

CHAPTER THREE

Antihypertensive agents

GENERAL INFORMATION ON TREATMENT OF HYPERTENSION

Hypertension is a disease characterized by an elevation of the blood pressure above values considered normal for patients of similar environmental and racial backgrounds. In North America statistics indicate that blood pressures above 140/90 to 150/90 mm Hg are associated with premature death resulting from accelerated vascular disease of the brain, heart, and kidneys.

Clinical classification usually divides this disease into primary (essential) hypertension and secondary hypertension. Secondary hypertension may be caused by renal or endocrine dysfunction or a number of other miscellaneous causes such as coarctation of the aorta, toxemia of pregnancy, and CNS disorders. Treatment of secondary hypertension is often unnecessary after controlling the underlying disorder.

Primary hypertension accounts for 80% to 90% of all clinical cases of high blood pressure. Its etiology is basically unknown; it is incurable at the present time, but certainly controllable. A vast array of statistical data indicates that 20 to 25 million Americans have hypertension. The prevalence rises steadily with advancing age; however, in every age group the incidence is higher for blacks than for whites of both sexes. In addition to the age-sex-race patterns, other factors associated with high blood pressure include a family history of hypertension, spikes of high blood pressure in young adult years, obesity, cigarette smoking, hypercholesterolemia, hyperglycemia, abnormal renal function, retinopathies, preexisting cardiovascular disease (that is, angina, congestive heart failure), and a previous history of stroke.

The landmark Veteran's Administration Cooperative Study on hypertension provided dramatic indications of the influence of adequate therapy on morbidity and mortality. Treatment of hypertension requires a multifaceted approach to delay progression of the disease. The ultimate goal of antihypertensive therapy is prolongation of a useful life by preventing cardiovascular complications. To accomplish this the blood pressure must be reduced and maintained at acceptable levels. *Acceptable levels* are variable, since they imply achieving and maintaining an acceptable blood pressure without the patient's neglecting therapy because of the side effects of treatment. Treatment regimens should be established that interfere as little as possible with the patient's life-style.

Patient education is extremely important in treating hypertension and maintaining compliance with the treatment regimen. Patients must be advised that their disease is progressive and that they cannot rely on symptoms to alert them of a higher blood pressure, since hypertension is notoriously asymptomatic until complications occur. Drug therapy is a mainstay of antihypertensive therapy, but ancillary measures are also important. Reduction of dietary sodium intake and weight (if necessary), regular times of relaxation, developing hobbies, and a plan of moderate exercise to improve the patient's physical condition should also be encouraged. Cigarette smoking should be stopped, since it is an added risk factor in coronary artery disease.

Before initiation of therapy the patient should undergo a thorough physical examination in an attempt to determine the cause and the severity of the hypertension as well as to establish baseline data to monitor both the benefits and the side effects of therapy. If no cause for the hypertension is found, it is assumed that the patient has essential hypertension.

Despite the large number of antihypertensive agents available, there are only three general classes of drugs: (1) diuretics—thiazides, furosemide (Lasix), ethacrynic acid (Edecrin), (2) direct vasodilators—hydralazine (Apresoline), minoxidil (Loniten), and (3) sympathetic nervous system inhibitors—reserpine, methyldopa (Aldomet), guanethidine (Ismelin), guanabenz (Wytensin), clonidine (Catapres), prazosin (Minipress), propranolol (Inderal). All of the above agents act either directly or indirectly to reduce the peripheral vascular resistance, therefore lowering blood pressure. Combination therapy using two or more antihypertensive agents is routine practice. (See Table 3-2 for the ingredients of combination antihypertensive products.) Using drugs that act by different mechanisms to reduce peripheral vascular resistance provides the benefit of using lower doses of each agent so that the patient suffers fewer adverse effects from the therapy.

A patient is classified as having mild hypertension if the diastolic blood pressure is between 90 and 105 mm Hg and if there is no indication of tissue damage (for example, retinopathies). Mild hypertension is usually treated with a thiazide diuretic, and, if necessary, reserpine, clonidine, or methyldopa may be added to the regimen.

Moderate hypertension exists when the diastolic pressure is between 105 and 130 mm Hg. Tissue damage may or may not be present. Treatment usually consists of methyldopa, hydralazine, clonidine, and/or propranolol in combination with an oral diuretic.

A patient may have severe hypertension if the diastolic blood pressure is above 130 mm Hg. These patients are symptomatic and do display tissue damage. The treatment regimen is initiated with an oral diuretic, hydralazine, and propranolol. Inadequate response might require the addition of guanethidine. Other combinations using clonidine, captopril, or methyldopa may also be successful.

Patients who suddenly develop hypertensive encephalopathy, indicated by neurologic signs and symptoms, require more rapid control of blood pressure. Boluses of diazoxide or a sodium nitroprusside infusion may be indicated to control the symptomatology.

Nurse and patient considerations

Recognize that the patient's cooperation in redirecting much of his or her life-style is a difficult task to achieve. Adherence to the treatment objectives will be more successful if the goals are realistic for the patient. Patient education with periodic encouragement and reinforcement will increase the patient's ability to maintain therapy.

Request the assistance of the patient and the spouse or a family member in planning a coordinated treatment guide that includes a dietary plan, a reduction in smoking, and a plan to lower stressful, emotional activities.

If feasible, teach the patient to monitor blood pressure at home. Inform the patient of the blood pressure readings that should be reported to the physician.

Plan a schedule so that medications are taken regularly at a proper but yet convenient time. Inform the patient of the side effects of the therapeutic medications and offer assistance in coping with these effects. The frequency of orthostatic hypotension is higher in the morning on arising, and the patient should be taught to get up slowly to offset the feeling of dizziness or to lie down immediately if feeling faint. Other bothersome side effects include nasal congestion, anorexia, loss of strength, and fatigue.

Inform the patient of conditions that will minimize an increased arterial pressure. Situations with associated feelings of anxiety, anger, or annoyance aggravate hypertension. Alterations in normal, ordinary functions such as eating, sleeping, and elimination also increase the physiologic stress response.

To effectively monitor the antihypertensive agents, consult the monographs on those specific medications.

Captopril
(Capoten)

AHFS 24:08
CATEGORY Antihypertensive agent

Action and use

Captopril is a competitive inhibitor of angiotensin I–coverting enzyme (ACE), the enzyme responsible for the conversion of angiotensin I to angiotensin II. The mechanism of antihypertensive activity is not completely known, but captopril appears to lower blood pressure by suppression of the renin-angiotensin-aldosterone system. Inhibition of ACE results in decreased plasma levels of angiotensin II (a potent vasoconstrictor). Blood pressure is thought to be reduced, at least in part, by decreased vasoconstriction, resulting in lower total peripheral resistance. There is no compensatory increase in heart rate, stroke volume, or cardiac output. Blood pressure is reduced to the same extent in both supine and standing positions. A few cases of orthostatic hypotension have been reported. Although captopril is effective in mild to severe hypertension, its side effects dictate that it be used only in those hypertensive patients in whom other multiple drug regimens have failed or were not tolerated.

Characteristics

Bioavailability: 75%; food diminishes absorption by 30% to 40%. Onset: 15 min. Peak activity: 1 to 2 hr. Duration: 2 to 6 hr, but increases with increasing doses, up to 12 hr. Protein binding: 25% to 30%. Half-life: normal renal function—

less than 2 hr; with creatinine clearance less than 20 ml/min—20 to 40 hr; anuria—6.5 days. Metabolism: yes. Excretion: 40% to 50% unchanged, remainder as metabolites in urine. Dialysis: yes, H. Breast milk: yes.

Administration and dosage

NOTE: Administer 1 hr before meals. Dosage must be individualized. Initiation of therapy requires consideration of recent antihypertensive drug treatment, the degree of blood pressure elevation, and salt restriction. If possible, discontinue the patient's previous antihypertensive drug regimen for 1 week before starting captopril.

Adult

PO 1. Initially, 25 mg 3 times daily. Increase to 50 mg 3 times daily in 1 to 2 weeks. If therapeutic goals are not achieved in another 1 to 2 weeks, add hydrochlorothiazide, 25 mg daily. The diuretic dose may be increased at 1- to 2-week intervals to 100 mg daily.
2. If further hypotensive activity is needed, continue the diuretic and increase captopril to 100 mg 3 times daily up to 150 mg 3 times daily. Do not exceed 450 mg daily.
3. For those patients for whom it is inappropriate to discontinue other antihypertensive medication the previous week, discontinue and start captopril 25 mg 3 times daily immediately under close medical supervision. Dosages may be increased every 24 hr to a maximum of 450 mg daily. A more potent diuretic, usually furosemide, may also be used.
4. For patients with renal impairment, lower initial doses should be used and smaller incremental changes made every 1 to 2 weeks.

Nurse and patient considerations

* Approximately 1.2% of patients receiving captopril develop proteinuria greater than 1 g/day during the first 8 months of therapy. About one fourth of these patients develop nephrotic syndrome. Patients with prior renal disease are predisposed to proteinuria. Patients receiving captopril should have urinary protein estimates (dipstick on first morning urine, or quantitative 24 hr urine) before therapy and at

monthly intervals for the first 9 months of treatment and periodically thereafter.

* Neutropenia (<300 neutrophils/mm^3) and agranulocytosis (drug-induced bone marrow suppression) have been observed in 0.3% of patients treated with captopril. The neutropenia appears within the first 3 to 12 weeks of therapy and develops slowly, the white count falling to its nadir in 10 to 30 days. The white count returns to normal in about 2 weeks after discontinuation of captopril therapy. Patients most susceptible are those with impaired renal function or serious autoimmune disease (particularly systemic lupus erythematosus) or those who are exposed to other drugs known to affect the white cells or immune response. Patients at risk should have differential and total white cell counts before initiation of therapy and then every 2 weeks thereafter for the first 3 months of therapy.

* Patients should be told to notify their physician promptly if any indication of progressive edema (which may be an indicator of proteinuria and nephrotic syndrome) or evidence of infection such as sore throat or fever (which may be an indicator of neutropenia) should develop.

* About 10% of patients receiving captopril will develop a rash, usually maculopapular in nature, usually in the first 4 weeks of therapy. The rash is often accompanied with pruritus and sometimes fever and eosinophilia. The rash is usually mild and disappears within a few days of dosage reduction, short-term treatment with an antihistaminic agent, and/or discontinuation of therapy. Remission may occur even if captopril is continued.

* Taste impairment manifested by loss of taste acuity, metallic taste, salty taste, or loss of taste perception occurs in 7% of patients. Taste impairment develops within the first 3 months of therapy and resolves within 2 to 3 months of continued therapy.

* Many other side effects including angina pectoris, palpitations, congestive heart failure, Raynaud's syndrome, headache, paresthesias, insomnia, gastric discomfort, constipation, and diarrhea have infrequently been reported in conjunction with captopril therapy.

* Captopril may cause false-positive results in urine acetone determinations using the sodium nitroprusside reagent.
* Captopril has been shown to be embryocidal in laboratory animals. Use in pregnancy is not recommended unless the benefits significantly outweigh the risks of therapy.

Drug interactions

Captopril may be used in combination with other antihypertensive agents to enhance hypotensive activity and allow a reduction in the dosages of the antihypertensive agents. Excessive hypotension may occur in patients on severe salt restriction or those with hypovolemia. It may also be exacerbated by vigorous use of diuretics.

Although both are antihypertensive agents, the combined effects of beta blockers (propranolol, others) and captopril are less than additive.

The sympathetic nervous system is especially important in supporting blood pressure in patients receiving captopril alone or with diuretics. Ganglionic blocking agents (trimethaphan camsylate) or adrenergic neuron-blocking agents (guanethidine sulfate) should be used with extreme caution in patients receiving captopril.

Since captopril decreases aldosterone secretion, small increases in serum potassium frequently occur. Potassium-sparing diuretics (triamterene, spironolactone, amiloride) or potassium supplements should be given only for documented hypokalemia. If a patient has received spironolactone up to several months before captopril therapy, the serum potassium level should be monitored closely because the potassium-conserving effect of spironolactone persists.

Clonidine hydrochloride (Catapres)

AHFS 24:08
CATEGORY Antihypertensive agent

Action and use

Clonidine is a potent antihypertensive agent that acts within the central nervous system to reduce both systolic and diastolic blood pressure. It also causes bradycardia, resulting in decreased cardiac output. After prolonged therapy the lowered blood pressure results primarily from reduced peripheral vascular resistance. Clonidine is now used in the treatment of mild to moderate hypertension. Its effectiveness is generally improved when used in combination with diuretics and/or other antihypertensive agents.

Characteristics

Onset: 30 to 60 min (PO). Peak activity: 2 to 4 hr (PO). Duration: 8 hr (PO). Half-life: 12 to 16 hr with normal renal function, 25 to 37 hr with impaired renal function. Metabolism: liver, to 4 metabolites. Excretion: 20% in feces, 32% unchanged in urine, 33% as metabolites in urine.

Administration and dosage
Adult

PO
1. Initial: 0.1 mg 2 times daily.
2. Maintenance: Add 0.1 to 0.2 mg daily until desired effect is achieved. Average daily doses range from 0.2 to 0.8 mg in divided doses. Maximum recommended daily dose is 2.4 mg.

Pediatric

No dosage recommendations are available.

Nurse and patient considerations

* Patients must be informed of the need for continuity of therapy. Abrupt discontinuance of therapy may result in a rapid increase in systolic and diastolic pressure. Patients may display such symptoms as nervousness, restlessness, agitation, tremor, headache, nausea, and increased salivation. These symptoms are more pronounced after 1 to 2 months of therapy and begin to appear a few hours after a dose is missed. Blood pressure rises significantly within 8 to 24 hr. When clonidine therapy is to be discontinued, dosage should be gradually reduced over 2 to 4 days, depending on the patient's response.

* The most frequent adverse effects reported with clonidine are dry mouth, drowsiness, and sedation (caution patients about performing hazardous tasks). Other side effects include constipation, dizziness, and headache. Numerous other gastrointestinal, metabolic, cardiovascular, dermatologic, and genitourinary effects have also been reported.

* Diuretic therapy is often beneficial in diminishing sodium and water retention, especially during the first few days of clonidine therapy.
* Periodic ophthalmologic examinations are recommended for patients on long-term clonidine therapy. Laboratory animals have developed degenerative retinal changes, although none have been reported in humans.
* Patients suffering from mental depression may be more susceptible to further depressive activity.
* Reproduction studies have found no teratogenic activity, but embryo toxicities have been found at doses within the normal therapeutic range. Clonidine should therefore not be used in pregnant women unless the potential benefit outweighs the potential risk. It is not known whether clonidine is found in breast milk.

Drug interactions

The sedative effects of clonidine may enhance the CNS depressant effects of alcohol, barbiturates, tranquilizers, and antihistamines.

Desipramine (Norpramin, Pertofrane) blocks the antihypertensive effects of clonidine. Other tricyclic antidepressants may also result in loss of hypertensive control.

Clonidine may be administered together with hydralazine, guanethidine, methyldopa, reserpine, spironolactone, furosemide, and the thiazide diuretics without interactions. However, the antihypertensive effects of all these agents will be enhanced, requiring careful adjustment of dosages.

The bradycardic effects of clonidine may be enhanced by guanethidine, propranolol, and digitalis glycosides.

If it should be decided to discontinue therapy in patients receiving beta blockers and clonidine concurrently, the beta blocker should be discontinued several days before the gradual withdrawal of clonidine.

Trazodone (Desyrel) may inhibit the antihypertensive properties of clonidine.

Diazoxide
(Hyperstat I.V.)

AHFS 24:08
CATEGORY Antihypertensive agent

Action and use

Diazoxide lowers blood pressure by a direct vasodilatory action on the smooth muscle of peripheral arterioles, thus reducing peripheral vascular resistance. Diazoxide is used for emergency reduction of blood pressure in hospitalized patients with severe hypertension when a rapid decrease in diastolic pressure is required.

Characteristics

Onset and peak: less than 5 min (IV). Duration: 4 to 12 hr. Protein-binding: more than 90%. Half-life: 28 hr. Metabolism: questionable. Excretion: urine, primarily unchanged. Dialysis: yes, H, P.

Administration and dosage
Adult

IV—300 mg in 30 sec or less. Monitor the blood pressure closely. A second dose may be required for a satisfactory reduction in blood pressure if the first injection fails to give an adequate response within 30 min.

Pediatric

IV—5 mg/kg in 30 sec or less. Monitor the blood pressure closely. A second dose may be needed within 30 min.

NOTE: Administer undiluted in a peripheral vein. As a result of the alkalinity of the solution, extravascular injection or leakage may be quite irritating and should be avoided.

Nurse and patient considerations

* Blood pressure must be monitored at frequent intervals, particularly during the first hour after administration. If hypotension occurs, it will usually respond to the administration of dopamine or levarterenol. Monitor input and output and pulmonary status closely.

* Diazoxide may caused marked sodium and water retention, particularly after repeated injections, resulting in edema and congestive heart failure. Potent diuretics such as furosemide (Lasix) or ethacrynic acid (Edecrin) may be required to diminish

the water retention. The diuretics may also potentiate the hypotensive and hyperglycemic properties of diazoxide.

* Hyperglycemia is a frequent adverse effect of diazoxide therapy. Treatment with insulin is occasionally required, especially in those patients with diabetes mellitus. Dipstick the urine for glucose.

* Diazoxide must be used with caution during pregnancy. Fetal abnormalities have been observed in animals. Diazoxide crosses the placental barrier, but its presence and content in human breast milk are not known.

Drug interactions

The anticoagulant activity of warfarin (Coumadin) may be increased as a result of the displacement from protein-binding sites by diazoxide.

The hyperglycemic potential of diazoxide may be enhanced by patients concurrently receiving diuretics, phenytoin (Dilantin), propranolol (Inderal), corticosteroids such as prednisone, and oral contraceptives.

Guanabenz acetate
(Wytensin)

AHFS 24:08
CATEGORY Antihypertensive agent

Action and use

Guanabenz is a centrally acting alpha$_2$-adrenergic receptor stimulant used to treat hypertension. It acts by stimulating alpha-adrenergic receptors in the brain to decrease sympathetic outflow to the peripheral circulatory system, causing a drop in peripheral vascular resistance. A decrease in blood pressure is seen in both supine and standing positions, without evidence of postural hypotension. It may be used alone or in combination with a thiazide diuretic.

Characteristics

Bioavailability: 75%. Onset: within 60 min. Peak activity: 2 to 5 hr. Duration: 8 to 12 hr. Half-life: 6 hr. Metabolism: extensive, sites unknown. Excretion: less than 1% excreted unchanged in urine. Dialysis: unknown. Breast milk: unknown.

Administration and dosage
Adult
PO—Initially, 4 mg 2 times daily, alone or in combination with a thiazide diuretic. Doses may be increased every 1 to 2 weeks in increments of 4 to 8 mg daily. Maximum dose is 64 mg/day.

Pediatric
Safe use in children under the age of 12 years has not been determined.

Nurse and patient considerations

* Patients must be informed of the need for continuity of therapy. Abrupt discontinuance of therapy may result in a rapid increase in systolic and diastolic pressure. If therapy is to be discontinued, the patient's dose should be tapered down over 1 to 2 weeks if possible.

* The most frequent side effects reported are drowsiness and sedation (20% to 40%). Patients should be cautioned about performing hazardous tasks. Other side effects include dry mouth, dizziness, weakness, and headache. Numerous other gastrointestinal, metabolic, cardiovascular, dermatologic, and genitourinary effects have rarely been reported.

* Guanabenz should not be administered to pregnant women. Teratogenic effects have been reported in laboratory animals.

Drug interactions
The sedative effects of guanabenz may enhance the CNS depressant effect of alcohol, barbiturates, phenothiazines, benzodiazepines, and antihistamines. Patients should be warned that their tolerance for alcohol and other CNS depressants may be diminished.

Guanethidine sulfate
(Ismelin)

AHFS 24:08
CATEGORY Antihypertensive agent

Action and use
Guanethidine sulfate acts both by blocking the release of norepinephrine from nerve endings in response to nerve

stimulation and by depleting norepinephrine from storage sites at adrenergic nerve endings. The effects of PO administration are cumulative over 10 days to 2 weeks and result in gradual reduction of both systolic and diastolic blood pressure. Guanethidine sulfate is a potent agent used in combination therapy with other antihypertensive agents to treat sustained moderate to severe hypertension.

Characteristics

Gastrointestinal absorption varies from 3% to 27% of the administered PO dose. Onset and duration: cumulative over several days. Metabolism: hepatic microsomal enzymes. Excretion: via urine as active and inactive metabolites.

Administration and dosage
Adult

PO 1. Initial: 10 mg daily. Increase the dose 10 mg every 5 to 7 days if the blood pressure measurements so indicate and side effects are tolerable.
2. Maintenance: 25 to 50 mg daily; however, much higher doses are occasionally required. The dose may be given once daily.

Pediatric

PO 1. Initial: 0.2 mg/kg/day.
2. Maintenance: increase every 7 to 10 days by 0.2 mg/kg. A final dose 6 to 8 times the initial dose may be required for optimal therapy.

NOTE: Take the blood pressure with the patient supine and after standing for 10 min. The dosage should be reduced if there is a normal supine pressure or an excessive fall in pressure on standing or if severe diarrhea is present.

Nurse and patient considerations

* Orthostatic hypotension occurs frequently, especially with sudden changes in posture. Patients must be taught to rise slowly from a horizontal position to a sitting position and then flex the arms and legs several times before standing. Orthostatic symptoms are more apparent in the morning and may also be aggravated by heavy exercise, hot weather, and ingestion of alcohol. Standing for prolonged periods may also make the patient feel dizzy and weak. The patient should be forewarned to sit or lie down with the onset of weakness and dizziness.

* Frequent adverse reactions include bradycardia, fluid retention, increased numbers of bowel movements and diarrhea. The diarrhea may be severe enough to result in discontinuance of the drug.
* Other side effects include fatigue, nausea, muscle tremor, mental depression, nasal congestion, blurred vision, dry mouth, angina, and asthma in susceptible patients. Genitourinary symptoms include impotence, nocturia, urinary incontinence, and retrograde ejaculation.
* Safe use has not been established in pregnancy.

Drug interactions

The following drugs may enhance the hypotensive effects of guanethidine:

Ethanol
Propranolol hydrochloride (Inderal) and other beta-adrenergic blocking agents
Quinidine*
Diuretics
Methotrimeprazine (Levoprome)
Reserpine

The following drugs may antagonize the hypotensive effects of guanethidine:

Amphetamines (Dexadrine, Benzadrine)
Methylphenidate (Ritalin)
Ephedrine
Tricyclic antidepressants
 Desipramine (Norpramin, Pertofrane)
 Imipramine (Tofranil)
 Protriptyline hydrochloride (Vivactil)
 Nortriptyline (Aventyl)
 Amitriptyline hydrochloride (Elavil)
 Doxepin (Sinequan)
Phenothiazines
Haloperidol (Haldol)
Monamine oxidase inhibitors
Oral contraceptives

The response from the following drugs would be expected to be enhanced by guanethidine as a result of increased sensitivity of receptor sites (initial therapy with very low doses):

---

*More hypotension observed after parenteral administration.

Levarterenol bitartrate (Levophed)
Dopamine hydrochloride (Intropin)
Phenylephrine (Neo-Synephrine)

Guanethidine may potentiate the hypoglycemic effects of oral hypoglycemic agents and insulin.

Hydralazine hydrochloride
(Apresoline)

AHFS 24:08
CATEGORY Antihypertensive agent

Action and use

Hydralazine is a hypotensive agent that acts on the smooth muscle in arteries and veins, causing vasodilatation. Hydralazine is used to treat moderate to severe hypertension, usually in combination with other agents. Propranolol is often used in combination with hydralazine to prevent the adverse hemodynamic effects of hydralazine.

Characteristics

Peak blood levels: 3 to 4 hr (PO). Duration: 24 hr. Metabolism: liver, by conjugation and acetylation. Excretion: urine as metabolites.

Administration and dosage
Adult

PO   1. Initial: 10 mg 4 times daily for the first 2 to 4 days, then 25 mg 4 times daily. The second week, increase the dosage to 50 mg 4 times daily as the patient tolerates the dosage and the blood pressure is brought under control.
2. Maintenance: adjust the dosage to the lowest effective levels.

IM or IV—20 to 40 mg repeated as necessary. Monitor blood pressures frequently. Results usually become evident within 10 to 20 min.

Pediatric

PO   1. Initial: 0.75 mg/kg/24 hr in 4 divided doses.
2. Maintenance: increase over 3 to 4 weeks to 10 times the initial dosage.

IM or IV—1.7 to 3.5 mg/kg/24 hr in 4 to 6 divided doses.
NOTE: Some patients may require 300 mg or more daily. Combination therapy with thiazides, reserpine, propranolol, or clonidine may allow a reduction in dosage of hydralazine. At these higher doses there is a greater incidence of an

arthritis-like syndrome that may lead to a syndrome indistinguishable from diseminated lupus erythematosus. The syndrome is reversible on discontinuance of hydralazine and may require months of corticosteroid therapy before elimination of the symptoms.

Nurse and patient considerations

* As with any antihypertensive therapy, patients should be advised concerning orthostatic hypotension.
* Headache, palpitations, tachycardia, angina pectoris, nausea, vomiting, and diarrhea are common side effects of hydralazine.
* During prolonged therapy, complete blood count determinations are indicated, as well as LE cell preparations and antinuclear antibody titer determination. Blood dyscrasias and rheumatoid disease have been reported during prolonged therapy.
* Peripheral neuritis, characterized by numbness and tingling, has been reported. Pyridoxine may be effective in treating these symptoms.
* Hydralazine may cause sodium and water retention. Diuretic therapy may be required to control the edema.

Drug interactions

Hydralazine is often used in combination with other antihypertensive medications to enhance the hypotensive activity and allow a reduction in the dosages of the antihypertensive agents. Propranolol is particularly useful in this respect.

Methyldopa
(Aldomet)

AHFS 24:08
CATEGORY Antihypertensive agent

Action and use

Methyldopa is a hypotensive agent whose mechanism of action has not been completely determined. It has several proposed mechanisms, but the major antihypertensive effects now appear to be caused by the formation of a metabolite, α-methylnorepinephrine, which acts predominantly within the central nervous system. There are some unexplained discrepancies in activity, however, and other mechanisms yet to be explained are involved. Methyldopa is recommended for sustained moderate to severe hypertension, usually in combination with other agents.

Characteristics

Fifty percent absorbed from GI tract. Onset: 6 to 12 hr. Peak plasma levels: 3 to 6 hr. Duration: 8 to 12 hr. Elimination: biphasic. Normal renal function: first half-life—approximately 100 min, 90% of unchanged drug in urine; second half-life—5 to 8 hr. Severely impaired renal function: first half-life—3½ hr, with only 50% excreted in early phase. Accumulation occurs with chronic administration. Metabolism: liver. Dialysis: yes, H, P.

Administration and dosage
Adult

PO 1. Initial: 250 mg 3 times daily for the first 48 hr. Add 250 to 500 mg every 2 to 3 days as indicated by blood pressure measurement and patient's tolerance.
2. Maintenance: the minimum effective dose. Combination therapy with thiazide diuretics often allows the use of lower doses of methyldopa with fewer side effects. The maximum daily dose is 3.0 g.

IV—250 to 500 mg every 6 hr as needed. Hypotensive effects are noted in 4 to 6 hr with a duration of 10 to 16 hr. Add the desired dose of methyldopa (50 mg/ml) to 100 ml of dextrose 5% and infuse IV over 30 to 60 min.

Pediatric

PO—10 to 20 mg/kg/24 hr in 2 to 4 divided doses. Adjust maintenance doses every 2 to 3 days for optimal effect. Maximum dosage is 65 mg/kg/24 hr or 3.0 g (whichever is less).
IV—20 to 40 mg/kg/24 in 4 divided doses.

Nurse and patient consideration

* Sedation, lethargy, and dizziness commonly occur when methyldopa therapy is initiated or during adjustment to higher doses. These effects are most notable during the first 2 to 3 days and tend to dissipate with time.

* Between 1% and 3% of patients develop a drug-induced fever during the first 2 to 3 weeks of therapy. It is often associated with muscle pain, malaise, nausea, vomiting, and diarrhea. Occasionally abnormal liver function tests, eosinophilia, and skin rashes have been reported. The symptoms are reversible on discontinuance of the drug, but the fever will redevelop 6 to 12 hr after a challenge dose.

* An average of about 20% of patients on methyldopa therapy for 6 to 12 months develop a positive reaction to the direct Coombs' test. The incidence is dose related. Which patients with a positive direct Coomb's test who may develop true hemolytic anemia secondary to methyldopa therapy cannot be predicted, but data indicate that only 0.1% to 0.2% of the patients will develop an autoimmune hemolytic anemia. It takes another 6 to 12 months after methyldopa is discontinued for the Coombs' test to revert to normal. Periodic blood counts should be determined during therapy to detect hemolytic anemia.

* Methyldopa may cause sodium and water retention with weight gain, especially when not used in conjunction with diuretic therapy. Patients should weigh themselves daily and report a weight gain of 5 lb or more.

* Other adverse effects that occur with methyldopa therapy include angina pectoris, bradycardia, nasal stuffiness, dry mouth and constipation.

* Methyldopa or its metabolites may discolor the urine, causing it to darken on exposure to air.

* Methyldopa crosses the placental barrier and is not recommended in pregnancy. Excretion in breast milk is unknown.

Drug interactions

The following drugs may enhance the hypotensive activity of methyldopa:

Diuretics
Propranolol (Inderal)
Procainamide (Pronestyl)
Quinidine
Levodopa (Dopar, Larodopa)
Phenothiazines

The following tricyclic antidepressants may antagonize the hypotensive effects of methyldopa:

Doxepin (Sinequan)
Imipramine (Tofranil)
Desipramine (Pertofrane, Norpramin)
Amitriptyline (Elavil)
Protriptyline hydrochloride (Vivactil)

Minoxidil
(Loniten)

AHFS 24:08
CATEGORY Antihypertensive agent

Action and use

Minoxidil is an antihypertensive agent that acts by direct relaxation of arteriolar smooth muscle. It decreases blood pressure in both the supine and standing positions, without evidence of postural hypotension. The drop in peripheral vascular resistance and blood pressure triggers compensatory sympathetic vagal inhibitory and renal homeostatic mechanisms that lead to increased heart rate and output and sodium and water retention. To control these adverse effects, minoxidil is usually administered concomitantly with a beta-adrenergic blocking agent and a potent diuretic (usually furosemide).

Because of its potency and frequency of adverse effects, minoxidil is used only for severely hypertensive patients who do not respond adequately to maximum therapeutic doses of a diuretic and 2 other antihypertensive agents.

Characteristics

Bioavailability: 90%. Onset: 30 min. Peak activity: 2 to 8 hr. Duration: 2 to 5 days. Half-life: 4.2 hr. Protein binding: none. Metabolism: 90%. Excretion: renal. Dialysis: yes, H, P. Breast milk: unknown.

Administration and dosage

NOTE: Before starting minoxidil therapy, the patient should already be stabilized on the equivalent of 160 to 320 mg of propranolol daily, methyldopa, 500 to 1500 mg daily, or clonidine, 0.2 to 0.4 mg daily, as well as a diuretic such as hydrochlorothiazide, 100 mg daily, chlorthalidone, 50 to 100 mg daily, or furosemide, 80 mg daily.

Adult

PO—Initially, 5 mg daily. Dosage may be gradually increased after at least 3-day intervals to 10 mg, 20 mg, and then

40 mg daily in 1 to 2 doses. Most patients' blood pressure is controlled in the 10 to 40 mg range. Do not exceed 100 mg daily.

Pediatric (under 12 years of age)

PO—Initially, 0.2 mg/kg/day (maximum = 5 mg), followed by gradual increases at least every 3 days of 50% to 100% until therapeutic goals are achieved. The usual effective range is 0.25 to 1 mg/kg/day. Do not exceed 50 mg daily.

Nurse and patient considerations

* Greater than 10% of patients will develop significant salt and water retention, causing edema and congestive heart failure, and tachycardia that may initiate or aggravate angina pectoris. Fluid and electrolyte balance and body weight should be monitored. Patients should be instructed to notify their physician if resting pulse rate increases by 20 or more beats/minute above normal, if breathing becomes more difficult (especially when lying down), or if dizziness, lightheadedness, fainting, symptoms of edema (rapid weight gain, swelling or puffiness of face, hands, ankles), or symptoms of angina occur.

* Pericardial effusion, occasionally with tamponade, has been observed in about 3% of patients. Those at greatest risk are patients with impaired renal function, connective tissue disease, uremic syndrome, congestive heart failure, or marked fluid retention. Patients should be observed closely for any suggestion of a pericardial complication, and echocardiograms should be performed if necessary.

* Within 3 to 6 weeks after initiating therapy, about 80% of patients will start developing hypertrichosis, an elongation, thickening, and increased pigmentation of fine body hair. It is usually noticed first on the face and later extends to the back, arms, legs, and scalp. Growth may be controlled with shaving or hair removers. On discontinuation of minoxidil therapy, new hair growth stops, but it may take up to 6 months for a complete return to the pretreatment appearance.

* Electrocardiographic abnormalities manifested by changes in direction and magnitude of the T waves appear in about 60% of patients being treated with minoxidil. No underlying pathologic conditions can be detected, and the ECG tracings gradually return to the pretreatment state on continued therapy or when minoxidil is discontinued.
* Other adverse effects that have been reported include breast tenderness and gynecomastia (1%), changes in skin pigmentation, polymenorrhea, thrombocytopenia, leukopenia, bullous lesions on the legs, and hypersensitivity rash.
* Minoxidil has been shown to be fetotoxic in laboratory animals. Use in pregnancy is not recommended unless the benefits significantly outweigh the risks of therapy.

Drug interactions

Minoxidil should be used in combination with other antihypertensive agents to enhance hypotensive activity and allow a reduction in the dosages of the antihypertensive agents.

Minoxidil should be administered with extreme caution to patients receiving guanethidine. Profound orthostatic hypotension frequently occurs. If possible, guanethidine should be discontinued 1 to 3 weeks before the initiation of minoxidil therapy. If guanethidine cannot be discontinued, therapy should be initiated in the hospital.

Nitroprusside sodium
(Nipride)

AHFS 24:08
CATEGORY Antihypertensive agent

Action and use

Nitroprusside is a potent vasodilator that acts directly on vascular smooth muscle to produce a peripheral vasodilation. It has been approved for use as an antihypertensive in hypertensive crisis. The drug is also being investigated for possible use in treating dissecting aneurysms, acute myocardial infarction, and low-output syndromes combined with increased peripheral resistance.

Text continued on p. 211.

Table 3-1. Nitroprusside administration*

amps/500 ml	1	2	4	6	8
mg/500 ml	50	100	200	300	400
µg/1 ml	100	200	400	600	800
50 kg µgtts/min	µg/kg/min	µg/kg/min	µg/kg/min	µg/kg/min	µg/kg/min
10	0.33	0.66	1.32	1.98	2.64
20	0.66	1.3	2.64	3.96	5.28
30	1.00	2.0	4.0	6	8
40	1.32	2.6	5.28	7.92	10.56
50	1.66	3.3	6.64	9.96	13.28
60	2.0	4.0	8	12	16
60 kg µgtts/min					
10	0.27	0.55	1.1	1.66	2.21
20	0.55	1.1	2.2	3.3	4.4
30	0.83	1.6	3.33	5.0	6.6
40	1.1	2.2	4.4	6.6	8.8
50	1.36	2.7	5.53	8.3	11.0
60	1.66	3.3	6.6	10	13.3

*Using a microdip administration set—60 gtts/ml.

Continued.

Table 3-1. Nitroprusside administration—cont'd

amps/500 ml	1	2	4	6	8
mg/500 ml	50	100	200	300	400
μg/1 ml	100	200	400	600	800
70 kg μgtts/min					
10	0.23	0.47	.95	1.42	1.9
20	0.47	0.94	1.88	2.82	3.77
30	0.71	1.4	2.85	4.3	5.7
40	0.94	1.9	3.77	5.65	7.5
50	1.16	2.4	4.74	7.11	9.5
60	1.4	2.8	5.7	8.57	11.4
80 kg μgtts/min					
10	0.2	0.41	0.83	1.24	1.66
20	0.41	0.82	1.65	2.5	3.3
30	0.62	1.25	2.5	3.75	5
40	0.82	1.6	3.3	4.95	6.6
50	1.0	2.0	4.15	6.22	8.3
60	1.25	2.5	5	7.5	10

Antihypertensive agents 209

90 kg

µgtts/min	µg/kg/min	µg/kg/min	µg/kg/min	µg/kg/min	µg/kg/min
10	0.18	0.36	0.73	1.10	1.5
20	0.36	0.74	1.46	2.2	2.93
30	0.55	1.1	2.2	3.3	4.4
40	0.73	1.5	2.93	4.4	5.86
50	0.92	1.8	3.7	5.5	7.37
60	1.11	2.2	4.4	6.6	8.88

100 kg

µgtts/min	µg/kg/min	µg/kg/min	µg/kg/min	µg/kg/min	µg/kg/min
10	0.16	0.33	0.66	1	1.33
20	0.33	0.66	1.32	2	2.64
30	0.5	1.0	2	3	4
40	0.66	1.3	2.64	4	5.32
50	0.83	1.6	3.3	5	6.64
60	1.0	2.0	4	6	8

Continued.

Table 3-1. Nitroprusside administration—cont'd

amps/500 ml	1	2	4	6	8
mg/500 ml	50	100	200	300	400
µg/1 ml	100	200	400	600	800
110 kg µgtts/min					
10	0.15	0.3	0.6	0.9	1.2
20	0.3	0.6	1.2	1.8	2.4
30	0.45	0.9	1.81	2.7	3.6
40	0.6	1.2	2.4	3.6	4.8
50	0.75	1.5	3	4.5	6.0
60	0.9	1.8	3.6	5.4	7.3
120 kg µgtts/min					
10	0.14	0.27	0.55	0.83	1.1
20	0.27	0.55	1.1	1.65	2.2
30	0.41	0.83	1.65	2.5	3.3
40	0.55	1.1	2.2	3.3	4.4
50	0.69	1.38	2.76	4.15	5.5
60	0.83	1.66	3.33	5	6.6

Characteristics

Onset: immediate. Duration: within minutes of discontinuance. Metabolism: in erythrocytes and tissues to cyanogen, which is then converted to thiocyanate in the liver (see Nurse and patient considerations).

Administration and dosage

IV—The usual initial infusion rate is between 0.5 to 1.5 μg/kg/min. The dosage must be carefully titrated with close monitoring of blood pressure in each patient. A dose of 1 μg/kg/min usually produces a prompt drop in pressure, although a dose required to produce a given hypotensive effect is variable. The average dose of nitroprusside is 3 μg/kg/min with a range of 0.5 to 8 μg/kg/min. For dosage adjustment see Table 3-1. Nitroprusside is highly light sensitive. A paper bag or foil wrap should be placed over the IV fluid container to protect against degradation. Label the preparation with date and time. At slow infusion rates the translucent plastic tubing should also be taped. Discard solutions over 24 hr old. With cessation of the drip, blood pressure promptly begins to rise, reaching control levels usually in 10 min or less.

NOTE: Safe use in children has not been established.

Nurse and patient considerations

* Adverse effects include nausea, retching, abdominal pain, diaphoresis, restlessness, apprehension, headache, muscle twitching, palpitations, and retrosternal discomfort. These symptoms are usually dose related and may be further minimized by keeping the patient supine.
* Thiocyanate is a metabolite of nitroprusside. Toxic symptoms (fatigue, anorexia, weakness, skin rashes, tinnitus, and mental confusion) begin to appear at thiocyanate plasma levels of 5 to 10 mg/100 ml, with fatalities occurring at 20 mg/100 ml. The half-life of thiocyanate in patients with normal renal function is 7 days but is prolonged in patients with impaired hepatic or renal function. Peritoneal dialysis and hemodialysis may be used to treat thiocyanate toxicities.
* The distribution of nitroprusside and its metabolites across the placenta and into breast milk has not been studied. Thus its safety for pregnant and lactating women has not been established.

Drug interactions

Thiocyanate inhibits both the uptake and binding of iodine. Symptoms of hypothyroidism have been reported after several days of nitroprusside therapy.

Phentolamine
(Regitine)

AHFS 24:08
CATEGORY Alpha-adrenergic blocking agent

Action and use

Phentolamine acts on vascular smooth muscle, blocking alpha-stimulated vasoconstriction. The resulting dilatation decreases the peripheral vascular resistance, usually causing a drop in blood pressure.

It is used as an adjunct in the diagnosis of pheochromocytoma, in the control of hypertensive episodes before and during surgical removal of a pheochromocytoma, and in the prevention and treatment of skin necrosis following IV administration or extravasation of levarterenol (Levophed).

Administration and dosage

PO—Control of hypertensive episodes prior to surgery, 50 mg 4 to 6 times daily. Higher doses may be required.

IM—Preoperative and operative reduction of blood pressure, 5 mg 1 to 2 hr before surgery and repeated as necessary.

IV—5 mg as needed.

NOTE: Prolonged hypotensive episodes may result, especially after parenteral use.

For dermal necrosis and sloughing following IV administration or extravasation of levarterenol (Levophed):

PREVENTION—Add 10 mg of phentolamine to each liter of solution containing levarterenol.

TREATMENT—Inject 5 to 10 mg of phentolamine diluted in 10 ml saline into the area of extravasation as soon as possible.

Nurse and patient considerations

* Phentolamine, both as an indirect cardiac stimulant and as a result of hypotensive episodes, may cause tachycardias, cardiac arrhythmias, anginal pain, myocardial infarction, cerebrovascular spasm, and cerebrovascular occlusion.

* Other adverse effects include nausea, vomiting, diarrhea, and exacerbation of peptic ulcer caused by gastrointestinal stimulation; weakness; dizziness; flushing; and nasal stuffiness.
* Safe use during pregnancy and lactation has not been established.

Drug interactions

No specific drug interactions have been reported with phentolamine.

Prazosin hydrochloride
(Minipress)

AHFS 24:08
CATEGORY Antihypertensive agent

Action and use

Prazosin is an antihypertensive medication structurally unrelated to other antihypertensive agents. Although the exact mechanism of action is unknown, prazosin is an alpha blocker that may also act directly on smooth muscle to produce peripheral dilation and a reduction in diastolic blood pressure. There is no significant change in heart rate or renal blood flow. Prazosin is now used in the treatment of mild to moderate hypertension. Prazosin's effectiveness is generally improved when the drug is used in combination with diuretics and/or other antihypertensive agents.

Characteristics

Onset: 2 hr. Peak activity: 2 to 3 hr. Duration: less than 24 hr. Protein binding: 97%. Half-life: 2 to 4 hr. Metabolites: hepatic, to several active and inactive metabolites. Excretion: 5% to 10% unchanged in urine, remainder in feces. Dialysis: unknown.

Administration and dosage

PO   1. Initial: 1 mg 3 times daily.
2. Maintenance: dosage may be gradually increased to 20 mg daily. For maintenance therapy, prazosin may be administered twice daily. Maximum recommended dosage is 40 mg daily.

When adding other antihypertensive agents, reduce the dose of prazosin to 1 to 2 mg 3 times daily, add other agents, and then readjust the prazosin dosage.

Nurse and patient considerations

* The initial doses of prazosin may cause tachycardia, followed by syncope and unconsciousness. This adverse effect occurs in about 1% of patients starting on the drug; symptoms develop 15 to 90 min after the initial dose. This effect may be minimized by giving the first dose with food and limiting it to 1 mg. Warn patients that this side effect may occur, that it is transient, and that they should lie down immediately if symptoms develop. This "first-dose response" is seen more frequently in patients who are receiving propranolol (and presumably other beta-adrenergic blocking agents). Patients should begin therapy at home with someone with them in case of a syncopal or unconscious episode.

* The most frequent adverse effects reported with prazosin include dizziness, headache, drowsiness, nausea, weakness, and lethargy. All are transient and rarely require discontinuation of therapy.

* Reproduction studies have not reported teratogenetic activity; however, prazosin is not recommended in pregnant women unless the potential benefit outweighs the potential risk. It is not known whether prazosin is secreted in breast milk.

Drug interactions

The sedative effects of prazosin may enhance the CNS depressant effects of alcohol, barbiturates, tranquilizers, and antihistamines.

The hypotensive effects of prazosin are enhanced by the concomitant administration of other antihypertensive agents and diuretics.

Reserpine
(Serpasil)

AHFS 24:08
CATEGORY Antihypertensive agent

Action and use

Reserpine lowers blood pressure by depleting stores of catecholamines at nerve endings. It prevents the reuptake of norepinephrine at storage sites, allowing enzymatic destruction of the neuronal transmitter. There is a gradual reduction over a few days to several weeks in peripheral vasoconstriction, resulting in a drop in blood pressure. It is used to treat mild essential hypertension and may be an effective adjunct to the treatment of more severe hypertension.

Administration and dosage

PO   1. Initial: 0.5 mg daily for 1 to 2 weeks.
     2. Maintenance: 0.1 to 0.25 mg daily.
IM—Hypertensive crises:
     1. Initial: 0.5 to 1 mg.
     2. Maintenance: 2 to 4 mg every 3 hr as needed.

Nurse and patient considerations

* Severe mental depression is the most dangerous side effect of reserpine. The onset of depression may be quite insidious and often difficult to relate to initiation of reserpine therapy. Chronic administration of low doses (0.25 mg) can produce nightmares and mental depression that may require hospitalization or result in suicide. It is recommended that therapy be discontinued at the first sign of despondency, early morning insomnia, loss of appetite, impotence, or self-deprecation. These effects may continue for several weeks after discontinuance, depending on the dosage used and the duration of therapy. Patient education is essential to alert the patient and significant others to early signs of depression or suicidal ideation.

* A pharmacologic action of reserpine is the stimulation of gastric hydrochloric acid. Although the doses required are usually higher than those used routinely for hypertension, patients should be observed for the development of gastric ulcers, and reserpine should be used with caution in patients with a history of ulcer disease. Patients should be instructed to report dark stools, "coffee ground" emesis, or continued nausea.

* Other side effects include nausea, vomiting, diarrhea, abdominal cramps, bradycardia, angina-like symptoms, arrhythmias, (particularly when used concurrently with digitalis or quinidine), nasal stuffiness, and dryness of the mouth.

* Reserpine is not recommended for pregnant or lactating women. It crosses the placental barrier and is secreted in breast milk. Increased respiratory tract secretions, nasal congestion, and cyanosis have been reported in neonates and nursing infants whose mothers had been treated with reserpine.

Drug interactions

The following drugs may add to the hypotensive effects of reserpine:

Diuretics
Phenothiazines
Procainamide (Pronestyl)

Quinidine
Thiothixene (Navane)
Methotrimeprazine
(Levoprome)

The following tricyclic acid antidepressants may antagonize the antihypertensive effects of reserpine:

Doxepin (Sinequan)
Amitriptyline hydrochloride
(Elavil)
Nortriptyline (Aventyl)

Imipramine (Tofranil)
Desipramine
(Norpramin)

Beta-adrenergic blocking agents
GENERAL INFORMATION

The beta-adrenergic blocking agents (beta blockers) are a class of compounds that are believed to act primarily by beta-adrenergic receptor blockade. Each individual agent has other pharmacologic properties in addition to its beta-adrenergic receptor-blocking capability. These properties include partial beta receptor stimulation, called "intrinsic sympathomimetic activity" (ISA), and direct actions on cell membranes, referred to as membrane stabilizing, local anesthetic, and quinidine-like activity. As a group, the beta blockers have little activity on the heart at rest but with exercise will attenuate increases in heart rate, systolic blood pressure, and cardiac output. They also decrease conduction velocity through the atrioventricular (AV) node and decrease myocardial automaticity.

The mechanism of the antihypertensive effects of beta-blocking agents has not been determined, but several mechanisms have been hypothesized: (1) an effect on the central nervous system resulting in a reduced sympathetic outflow to the periphery, (2) competitive antagonism of catecholamines at peripheral (especially cardiac) adrenergic receptor sites, leading to decreased cardiac output, and (3) an inhibition of renin release. It is certainly possible that more than one mechanism contributes to the antihypertensive effects of the beta blockers. Beta blockers decrease both standing and supine blood pressure.

The beta-adrenergic blocking agents can be subdivided into the nonselective and selective blocking agents. The nonselective blocking agents have an equal affinity for and inhibit both beta$_1$ and beta$_2$ receptors. These agents are propranolol, nadolol, pindolol, and timolol. Selective beta$_1$ (cardioselective)-adrenergic blocking agents that are available are metoprolol and atenolol. Metoprolol has a tenfold to twentyfold affinity for beta$_1$ receptors, while atenolol has a threefold affinity for beta$_1$ receptors. The selectivity of the beta$_1$ blockers is only relative, however. In larger doses, these selective agents will also inhibit the beta$_2$ receptors. There are no selective beta$_2$ receptor antagonists available.

The beta-adrenergic blocking agents are used primarily to treat hypertension, angina pectoris, and cardiac arrhythmias. See the individual monographs on these agents for descriptions and additional uses of each drug.

Administration and dosage

There is great interpatient variation in response to given dosages of the beta blockers. Dosages must be individualized according to the pathologic condition being treated and the response of the patient. Although the onset of activity is fairly rapid, it may often take several days to weeks for a patient to show optimal improvement and to become stabilized on an adequate maintenance dosage. As a result of the side effects often associated with beta inhibition, patients must be periodically reevaluated to determine the lowest effective dosage necessary to control the disorder being treated. Combination therapy with other antihypertensive, antianginal, or antiarrhythmic agents will frequently allow a reduction of dosage of all medications, thus minimizing side effects of therapy while maintaining therapeutic goals.

It is extremely important that beta blocker therapy *not* be discontinued abruptly, especially in patients who are being treated for angina pectoris. Sudden discontinuation of therapy has resulted in an exacerbation of anginal symptoms followed in some cases by myocardial infarction. When discontinuing chronically administered beta blockers, the dosage should be gradually reduced over a period of 1 to 2 weeks with careful monitoring of the patient. If anginal symptoms develop or become more frequent, beta-blocker therapy should at least temporarily be reinitiated until the angina is controlled by other means. Patients must be counseled against poor compliance or sudden discontinuation of therapy without a physician's advice.

It is usually recommended that beta-blocker therapy be discontinued a few days before surgery, if possible, because beta blockade impairs the ability of the heart to respond to reflex stimuli increasing the risk of general anesthesia and surgery. If beta-blocker therapy cannot be discontinued before surgery, the effects of the beta blockers can be reversed by administration of beta-receptor stimulants such as isoproterenol, dopamine, or dobutamine.

To treat overdosage or exaggerated response (in addition to gastric lavage):

Bradycardia: atropine, 0.6 to 1 mg IV or IM. If there is no response to vagal blockade, administer isoproterenol (Isuprel) cautiously.

Hypotension: levarterenol (Levophed) or epinephrine.

Bronchospasm: a beta$_2$ stimulant such as terbutaline (Brethine), isoproterenol (Isuprel), or aminophylline.

Cardiac failure: digitalization and diuretics.

Nurse and patient considerations

1. All the beta-adrenergic blocking agents have the potential for similar adverse effects. The major adverse effects of these agents are usually related to the pharmacologically induced beta blockade.

   a. Hypotension, bradycardia, and/or congestive heart failure may develop, usually in patients whose hearts are severely compromised by disease or other drugs (See Drug interactions). Although beta blockers should be avoided in overt congestive heart failure, they may be used with caution in patients with a history of failure who are well compensated, usually with digitalis glycosides and diuretics.

   b. Beta-adrenergic blocking agents must be used with extreme caution in patients with respiratory conditions such as bronchitis, emphysema, bronchial asthma, or allergic rhinitis. Beta blockade will produce severe bronchoconstriction and may aggravate wheezing, especially during the pollen season. Low doses of the selective beta$_1$ agents (metoprolol, atenolol) may be cautiously tried in patients whose bronchopulmonary status is controlled by theophylline derivatives or selective beta$_2$-stimulants (terbutaline, albuterol) if beta blockers are deemed necessary.

   c. Use beta blockers with caution in diabetic patients and patients susceptible to hypoglycemia. The nonselective beta blockers will augment the hypoglycemic effects of insulin by blocking epinephrine-induced glycogenolysis. Beta blockade also reduces the release of insulin in response to hyperglycemia, thus requiring a possible adjustment in dosages of antidiabetic agents. All the beta blockers will mask the signs and symptoms of acute hypoglycemia (tachycardia and changes in blood pressure, but not sweating). If possible, beta blockers should not be administered to diabetic patients who are being treated with insulin or oral hypoglycemic agents.

2. Other adverse effects (the frequency of which may vary somewhat, based on the individual agent and dosages used and tolerance of the patient), listed according to organ systems involved, include those listed below.

   a. Cardiovascular: bradycardia, with heart rates of 40 to 60 beats/min occur fairly frequently, in up to 6% of patients. Symptoms of peripheral vascular insufficiency, usually of the Raynaud type, occur in up to 2% of patients.

   b. Gastrointestinal: diarrhea, nausea, vomiting, constipation, abdominal discomfort, anorexia, and flatulence have infrequently been reported.

   c. Central nervous system: dizziness, insomnia, and fatigue have each been reported in 2% to 5% of patients taking beta-blocker therapy. Sedation, paresthesias, hallucinations, changes in behavior, and mental depression have been reported much less frequently (<1%).

   d. Hematologic: agranulocytosis and thrombocytopenic and nonthrombocytopenic purpura have been reported very rarely.

   e. Allergic: erythematous rash, fever combined with aching and sore throat, laryngospasm, and respiratory distress have all been reported.

   f. Other: headache, dry mouth, eyes or skin, impotence or decreased libido, nasal stuffiness, sweating, tinnitus, and blurred vision have all been reported.

Drug interactions

All the beta-blocking agents have hypotensive properties that are additive with antihypertensive agents: guanethidine (Ismelin), methyldopa (Aldomet), hydralazine (Apresoline), clonidine (Catapres), prazocin (Minipress), minoxidil (Loniten), captopril (Capoten), saralasin (Sarenin), and reserpine. If it is decided to discontinue therapy in patients receiving beta blockers and clonidine concurrently, the beta blocker should be gradually withdrawn and discontinued several days before the gradual withdrawal of the clonidine.

Phenothiazines and beta-blocking agents have additive hypotensive activity.

The inotropic activity of the digitalis glycosides is not prevented by the beta blockers, but both classes of drugs depress atrioventricular conduction, resulting in partial or complete heartblock manifested by bradycardia.

When beta blockers are administered with other antiarrhythmic agents such as lidocaine (Xylocaine), phenytoin (Dilantin), procainamide (Pronestyl), or quinidine, the cardiac effects may be additive or antagonistic, and toxic effects may be cumulative.

Beta-blocking agents may potentiate and prolong the effects of neuromuscular blocking agents (tubocurarine).

Depending on the dosages used, beta blockers inhibit the activity of beta-adrenergic stimulants such as isoproterenol (Isuprel), metaproterenol (Alupent), terbutaline (Brethine), albuterol (Ventolin), and ritodrine (Yutopar).

Use epinephrine with caution in patients receiving beta blockers. Vagal reflex activity may result in marked bradycardia. Atropine may counteract the bradycardia. Cases have also been reported where patients taking beta blockers have developed acute, severe hypertension when epinephrine was administered. The mechanism for this interaction is that the beta blocker blocked the beta-adrenergic effect of epinephrine, leaving relatively unopposed the alpha-adrenergic vasoconstrictive activity. When epinephrine is administered on an emergency basis, be observant for sudden hypertension. Administration of phentolamine (Regitine), nitroprusside (Nipride), or diazoxide (Hyperstat) may be necessary to control the hypertension.

Enzyme-inducing agents such as phenobarbital, nembutal, and phenytoin enhance the metabolism of propranolol and metoprolol (and presumably pindolol and timolol), reducing therapeutic activity. Increases in dosage may be necessary. Nadolol and atenolol are not affected, since they are not metabolized.

See individual agents for other specific drug interactions.

Atenolol
(Tenormin)

AHFS 24:04
CATEGORY Beta-adrenergic blocking agent

Action and use

Atenolol is a beta$_1$ selective (cardioselective) beta-adrenergic blocking agent that has no intrinsic sympathomimetic activity or membrane-stabilizing property. It is used to treat mild to severe hypertension, usually in conjunction with other antihypertensive agents and thiazide diuretics. The antihypertensive action appears to be quantitatively similar to those of other beta blockers, methyldopa, and thiazide diuretics. As with other beta blockers the reduction in blood pressure with atenolol is accompanied by a 20% reduction in heart rate and cardiac output. Advantages of atenolol are its long duration of action, allowing once-daily administration, and its relative beta$_1$ blocking selectivity. Atenolol may be used with caution in patients with bronchospastic disease who do not respond to or do not tolerate other antihypertensive therapy.

Characteristics

Bioavailability: 50% (PO). Peak serum levels: 2 to 4 hr. Duration: at least 24 hr. Protein binding: 6% to 16%. Half-life: 6 to 9 hr. Metabolism: no. Excretion: absorbed fraction, renal. Dialysis: yes, H. Breast milk: yes.

Administration and dosage

NOTE: See General information on beta-adrenergic blocking agents (p. 216).

Adult

PO 1. Initially, 50 mg daily, alone or in combination with a diuretic. Full therapeutic activity will be observed within 1 to 2 weeks. If therapeutic goals are not achieved, increase to 100 mg daily. Increasing the dosage beyond 100 mg daily is unlikely to produce any further benefit.
2. Dosage adjustment is necessary if the patient's creatinine clearance is less than 35 ml/min/1.73 m^2 (see chart below).

Creatinine clearance (ml/min/1.73 m^2)	Maximum dosage
15 - 35	50 mg daily
<15	50 mg every other day

Pediatric:

Safety has not been established in pediatric patients.

Nurse and patient considerations

* See General information on beta-adrenergic blocking agents (p. 216).
* Atenolol therapy is not recommended in pregnant patients. Embryo and fetotoxic effects have been reported in laboratory animals.

Drug interactions

See General information on beta-adrenergic blocking agents (p. 216).

Metoprolol tartrate
(Lopressor)

AHFS 24:08
CATEGORY Antihypertensive,
beta-adrenergic blocking agent

Action and use

Metoprolol is a synthetic antihypertensive agent that acts by selectively blocking beta$_1$-adrenergic receptors. As a beta$_1$-adrenergic blocking agent it has an inhibitory effect on cardiac muscle, resulting in a reduction of heart rate and cardiac output both at rest and during exercise. At higher doses metoprolol also blocks beta$_2$-adrenergic receptors, which are located in bronchial and vascular smooth muscle. Metoprolol is now used in the treatment of mild to moderate hypertension. Its effectiveness is generally improved when used in combination with thiazide diuretics and/or other antihypertensive agents.

Characteristics

Onset: 60 min (PO). Peak activity: 1½ hr (PO). Duration: dose related. Half-life: 3 to 4 hr. Metabolism: liver to several metabolites. Excretion: 95% excreted in urine, 3% to 10% unchanged.

Administration and dosage

NOTE: See General information on beta-adrenergic blocking agents (p. 216)

Adult

PO 1. Initial: 50 mg 2 times daily. Increase the dosage by 50 mg every 7 to 10 days until desired blood pressure is obtained.
2. Maintenance: usually 100 mg 2 times daily. Dosage range: 100 to 450 mg daily.

Pediatric

Safety in children has not been established.
NOTE: Bradycardia may occur. Therefore do not administer to patients with heart disease or a heart rate of less than 60 beats/min unless the patient uses a pacemaker.

Nurse and patient considerations

✻ See General information on beta-adrenergic blocking agents (p. 216).

✻ The risk to the human fetus during metoprolol therapy is unknown. It is not known whether metoprolol is excreted in breast milk.

Drug interactions

See General information on beta-adrenergic blocking
agents (p. 216).

Nadolol
(Corgard)

AHFS 24:04
CATEGORY Beta-adrenergic blocking agent

Action and use

Nadolol is a nonselective, beta-adrenergic blocking
agent that has essentially no agonist (ISA) or local anesthetic, membrane-stabilizing properties and is nearly as potent
as propranolol. It is used to treat mild to severe hypertension
(usually in conjunction with other antihypertensive agents),
angina pectoris, sinus tachycardia, paroxysmal atrial tachycardia, premature ventricular contractions, and tachycardia
associated with atrial flutter or fibrillation. The primary
advantage of nadolol is that it has a long half-life and is not
metabolized, allowing once-daily administration.

Characteristics

Bioavailability: 30% to 40% (PO). Peak serum levels: 2
to 4 hr. Duration of antihypertensive and antianginal effects:
at least 24 hr. Protein binding: 30%. Half-life: normal renal
function—20 to 24 hr; renal impairment—prolonged.
Metabolism: none. Excretion: unchanged, urine 25%, feces
75% (includes portion not absorbed). Dialysis: yes, H. Breast
milk: unknown.

Administration and dosage

NOTE: See General information on beta-adrenergic blocking
agents (p. 216).

Adult

HYPERTENSION

PO—Initially, 40 mg daily, alone or in combination with a
diuretic. Increase by 40 to 80 mg daily at 2- to 14-day

intervals until the therapeutic goal is achieved. The usual maintenance dose is 80 to 320 daily. Dosages up to 640 mg may be used.

ANGINA PECTORIS

PO—Initially, 40 mg daily. Increase by 40 to 80 mg daily at 3- to 7-day intervals until therapeutic goal is achieved or bradycardia (less than 55 beats/min) develops. The maintenance dosage range is 80 to 240 mg once daily. When the drug is to be discontinued, reduce the dosage gradually over 1 to 2 weeks.

DOSAGE ADJUSTMENT IN RENAL IMPAIRMENT

The dosage remains constant, but the dosing interval is prolonged, based on the creatinine clearance. (see chart).

Creatinine clearance (ml/min/1.73 m^2)	Dosing interval (hr)
> 50	24
31-50	24-36
10-30	24-48
< 10	40-60

Pediatric:

Safety has not been established in pediatric patients.

Nurse and patient considerations

＊ See General information on beta-adrenergic blocking agents (p. 216).
＊ Nadolol therapy is not recommended in pregnant patients. Embryocidal and fetotoxic effects have been reported in laboratory animals.

Drug interactions

See General information on beta-adrenergic blocking agents (p. 216).

Pindolol
(Visken)

AHFS 24:04
CATEGORY Beta-adrenergic blocking agent

Action and use

Pindolol is a nonselective beta-adrenergic blocking agent that also has "intrinsic sympathomimetic activity"

(ISA). The ISA or partial beta-stimulant activity occurs directly on the beta receptor and can be blocked by other beta blocking agents without intrinsic sympathomimetic activity. The ISA shown by pindolol is manifested by a smaller reduction in the resting heart rate and resting cardiac output than is seen with drugs lacking ISA. The clinical significance of ISA is yet to be determined. Pindolol is used to treat mild to severe hypertension, usually in conjunction with diuretics and other antihypertensive agents.

Characteristics

Bioavailability: 95% (PO). Peak serum levels: 60 min. Protein binding: 40%. Half-life: 3 to 4 hr; elderly, hypertensive patients with "normal" renal function—7 to 15 hr. Metabolism: hepatic, extensive, no first-pass effect, to glucuronides and sulfates. Excretion: 74% urinary, 26% fecal; 35 to 40% unchanged in urine; 60 to 65% as inactive metabolites. Dialysis: unknown. Breast milk: yes.

Administration and dosage

NOTE: See General information on beta-adrenergic blocking agents (p. 216).

Adult

PO—Initially, 10 mg 2 times daily alone or in combination with other antihypertensive agents. Many patients respond adequately to 5 mg 3 times daily. The antihypertensive effects usually are maximal in about 1 week. If therapeutic goals are not met within 2 to 3 weeks, adjust in increments of 10 mg/day at 2- to 3-week intervals up to 60 mg/day.

Pediatric:

Safety in children has not been established.

Nurse and patient considerations

* See General information on beta-adrenergic blocking agents (p. 216).
* Due to extensive hepatic metabolism and renal excretion, use with caution in patients with significant hepatic and renal impairment.
* An average 3 lb weight gain has been noted in patients taking pindolol. This gain is greater than that observed with propranolol or placebo.

> * No embryocidal or fetotoxic activity has been reported in laboratory animals, but use in pregnancy should be limited to those patients for whom the benefits of therapy significantly outweigh the risk to the fetus.

Drug interactions

See General information on beta-adrenergic blocking agents (p. 216).

Propranolol hydrochloride
(Inderal)

AHFS 24:04
CATEGORY Beta-adrenergic blocking agent

Action and use

Propranolol nonselectively blocks the beta-adrenergic stimulating action of the catecholamines (isoproterenol, epinephrine, and norepinephrine). It causes lowered heart rate, reduced cardiac output, reduced resting stroke volume, reduced oxygen consumption, and increased left ventricular end diastolic pressure.

It is indicated in the treatment of angina pectoris caused by coronary atherosclerosis, supraventricular arrhythmias, and ventricular tachycardias. Propranolol is also being used for antihypertensive therapy, various types of tremors, anxiety, migraine, and supraventricular and ventricular arrhythmias associated with acute myocardial infarction, overdoses of tricyclic antidepressants and digitalis glycosides, and hyperthyroidism.

Characteristics

Onset: 30 min (PO), immediate (IV). Peak plasma levels: 60 to 90 min (PO). Peak response: 15 min (IV). Duration: 3 to 6 hr (IV). Protein binding: 90%. Half-life: 10 min (IV) caused by distribution, $3\frac{2}{5}$ to 6 hr (PO) after chronic administration. Metabolism: liver, active, and inactive metabolites. Excretion: several metabolites in urine, 1% to 4% in feces as unchanged drug and metabolites. Dialysis: no, H.

Administration and dosage

NOTE: See General information on beta-adrenergic blocking agents (p. 216).

Adult

PO—10 to 80 mg 3 to 4 times daily. When the drug is to be discontinued after chronic administration, therapy should be reduced slowly as tolerated.

IV—The usual dose is from 1 to 5 mg at a rate not to exceed 1 mg/min every 2 to 3 min under close monitoring of ECG.

Pediatric

PO 1. Cardiac arrhythmias: 0.5 to 1 mg/kg in 3 to 4 divided doses daily. Maximum dose is 60 mg.
    2. Maintenance dose: 1 to 2 mg/kg every 6 hr.

IV—0.01 to 0.15 mg/kg/dose by slow IV push. Repeat as needed every 6 to 8 hr. Maximum single dose is 10 mg.

Nurse and patient considerations

* See General information on beta-adrenegic blocking agents. (p. 216).
* The pharmacologic activity of propranolol may produce hypotension and/or marked bradycardia. This is the most common cardiovascular side effect; it may be accompanied by syncope, shock, and angina pectoris.
* Other side effects include exacerbation of congestive heart failure, confusion, giddiness, visual disturbances, hallucinations, mental depression, skin rashes, and hematologic effects (eosinophilia, thrombocytopenia, agranulocytosis).
* The risk to the human fetus during propranolol therapy is unknown. Propranolol readily crosses the placental barrier and may appear in breast milk.

Drug interactions

See General information on beta-adrenergic blocking agents (p. 216).

Cimetidine has been shown to inhibit the hepatic metabolism of propranolol, resulting in accumulation of propranolol with excessive pharmacologic activity. A reduction in propranolol dosage may be necessary.

Indomethacin (Indocin) and possibly other prostaglandin inhibitors inhibit the antihypertensive activity of propranolol and pindolol, resulting in loss of hypertensive control. The dosage of the beta blocker may need to be increased if long-term concomitant therapy is planned.

Propranolol significantly reduces excretion of lidocaine, resulting in accumulation during lidocaine infusions. Observe closely for lidocaine toxicity and reduce the dosage if necessary.

Long-term propranolol therapy increases the half-life and decreases the elimination of procainamide. Observe patients for possible toxicity and reduce the procainamide dose if necessary.

Timolol
(Blocadren)

AHFS 24:04
CATEGORY Beta-adrenergic blocking agent

Action and use

Timolol is a nonselective beta-adrenergic blocking agent that lacks both intrinsic sympathomimetic activity (ISA) and membrane stabilizing properties and is 5 to 10 times more potent than propranolol as a beta antagonist. Timolol is approved for use as an antihypertensive agent (usually in combination with other antihypertensive agents) and is the first beta blocker to be approved for use to reduce the long-term risk of cardiovascular mortality and reinfarction in stablized survivors of acute myocardial infarction.

Characteristics

Bioavailability: 90% (PO). Peak serum levels: 1 to 2 hr. Protein binding: 10%. Half-life: 3 to 4 hr. Metabolism: liver, 80%; 50% first-pass hepatic metabolism. Excretion: renal. Dialysis: yes, H. Breast milk: unknown.

Administration and dosage

NOTE: See General information on beta-adrenergic blocking agents (p. 216).

Adult

POSTMYOCARDIAL INFARCTION

PO— 10 mg 2 tmes daily. The drug should be started 7 to 28 days after infarction in patients who have no contraindications to beta-adrenergic blockade.

HYPERTENSION

PO—Initially, 10 mg twice daily, alone or in combination with a thiazide diuretic. The usual maintenance dose is
Text continued on p. 234.

Table 3-2. Ingredients of antihypertensive combination products

Product	Diuretic (mg)											Antihypertensive (mg)							Other (mg)
	Bendroflumethiazide	Benzthiazide	Chlorothiazide	Chlorthalidone	Cyclothiazide	Flumethiazide	Hydrochlorothiazide	Hydroflumethiazide	Methyclothiazide	Polythiazide	Trichlormethiazide	Clonidine	Deserpidine	Guanethidine	Hydralazine	Methyldopa	Rauwolfia	Reserpine	
Aldochlor-150			150													250			
Aldochlor-250			250													250			
Aldoril-15							15									250			
Aldoril-25							25									250			
Apresazide 25/25							25								25				
Apresazide 50/50							50								50				
Apresazide 100/50							50								100				

Continued.

Table 3-2. Ingredients of antihypertensive combination products—cont'd

Product	Diuretic (mg)											Antihypertensive (mg)							Other (mg)
	Bendroflumethiazide	Benzthiazide	Chlorothiazide	Chlorthalidone	Cyclothiazide	Flumethiazide	Hydrochlorothiazide	Hydroflumethiazide	Methyclothiazide	Polythiazide	Trichlormethiazide	Clonidine	Deserpidine	Guanethidine	Hydralazine	Methyldopa	Rauwolfia	Reserpine	
Apresoline-Esidrix							15								25				
Butiserpazide-25							25											0.1	Butabarbital, 30
Butiserpazide-50							50											0.1	Butabarbital, 30
Combipres 0.1 mg				15								0.1							
Combipres 0.2 mg				15								0.2							
Demi-Regroton				25														0.125	
Diupres-250			250															0.125	
Diupres-500			500															0.125	

									Pargyline, 25	Cryptenamine, 2
Diutensen				2.5						2
Diutensen-R				2.5				0.1		
Dralserp							25	0.1		
Enduronyl				5	0.25					
Enduronyl Forte				5	0.5					
Esimil		25		5		10				
Eutron Filmtab				5					25	
Exna-R	50							0.125		
Hydropres-25		25						0.125		
Hydropres-50		50						0.125		
Hydrotensin-25		25						0.125		
Hydrotensin-50		50						0.125		
Hydrotensin-Plus		15					25	0.1		
Hystol		15					25			
Metatensin			2/4					0.1		

Continued.

Table 3-2. Ingredients of antihypertensive combination products—cont'd

Product	Diuretic (mg)											Antihypertensive (mg)							Other (mg)
	Bendroflumethiazide	Benzthiazide	Chlorothiazide	Chlorthalidone	Cyclothiazide	Flumethiazide	Hydrochlorothiazide	Hydroflumethiazide	Methyclothiazide	Polythiazide	Trichlormethiazide	Clonidine	Deserpidine	Guanethidine	Hydralazine	Methyldopa	Rauwolfia	Reserpine	
Naquival											4							0.1	
Naturetin W/K	25/5																		Potassium chloride, 500
Oreticyl							25 50											0.125	
Oreticyl Forte							25											0.25	
Rautrax						400											50		Potassium chloride, 400
Rautrax-N	4																50		Potassium chloride, 400
Rautrax-N Modified	2																50		Potassium chloride, 400
Rauzide	4																50		

Regroton	50					0.25	
Renese-R				2		0.25	
Ro-Chloro-Serp 250	250					0.125	
Ro-Chloro-Serp 500	500					0.125	
Salutensin			50			0.125	
Ser-Ap-Es		15			25	0.1	
Serpasil-Apresoline #1					25	0.1	
Serpasil-Apresoline #2					50	0.2	
Serpasil-Esidrix #1		25				0.1	
Serpasil-Esidrix #2		50				0.1	
Thia-Serp-25		25				0.125	
Thia-Serp-50		50				0.125	
Thia-Serpa-Zine		15			25	0.1	
Thia-zine		15			25		
Timolide		25					Timolol, 10
Unipres		15			25	0.1	

10 to 20 mg twice daily. There should be an interval of at least 7 days between dosage adjustments. Maximum dosage is 30 mg 2 times daily.

Pediatric

Safety has not been established in pediatric patients.

Nurse and patient considerations

* See General information on beta-adrenergic blocking agents (p. 216).
* Timolol may produce slight increases in BUN, serum potassium, and serum uric acid levels and slight decreases in hemoglobin and hematocrit. Changes in these levels are not progressive and are generally not clinically significant.
* Timolol therapy is not recommended in pregnant patients. Embryo and fetotoxic effects have been reported in laboratory animals.

Drug interactions

See General information on beta-adrenergic blocking agents (p. 216).

CHAPTER FOUR

Diuretic agents

GENERAL INFORMATION ON DIURETICS

Diuretics act primarily on the kidneys to promote excretion of excess fluid. Appropriate selection of a diuretic agent to treat edema (excessively increased fluid volume in the interstitial compartment) or hypertension (elevated blood pressure) depends on the pathophysiology of the disease creating the edema or hypertension, the mechanism of action and characteristics of the diuretics, and the physiologic side effects that the diuretics may produce. Diuretics act primarily by enhancing sodium excretion, but they may also alter electrolyte balance, acid-base equilibrium, renal perfusion, and the effect of hormones on the kidneys. See Fig. 1 for the sites of actions of diuretics and Tables 4-2 and 4-3 for the characteristics and dosages of diuretic agents.

Nurse and patient considerations

Weigh the patient before drug therapy begins and daily during therapy. Maintain consistency of measurement by calibrating and using the same scales. Weigh the patient at the same time daily and with the same type of clothing. Measuring the circumference of edematous extremities or an abdomen filled with ascitic fluid is also a worthwhile parameter for fluid control. Use guideline marks to ensure measurement in the same location.

Record the daily input and output. Be conscious of output from wounds and drainage and insensible losses by perspiration and respiration.

Dehydration, possibly secondary to overzealous diuretic therapy, may be monitored by decreased skin turgor, thirst, hypotension, and elevated hemoglobin, hematocrit, and BUN levels.

Diuretics, as a result of multiple mechanisms, can cause hypotension. Patients should be advised of orthostatic hypotension and how to avoid excessive dizziness. The blood

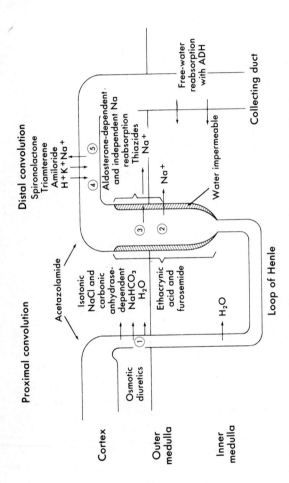

Fig. 1. Sites of actions of diuretics. (Adapted from Melmon, K.L., and Morrelli, H.F., editors: Clinical pharmacology: basic principles in therapeutics, New York, 1972, Macmillan Publishing Co., Inc.)

Table 4-1. Indications of electrolyte imbalance

	Excess	Deficit
Extracellular fluid volume	Puffy eyelids Peripheral edema Ascites Acute weight gain Pleural effusion Moist rales in lungs ↑ Central venous pressure Pulmonary edema Jugular venous distension	Dry skin and mucous membranes Thirst Fatigue Poor skin turgor Systolic BP 10 mm ↓ standing than supine Rapid pulse Subnormal temperature Elevated respiration ↓ Central venous pressure Body weight loss Urine flow rate under 20 to 40 ml/hr Longitudinal wrinkles in tongue Depressed fontanel (infant) "Heat prostration," apprehension, feeling of "impending doom," weak, confused, stuporous, convulsions Abdominal cramps, muscle twitching Diarrhea
Sodium (hyponatremia, hypernatremia)	Agitation → mania → convulsions Dry, sticky mucous membranes; rough, dry tongue Oliguria → anuria Firm rubbery tissue turgor Thirst → fever	

Continued.

Table 4-1. Indications of electrolyte imbalance—cont'd

	Excess	Deficit
Potassium (hypokalemia, hyperkalemia)	Irritability, nausea, diarrhea Oliguria progressing to anuria Weakness and flaccid paralysis Cardiac conduction abnormalities: elevated, peaked T waves; may also develop lowering of R wave, deeper S wave, widening of P wave and QRS complex, prolonged PR interval, ST depression	Muscular flaccidity and weakness, malaise Cardiac arrhythmias, ↓ BP, weak pulse Intestinal muscular weakness: anorexia, vomiting, distension, paralytic ileus Cardiac conduction: T wave becomes flat, can possibly become inverted; a U wave develops and becomes more prominent as hypokalemia becomes severe

pressure should be monitored routinely and vital signs taken, especially during dosage adjustment periods to prevent significant hypotension.

Signs of possible hypokalemia include weakness, hyporeflexia, tingling or numbness in extremities, arrhythmias (particularly with those patients on digitalis), irritability, stupor, muscle cramps, muscle weakness, increased thirst, anorexia, and vomiting (Table 4-1). Supplemental potassium chloride intake may be required.

Patients particularly susceptible to the clinical effects of hypokalemia and hypochloremia include the elderly; the debilitated; those patients losing body fluids through gastric suction, drainage, diaphoresis, vomiting, or diarrhea; and those patients receiving digitalis, diuretics, and adrenocorticosteroids.

Drug interactions

Nonsteroidal, antiinflammatory agents (e.g., indomethacin, ibuprofen, phenylbutazone) may reduce the diuretic, antihypertensive, and natriuretic response to diuretics. Dosages of diuretics may need to be increased to maintain diuretic activity. Renal impairment may predispose to this interaction.

Amiloride
(Midamor)

AHFS 40:28
CATEGORY Diuretic

Action and use

Amiloride is a potassium-sparing agent that has weak diuretic and antihypertensive activity. It is chemically unrelated to any of the other diuretic agents. The exact mechanism of action is unknown, but its primary site of diuretic activity is in the distal renal tubule, where it blocks the exchange of sodium in the urine for potassium within the cells lining the distal nephron. There is no inhibition of aldosterone. Amiloride is rarely used alone, but rather in combination with other diuretics in patients with congestive heart failure or hypertension to help prevent hypokalemia that may result from the use of other diuretics.

Characteristics

Onset: 2 to 3 hr. Peak activity: 6 to 10 hr. Duration: about 24 hr. Half-life: 6 to 9 hr. Metabolism: none. Excretion: renal, 50% unchanged, 40% unchanged in feces within 72 hr. Dialysis: unknown. Breast milk: unknown.

Administration and dosage
Adult

PO 1. Initially, 5 mg daily. The dosage may be increased to 10 mg daily if necessary. If hypokalemia persists, the dosage may be increased to 15 mg and then to 20 mg daily with close monitoring of electrolytes.
2. Administer with food.

Pediatric

Safety and effectiveness in children have not been determined.

NOTE: Hyperkalemia (serum potassium levels greater than 5.5 mEq/L) occurs in about 10% of patients when amiloride is used without a potassium-losing diuretic. When used in conjunction with a thiazide diuretic, the frequency of hyperkalemia is about 1% to 2%. Serum potassium levels must be monitored carefully, especially when therapy is initiated, at the time of diuretic dosage adjustments, and during any illness.

Amiloride should not be given to any patient with hyperkalemia or to patients taking potassium supplements or other potassium-sparing drugs (spironolactone, triamterene).

Nurse and patient considerations

* Side effects of amiloride therapy are generally quite mild, including anorexia, nausea, abdominal pain, flatulence, headache, and skin rash. Other side effects infrequently reported include muscle cramps, dizziness, constipation, fatigability, elevation of BUN, and impotence.
* Electrolyte abnormalities including hyponatremia, hypochloremia, hyperkalemia, and hypokalemia may result when amiloride is used in conjunction with other diuretics. See Table 4-1 for the signs and symptoms associated with electrolyte imbalance.
* Amiloride should be administered with extreme caution to the elderly or to any patients with impaired renal function, cirrhosis, or diabetes mellitus. These types of patients are at greater risk for developing hyperkalemia. If amiloride is used in such conditions, closely monitor renal and hepatic function and blood glucose levels.

* No evidence of teratogenicity has been found to be associated with amiloride; however, its use in pregnancy is not recommended unless the benefits significantly outweigh the risk of therapy.
* See General information on diuretics (p. 235).

Drug interactions

Amiloride may inhibit excretion of lithium carbonate, resulting in toxicity. Lithium serum levels should be closely monitored.

Ethacrynic acid
(Edecrin)

AHFS 40:28
CATEGORY Diuretic

Action and use

Ethacrynic acid exerts its major effect by blocking the reabsorption of sodium along the ascending branch of the loop of Henle. Additional effects probably occur in the proximal and distal convoluted tubules where the drug may exert a direct effect on electrolyte transport.

Characteristics

Onset: 30 min. (PO). Peak activity: 2 hr. Duration: 6 to 8 hr. Excretion: 33% fecal, 22% unchanged in urine, 44% metabolites. Dialysis: unknown.

Administration and dosage
Adult

PO—50 to 100 mg initially, followed by 50 to 200 mg daily.

IV—50 mg or a calculated dose of 0.5 to 1 mg/kg. Add 50 ml of dextrose 5% or saline solution to 50 mg of ethacrynic acid. Occasionally the addition of a diluent may result in an opalescent solution. These solutions should not be used.

Pediatric

NOTE: Safe use in infants has not been established. Dosage recommendations are unavailable.

PO 1. Initial: 25 mg daily
2. Maintenance: increase the dosage in increments of 25 mg to desired effect.

IV—1 mg/kg. Dilute with dextrose 5% and administer over 5 min.

Nurse and patient considerations

* If given in excessive dosage or in patients with massive fluid accumulation, treatment with ethacrynic acid may lead to excessive diuresis with water and electrolyte depletion. (see Table 4-1).
* Vertigo, deafness, and tinnitus with a sense of fullness in the ears have occurred, most frequently in patients with severe impairment of renal function.
* The drug should be discontinued and should not be readministered if increasing azotemia and/or oliguria occur during treatment of severe progressive renal disease or if severe watery diarrhea occurs.
* Gastrointestinal bleeding may result, especially in patients receiving IV therapy.
* See General information on diuretics (p. 235).

Drug interactions

Ethacrynic acid can produce ototoxicity, which may add to or potentiate the ototoxicity of aminoglycoside antibiotics (kanamycin, gentamicin, neomycin, and streptomycin).

Potassium-losing diuretics produce a predisposition to digitalis toxicity.

Ethacrynic acid may displace warfarin from protein-binding sites, resulting in overanticoagulation and spontaneous bleeding.

Furosemide
(Lasix)

AHFS 40:28
CATEGORY Diuretic

Action and use

Furosemide exerts its major effect by blocking the reabsorption of sodium along the ascending branch of the loop of Henle. Additional effects probably occur in the proximal and distal convoluted tubules. After PO administration the diuretic effect usually begins within 1 hr, peaks in the first or second hour, and lasts 6 to 8 hr. After IV injection the diuretic effect begins within 15 min and lasts about 2 hr. Maximum diuresis usually occurs within 30 min.

Characteristics

Onset: 5 min (IV), 30 to 60 min (PO, IM). Peak activity: 15 to 30 min (IV), 1 to 2 hr (PO, IM). Duration: 2 hr (IV), 6 to 8 hr (PO, IM). Half-life: biphasic, $\frac{1}{5}$ to $\frac{2}{5}$ hr, and 2 hr. Metabolism: hepatic. Excretion: 33% in feces, 66% in urine unchanged and as metabolites. Dialysis: unknown.

Administration and dosage
Adult

PO—20 to 80 mg given as a single dose preferably in the morning; a second dose can be administered 6 to 8 hr later.

IV—20 to 40 mg given over 1 to 2 min. Much larger doses are frequently administered IV. The rate of administration should be proportional to the dose administered.

Pediatric

PO—Initially, 2 mg/kg. If response is not satisfactory, increase by 1 to 2 mg/kg every 6 hr.

IV—Initially, 1 mg/kg. If diuresis is not satisfactory, increase by 1 mg/kg every 2 hr to a maximum of 6 mg/kg.

Nurse and patient considerations

∗ Furosemide is a potent diuretic that if given in excessive amounts can lead to a profound diuresis with water and electrolyte depletion (see Table 4-1). Therefore careful medical supervision is required, and the dosage schedule has to be adjusted to the individual patient's need.

∗ The most commonly reported side effects are related to the GI tract. Flushing, pruritus, postural hypotension, weakness, dizziness, blurred vision, and various forms of dermatitis may occur.

∗ With long-term use, serum uric acid excretion is diminished, resulting in hyperuricemia.

∗ Patients with known sulfonamide hypersensitivity may manifest an allergic reaction to furosemide.

∗ See General information on diuretics (p. 235).

Drug interactions

Excessive loss of potassium in patients receiving digitalis may precipitate digitalis toxicity.

Furosemide may enhance the beta-blocking effects of propranolol (Inderal). Monitor blood pressure and heart rate. Dosage adjustment of propranolol may be necessary, depending on the response of the patient.

Hydrochlorothiazide
(Hydro-Diuril, Esidrix)

AHFS 40:28
CATEGORY Thiazide diuretic

Action and use

Thiazide diuretics inhibit the reabsorption of sodium in the distal portion of the loop of Henle and the proximal portion of the distal tubule. Relaxation of peripheral vascular smooth muscle provides at least part of an explanation for the antihypertensive properties of thiazides.

Characteristics

Onset: 2 hr. Peak activity: 4 hr. Duration: 6 to 12 hr. Half-life: 3 hr. Dialysis: unknown.

Administration and dosage
Adult

PO—25 to 200 mg/day as a diuretic, 25 to 100 mg/day as an antihypertensive.

Pediatric
Under 6 months of age

PO—0.4 to 0.6 mg/kg/24 hr in 2 divided doses.

Over 6 months of age

PO—Usual dose: 0.4 mg/kg (1 mg/lb)/24 hr in 2 divided doses.

Nurse and patient considerations

* Thiazide diuretics cause a loss of potassium that may be of clinical significance; therefore electrolyte balance must be monitored and maintained.
* Thiazides may cause hyperglycemia in susceptible individuals, requiring alterations in insulin or oral hypoglycemic doses. Glycosuria may also increase.
* Long-term use of thiazides may block uric acid excretion, possibly resulting in an acute attack of

Table 4-2. Comparison of thiazide diuretics

Thiazide	Brand name	Dosage range (mg)	Onset (PO, hr)	Peak (PO, hr)	Duration (PO, hr)
Bendroflumethiazide	Naturetin	2.5-15	1-2	6-12	18-24
Benzthiazide	Exna, Hydrex	50-150	2	4-6	12-18
Chlorothiazide	Diuril	1000-2000	2	4	6-12
Cyclothiazide	Anhydron	1-2	6	7-12	18-36
Hydrochlorothiazide	Esidrix, Hydro-Diuril	25-100	2	4	6-12
Hydroflumethiazide	Saluron, Diucardin	25-100	1-2	3-4	12-24
Methyclothiazide	Aquatensen, Enduron	2.5-5	2	6	24
Polythiazide	Renese	1-4	2	6	24-36
Trichlormethiazide	Metahydrin, Naqua	1-4	2	6	24

Table 4-3. Comparison of other diuretics

Diuretic	Brand name	Dosage range (mg)	Onset (PO, hr)	Peak (PO, hr)	Duration (PO, hr)
Chlorthalidone	Hygroton	50-200	2	—	24-72
Metolazone	Zaroxolyn, Diulo	2.5-10	1	2	12-24
Quinethazone	Hydromox	50-100	2	6	18-24

gout in susceptible patients. Monitor serum uric acid levels. Signs and symptoms of impending gout attack include joint pain, heat, tenderness, and swelling.

∗ See General information on diuretics (p. 235).

Drug interactions

Excess loss of potassium may result in digitalis toxicity.

Thiazides may be additive or potentiate the action of other antihypertensive drugs.

Thiazides may antagonize the activity of oral anticoagulants.

Hypokalemia may develop with use of thiazides during concomitant use of corticosteroids.

Thiazides may inhibit excretion of lithium carbonate, resulting in toxicity. Lithium serum levels should be closely monitored.

Mannitol
(Osmitrol)

AHFS 40:28
CATEGORY Osmotic diuretic

Action and use

Mannitol is a hypertonic solution that when injected, draws water from the cells and extracellular spaces into the intravasculature. Plasma volume is increased, potentially enhancing renal blood flow and diuresis by increasing the osmotic pressure of the glomerular filtrate so that tubular reabsorption of water is diminished. Potassium, chloride, calcium, phosphorus, lithium, magnesium, urea, and uric acid are excreted in addition to sodium and water.

It is used as a diuretic to help prevent and/or treat the oliguric phase of acute renal failure. It is also used to reduce the pressure of intraocular and cerebrospinal fluids.

Characteristics

Onset: 1 to 3 hr (IV). Half-life: 100 min. Metabolism: minimal, to glycogen in liver. Excretion: 80% unchanged in urine in 3 hr.

Administration and dosage

IV—Oliguria and acute renal failure:
 1. Test dose: 12.5 g of mannitol in 50 to 60 ml over 3 to

5 min. A successful response is indicated by a urine
output of 30 to 50 ml/hr over the next 2 to 3 hr. If
unsuccessful, a second test dose may be given.
2. Prevention: 100 g of mannitol in 500 ml over 90 min
to several hours.
IV—Reduction of pressure of intraocular and cerebrospinal
fluids: 1 to 3 g/kg as a 15% to 25% solution over 30 to 60
min.

NOTE: As a result of high concentration the drug usually
appears in the ampule in crystalline form. Heating to greater
than 50 C will dissolve the crystals. After cooling to body
temperature the solution may be infused. The use of an in-
line filter is strongly recommended.

NOTE: Dosages for patients under 12 years of age have not
been established.

Nurse and patient considerations

* Renal function, urine output, serum electrolytes,
  and central venous pressure must be monitored
  during mannitol administration.
* Rapid infusion of large doses or accumulation of
  mannitol resulting from inadequate urine output
  may result in fluid overload and pulmonary edema.
  It is recommended that if the central venous pressure rises, but changes in urinary output remain
  minimal, the infusion should be slowed or
  stopped.
* Mannitol may also promote tissue dehydration and
  hypovolemia as a result of sustained diuresis,
  enhancing sodium and water retension leading to
  oliguria. Monitor skin turgor and blood pressure
  closely.
* Other side effects are acidosis, nausea, vomiting,
  thrombophlebitis, chills, dizziness, hypotension,
  hypertention, tachycardia, and angina-like chest
  pain. Hypersitivity reactions have also occurred.
* Safe use in pregnancy has not been established.
* See General information on diuretics (p. 235).

Drug interactions

Mannitol enhances the urinary excretion of lithium,
potentially diminishing the response to lithium carbonate
therapy.

Spironolactone
(Aldactone)

AHFS 40:28
CATEGORY Diuretic

Action and use

Spironolactone is a competitive antagonist of aldosterone. It is structurally related to aldosterone and binds to the receptor sites normally occupied when the mineralocorticoid is secreted. Inhibition of aldosterone results in diminished exchange of sodium for potassium in the distal convoluted renal tubule. Potassium elimination is spared and sodium, chloride, and water are excreted, promoting a weak diuresis.

Spironolactone is a mild diuretic that may be used in the treatment of essential hypertension, the edema of congestive heart failure, and nephrotic syndrome. It is also effective in promoting the slow excretion of ascitic and edematous fluid in patients who retain sodium as a result of hyperaldosterone secondary to hepatic cirrhosis.

When administered in combination with thiazide diuretics, spironolactone exerts a supplementary diuretic effect and offsets the usual potassium loss induced by other diuretics (see Table 4-4).

Characteristics

Onset: 48 to 72 hr. Metabolism: primarily to active canrenone, other inactive metabolites. Half-life: spironolactone, 10 min; canrenone, 13 to 24 hr. Excretion: metabolites in urine and feces. Dialysis: unknown.

Administration and dosage
Adult

PO—25 to 50 mg 4 times daily.

Pediatric

PO—3 mg/kg/day. Readjust dosage every 3 to 5 days.

Nurse and patient considerations

* Serum electrolytes should be monitored routinely. Spironolactone, because of its potassium-sparing effect, should be used with caution in patients with hyperkalemia and in patients with concomitant potassium supplementation and renal insufficien-

cy. Dehydration and hyponatremia may also result
from spironolactone therapy, especially when used
in combination with other diuretics.
* Hormonal irregularities such as gynecomastia,
diminished erectile capabilities, and decreased libido in men and breast soreness and menstrual irregularities in women have resulted as a result of ste-
roidlike structural similarities.
* See General information on diuretics (p. 235).

Drug interactions

Spironolactone may promote the systemic acidosis produced by ammonium chloride.

Spironolactone spares potassium excretion. Potassium
supplementation may result in hyperkalemia.

Triamterene
(Dyrenium)

AHFS 40:28
CATEGORY Diuretic

Action and use

The exact mechanism of action of triamterene is
unknown, but its primary site of diuretic activity is in the
distal renal tubule, where it blocks the exchange of sodium
in the urine for potassium within the cells lining the distal
nephron. It is a potassium-sparing agent used most effectively in conjunction with diuretics acting at other sites within the nephron. (See Table 4-4.)

Characteristics

Onset: 2 to 4 hr. Duration: 7 to 9 hr. Protein binding:
approximately 66%. Excretion: renal. Dialysis: unknown.

Administration and dosage

PO—100 to 300 mg daily.

Nurse and patient considerations

* Triamterene should not be administered to patients
with elevated serum potassium levels.
* Side effects of triamterene are generally quite mild.
Those reported include nausea, vomiting, diarrhea,

headache, weakness, dry mouth, leg cramps, photosensitivity, and rash.
* See General information on diuretics (p. 235).

Drug interactions

Potassium supplements must be used with caution in patients receiving triamterene.

A preliminary study indicates that the concomitant use of indomethacin and triamterene may cause a significant reduction in renal function. If the two drugs are used concomitantly, renal function must be monitored carefully.

Table 4-4. Diuretic combination products   AHFS 40:28

Product	Diuretic	Dosage
Aldactazide	Spironolactone, 25 mg; hydrochlorothiazide, 25 mg	2 to 4 tablets daily
Dyazide	Triamterene, 50 mg; hydrochlorothiazide, 25 mg	1 to 2 capsules daily after meals
Moduretic	Amiloride, 5 mg; hydrochlorothiazide, 50 mg	1 to 2 tablets daily with meals
Spiractazide	Spironolactone, 25 mg; hydrochlorothiazide, 25 mg	2 to 4 tablets daily
Spironazide	Spironolactone, 25 mg; hydrochlorothiazide, 25 mg	2 to 4 tablets daily

CHAPTER FIVE

Anticoagulant agents

Heparin
Warfarin sodium

Heparin
**(Liquaemin,
Panheprin)**

AHFS 20:12.04
CATEGORY Anticoagulant

Action and use

Heparin is a naturally occurring, high molecular weight mucopolysaccharide. It acts directly on various plasma protein molecules (heparin co-factors) within the blood. Heparin does not affect the hepatic biosynthesis or the plasma levels of any coagulation factor.

In low concentrations, heparin inhibits the interactions of factors IX_a, VIII_a, and X_a. In higher concentrations it enhances fibrinolysis.

The action of heparin on platelets is variable and dose related. The aggregation and adhesiveness of platelets may be reduced, but other clinical factors make this activity difficult to predict.

Heparin anticoagulant therapy is indicated in the treatment of pulmonary embolism, deep venous thrombosis, cerebral embolism, heart valve prosthesis, and acute peripheral arterial embolism. It is also used prophylactically before and during cardiovascular surgery and hemodialysis procedures.

Characteristics

Heparin has no anticoagulant activity with PO administration, but is well absorbed after SC, IM, and IV injection. When administered IV in therapeutic doses, there is rapid clearance from circulation at a rate dependent on the dose. Onset of activity is immediate (IV). The half-lives of 100, 200, and 400 units/kg are 56, 96, and 152 min, respectively. Heparin is bound to plasma proteins at concentrations up to 2 units/ml of blood. Higher concentrations of heparin result in greater quantities of unbound heparin, which pass into other tissue spaces and appear in the lymphatic system. At concentrations above 7 units/ml, unchanged heparin is excreted in the urine (up to 50%). Heparin may have cumulative effects in patients with renal impairment. Heparin is metabolized in the liver and about 20% of a normal dose appears in the urine as uroheparin, which has about 50% of the anticoagulant activity of heparin. No dosage adjustment is required for hemodialysis.

Administration and dosage
Adult

sc 1. Prophylactic: 5000 units every 8 to 12 hr.
2. Therapeutic: initial: 10,000 to 15,000 units; maintenance: 6000 to 10,000 units every 8 to 12 hr.
   Do not pinch the site or rub excessively. An ice pack applied on the site 5 minutes before and after administration will help prevent the formation of hematomas.

IM—Not recommended because of the development of hematomas.

IV 1. Intermittent—initial, 10,000-unit bolus; maintenance, 5000 to 10,000 units every 4 to 6 hr. A "heparin-lock," consisting of a 20-gauge scalp vein needle attached to 3½-inch tubing ending in a resealing rubber diaphragm, may be used to administer intermittent IV doses of heparin. Advantages of a heparin-lock are the mobility that it provides the patient and the fewer venipunctures needed. After injecting the bolus of heparin through the rubber diaphragm, flush the line with 1 ml of a solution containing 10 units of heparin/ml of saline solution. The heparin flush solution ensures that the patient will receive the entire heparin bolus and prevents the formation of a clot in the scalp vein needle.
2. Continuous infusion—initial, 5000-unit bolus; maintenance, 700 to 1200 units/hr. (Patient variation may require as little as 200 units/hr or as much as 2000 or more units/hr.) (See Table 5-1).

Pediatric

IV—Intermittent—initial, 50 units/kg; maintenance, 50 to 100 units/kg every 4 hr.
   Dosage is considered adequate when the partial thromboplastin time (PTT) is elevated 1½ to 2½ times the control value. (An exception is minidose heparin prophylactic therapy where changes in the PTT are minimal.) During intermittent IV therapy the PTT should be drawn 1 hr before the next dosage administration. During continuous IV therapy the PTT may be drawn at any time.

Table 5-1. Heparin infusion*

Units/500 ml	5000	10,000	15,000	20,000	25,000
Units/ml	10	20	30	40	50
ml/hr	Units/hr	Units/hr	Units/hr	Units/hr	Units/hr
5	50	100	150	200	250
10	100	200	300	400	500
15	150	300	450	600	750
20	200	400	600	800	1000
25	250	500	750	1000	1250
30	300	600	900	1200	1500
35	350	700	1050	1400	1750
40	400	800	1200	1600	2000
45	450	900	1350	1800	2250
50	500	1000	1500	2000	2500
55	550	1100	1650	2200	2750
60	600	1200	1800	2400	3000

*Using a microdrip administration set—60 gtts/ml.

Nurse and patient considerations

* Firm, prolonged pressure must be applied following any venipuncture in a heparinized patient to avoid extravasation and the development of hematomas.

* Factors that can influence the incidence of complications include age, weight, sex, and recent trauma. Spontaneous bleeding, such as hematomas, petechiae, hematuria, bleeding gums, and melena, after the administration of standard dosages is more frequent in women and occurs with increased incidence in those over 60 years of age. Hemorrhage is also more frequent in fully heparinized patients who have had recent trauma or who have undergone recent surgical procedures than in nontraumatized patients. Guaiac-test all stools, emesis, and urine.

* An infrequent adverse effect, but one with potentially serious complications, is heparin-induced thrombocytopenia. The thrombocytopenia of less than 70,000 platelets/cu mm occurs 1 to 3 weeks after the initiation of heparin therapy. Patients that develop hemorrhagic symptoms during heparin therapy should be reevaluated not only for an abnormal PTT, but also for an abnormally low platelet count. The thrombocytopenia resolves over the next 1 to 3 weeks following discontinuation of heparin therapy.

* USP standards require that the potency is not less than 120 USP units in each milligram of heparin when derived from lungs and not less than 140 USP units in each milligram when derived from other tissues. Most commercial preparationis exceed these standards with a higher degree of purification (up to 170 units/mg). Consequently it is clinically safer and far more accurate to base the dose on units, rather than the old method of using milligrams.

* Heparin therapy may be continued during menstruation unless bleeding becomes excessive.

* Heparin must be used with caution during pregnancy and the immediate postpartum period.

Antidote

One mg of protamine sulfate will neutralize approximately 120 units of heparin. If protamine sulfate is given more than ½ hr after the heparin was administered, then give only ½ the dose of protamine sulfate.

Drug interactions

Aspirin, dipyridamole (Persantin) and glyceryl guiacolate should be used cautiously in patients receiving heparin. These agents inhibit platelet aggregation, thus predisposing a heparinized patient to hemorrhage.

Warfarin sodium
(Coumadin, Panwarfin)

AHFS 20:12.04
CATEGORY Anticoagulant

Action and use

Warfarin inhibits the activity of vitamin K, which is required for the normal synthesis of blood coagulation factors II (prothrombin), VII (proconvertin), IX (Christmas factor), and X (Stuart-Prower factor). There is no direct effect on circulating coagulation factors.

Warfarin is indicated in the prophylaxis and treatment of venous thrombosis, atrial fibrillation with embolism, pulmonary embolism, and as an adjunct in the treatment of coronary occlusion.

Characteristics

Onset of anticoagulation: Dependent on the half-lives of the individual coagulation factors whose synthesis is suppressed. Peak prothrombin time effect: 24 to 96 hr. Duration: 1 to 5 days. Protein-binding: 97%. Half-life: 48 hr (15 to 55 hr). Metabolism: hapatic microsomal enzymes. Excretion: active and inactive metabolites in urine. Therapeutic level: 0.1 mg/100 ml to 1 mg/100 ml.

Administration and dosage

PO—10 to 15 mg daily for 3 days, then 2 to 15 mg daily maintenance.

IV—As for PO administration; onset of action is similar to that of PO administration because of dependence on individual coagulation factor synthesis. Punctures should be followed by firm pressure and be rechecked periodically for hematoma formation.

NOTE: Dosage can be controlled only by determining the prothrombin time on a routine basis. Dosage is considered adequate when the prothrombin time is elevated 1½ to 2½ times the control value. For the patient's safety the prothrombin time should be drawn daily for the first week, weekly for the first 1 to 2 months, and monthly once the dosage has been safely established.

Nurse and patient considerations

* Hemorrhage is the principal adverse reaction to overdosage. Hemorrhagic tendency may be manifested by hematuria, petechiae in the skin, hemorrhage into or from a wound, or petechial and purpuric hemorrhages throughout the body. Patients receiving warfarin should be examined daily for evidence of these complications, and the urine should be tested routinely to detect hematuria. Patients should be counseled to report any excessive bleeding following shaving, oral hygiene, menstruation, or minor trauma.
* Patients with impaired liver function may be more sensitive and require less warfarin for anticoagulation.
* IM injections should be avoided in patients receiving anticoagulants.
* Patients should be warned against self-medication with any over-the-counter product, especially those containing aspirin or other salicylates.
* Warfarin crosses the placental barrier and is excreted in breast milk. Warfarin should be used in pregnant or nursing women only when the benefits outweigh the risk. The nursing infant should also be monitored with routine coagulation studies.

Antidote

The antidote to overdosage is vitamin K (Aquamephyton), 5 to 25 mg IM or IV. Following IV administration the effects of Aquamephyton appear within 15 min; bleeding is usually controlled within 6 hr, and normal prothrombin level may be obtained in 12 to 14 hr.

The following drugs are reported to increase anticoagulant activity:

Allopurinol
Aminoglycoside
  antibiotics
Amiodarone
Anabolic steroids
Cephalosporins
Chloral hydrate
Chloramphenicol
Cimetidine
Clofibrate
Co-trimoxazole
Danazol
Dextrothyronine
Diazoxide
Diflunisal

Disulfiram
Erythromycin
Ethacrynic acid
Ethanol
Glucagon
Indomethacin
Isoniazid
Meclofenamate
Mefenamic acid
Metronidazole
Miconazole ni-
  trate
Nalidixic acid

Oxyphenbutazone
Phenylbutazone
Phenytoin
Propoxyphene hy-
  drochloride
Quinidine
Salicylates
Sulfinpyrazone
Sulfonamides
Sulindac
Tetracyclines
Thyroid hormones
Vitamin E

The following drugs are reported to decrease anticoagulant activity:

Barbiturates
Carbamazepine
Cholestyramine
Cyclophospha-
  mide

Disopyramide
  phosphate
Ethchlorvynol
Glutethimide
Griseofulvin

Mercaptopurine
Rifampin
Spironolactone
Vitamin K

CHAPTER SIX

Respiratory agents

Acetylcysteine
Albuterol
Cromolyn sodium
Epinephrine
Isoproterenol
    hydrochloride
Pseudoephedrine
    hydrochloride

Terbutaline
Theophylline derivatives
    General information
    Aminophylline, USP
    Dyphylline
    Oxtriphylline

Acetylcysteine
(Mucomyst)

AHFS 48:00
CATEGORY Mucolytic

Action and use

Acetylcysteine reduces the viscosity of purulent and nonpurulent pulmonary secretions by breaking disulfide bonds. This facilitates their removal by coughing, postural drainage, or mechanical means.

Acetylcysteine is used as an adjunct in the treatment of acute and chronic bronchopulmonary disorders such as pneumonia, bronchitis, emphysema, atelectasis caused by mucous obstruction, tuberculosis, and pulmonary complications of cystic fibrosis.

Characteristics

Liquifaction after inhalation is apparent within 1 min; maximal effects occur in 5 to 10 min.

Administration and dosage

Acetylcysteine may be administered by nebulization, direct application, or intratracheal instillation.

When nebulized into a face mask, mouthpiece, or tracheostomy, 1 to 10 ml of the 20% solution or 2 to 20 ml of the 10% solution may be given every 2 to 6 hr.

The recommended dosage for most patients is 3 to 5 ml of the 20% solution 3 to 4 times daily.

NOTE: After administration an increased volume of bronchial secretions may occur. Some patients with inadequate cough reflex may require mechanical suctioning to maintain an open airway.

Nurse and patient considerations

* Common side effects may include stomatitis, hemoptysis, nausea, severe rhinorrhea, and an unpleasant transient odor.
* Bronchospasm is most likely to occur in asthmatic patients. To prevent spasm and to maximize bronchodilatation, nebulize 0.5 ml 1:200 isoproterenol or 1% Bronkosol-2 in 5 ml of saline solution with or just before the use of acetylcysteine.
* Adjunct measures to aid in the removal of any pulmonary secretions include increasing hydration and humidifying the environment.

Drug interactions

Acetylcysteine inactivates a number of antibiotics, including the penicillins; therefore it should not be mixed with them for aerosol administration.

Albuterol
(Proventil, Ventolin)

AHFS 12:12
CATEGORY Beta stimulant

Action and use

Albuterol selectively stimulates beta$_2$ receptors, causing dilatation of bronchial, vascular, and uterine smooth muscle. This selective activity makes albuterol a useful agent in the treatment of symptoms of bronchial asthma and reversible bronchospasm that may occur in bronchitis and emphysema. When administered in usual dosages, albuterol is equally as effective as a bronchodilator as metaproterenol and has similar side effects and has a longer duration of action with fewer cardiac side effects than isoproterenol.

Characteristics
ORAL TABLETS

Onset: 30 min. Peak activity: 2 to 3 hr. Duration: 6 hr. Half-life: 2.7 to 5 hr. Excretion: renal—76% within 24 hours, 16% active, 60% metabolites; fecal—4% in 24 hr. Breast milk: unknown.

INHALATION

Albuterol appears to be absorbed from the respiratory tract over several hours following oral inhalation. Onset of bronchodilatation: 5 to 15 min. Peak effect: 0.5 to 2 hr. Duration: 3 to 4 hr. There is no apparent correlation between serum levels and peak bronchodilatory effect, indicating direct action on bronchial receptors. Metabolism: liver, to inactive metabolites. Excretion: urine, 30% unchanged in 24 hr; 10% in feces; remainder in urine as metabolites. Breast milk: unknown.

Administration and dosage
Adult and pediatric (over 12 years of age)

PO   1. Initial dose: 2 to 4 mg 3 to 4 times daily. The total daily dose should not exceed 32 mg.

      2. Elderly patients and those patients sensitive to beta-adrenergic stimulants should start at 2 mg 3 to 4 times daily as tolerated.

ORAL INHALATION—Usual dosage: 1 to 2 inhalations (180 to 360 μg) every 4 to 6 hr.

NOTE: Albuterol therapy is currently not recommended in children under 12 years of age.

NOTE: Patients must be well informed on the use of the inhaler.

1. The inhaler must be shaken well.
2. After exhaling as completely as possible, place the inhaler well into the mouth and close lips firmly around it.
3. Inhale deeply through the mouth while activating the inhaler.
4. After holding the breath for as long as possible, remove the mouthpiece and exhale the breath slowly.
5. The manufacturer recommends waiting at least 1 min between inhalations, whereas some investigators recommend waiting 10 to 20 min between inhalations to improve clinical response.
6. The plastic case and inhaler should be removed from the metal canister, washed in warm water, and thoroughly dried once daily.

NOTE: Excessive or prolonged use of albuterol inhalers may lead to tolerance. Patients should be instructed to contact their physician for reevaluation of the disease and therapy if decreased effectiveness occurs rather than increase the dose or frequency of administration.

    Paradoxic bronchoconstriction has occurred after repeated or excessive use of albuterol inhalers. Albuterol must be discontinued immediately if bronchoconstriction develops.

Nurse and patient considerations

* Most side effects are dose related. Most common, although infrequent, are tachycardia and palpitations, tremor, nervousness, and dizziness. Nausea, vomiting, increased or decreased blood pressure, CNS stimulation, and angina may occur rarely. Albuterol should be used with caution in patients with cardiovascular disorders, hypertension, hyperthyroidism, or diabetes mellitus and in patients who are unusually responsive to sympathomimetic amines.

* Unusual taste, heartburn, throat dryness, and irritation may occur with inhalation therapy.

* Patients known to have hypertension, hyperthyroidism, diabetes mellitus, or cardiac disease with arrhythmias may be particularly sensitive to adverse reactions and must be observed closely.

* Safe use in pregnancy has not been established. Albuterol should be used only on a risk versus benefit basis, since albuterol has been reported to be teratogenic in mice and rabbits when administered in very large doses.

Drug interactions

Beta-adrenergic blocking agents (atenolol, timolol, propranolol, nadolol) may inhibit the pharmocologic effects of albuterol.

The cardiovascular effects of albuterol may be potentiated in patients receiving epinephrine or other sympathomimetic agents (isoproterenol, metaproterenol), monoamine oxidase inhibitors (tranylcypromine, isocarboxazid, pargyline), or tricyclic antidepressants (imipramine, amitriptyline, nortriptyline, doxepine). Administer albuterol with caution in these patients.

Cromolyn sodium
(Intal)

AHFS 92:00
CATEGORY Unclassified

Action and use

Cromolyn sodium blocks the release of histamine and slow-reacting substance of anaphylaxis (SRS-A) from sensitized mast cells after the formation of specific antigen-antibody complexes. Cromolyn has no direct bronchodilator, antihistaminic, anticholinergic, or antiinflammatory activity. Cromolyn is recommended as an adjunct in the management of patients with severe perennial bronchial asthma. Cromolyn is effective only as a prophylactic agent and has no role in the treatment of an acute asthmatic attack.

Characteristics

Between 5% and 10% absorbed from inhaler. Peak blood levels: 15 min. Half-life: about 80 min. Metabolism: insignificant. Excretion: equal quantities in urine and feces unchanged.

Administration and dosage

NOTE: Not recommended in children under 5 years of age.

Adult and pediatric

PO—Patients must be advised that cromolyn sodium capsules are not absorbed when swallowed and that the drug is inactive when administered by this route.

INHALATION—20 mg (1 capsule) via inhaler 4 times daily. Patient education on proper use of the inhaler is particularly important to the therapeutic benefit of this agent.

1. Load the inhaler with a capsule and pierce (only once) the capsule immediately before use.
2. Holding the inhaler away from the mouth, exhale, emptying the air from lungs as much as possible.
3. With the head tilted backward and teeth apart, close lips around the mouthpiece.
4. Inhale deeply and rapidly through the inhaler with a steady, even breath.
5. Remove the inhaler and hold the breath for a few seconds, then exhale. (Do not exhale through the inhaler, because moisture from the breath will interfere with proper function of the inhaler.)
6. Repeat several times until the powder is inhaled. A light dusting of powder remaining in the capsule is normal.

A 2- to 4-week course of therapy is usually required to determine clinical response. Therapy should only be continued if there is a decrease in the severity of clinical symptoms of asthma and/or requirements for concomitant drug therapy.

Nurse and patient considerations

* The most common side effect of cromolyn therapy is irritation of the throat and trachea caused by inhalation of the dry powder, resulting in cough and/or bronchospasm.
* If the patient is being treated with steroids and/or bronchodilators when cromolyn therapy is initiated, therapy should be continued. If the patient shows clinical signs of improvement, an attempt should be made to reduce the corticosteroid dosage. Reduction should be gradual and with close supervision to avoid an exacerbation of the asthma. Alternate-day steroid therapy may also be considered.
* Caution should be used when decreasing the dosage of cromolyn because asthmatic symptoms may recur.
* Use in pregnancy is not recommended, as its safety has not been established.

Epinephrine
(Adrenalin, Sus-Phrine)

AHFS 12:12
CATEGORY Bronchodilator

Action and use

Epinephrine is one of the primary catecholamines of the body, stimulating both alpha- and beta-receptor cells. It is a potent bronchodilatory agent, acting directly on the beta cells of the bronchi. It also increases the respiratory tidal volume by stimulating the alpha-receptor cells, relieving congestion within the bronchial mucosa, and constricting pulmonary vessels. Epinephrine may also block the antigen-induced release of histamine, making it an effective agent in the treatment of asthma and anaphylactic reactions.

Administration and dosage

For anaphylaxis and asthmatic attacks:

Adult

sc—Epinephrine aqueous suspension 1:200 (Sus-Phrine): initial test dose: 0.1 ml (0.5 mg). Subsequent doses of 0.1 to 0.3 ml (0.5 to 1.5 mg) may be given only when necessary and not within 4 hr.

NOTE: Shake vial to disperse the suspension before drawing dose into syringe. A tuberculin syringe with a 26 gauge ½ inch needle is recommended. Do *NOT* administer the suspension IV. Refrigerate.

sc—Epinephrine 1:1000: 0.3 to 1 ml (0.3 to 1 mg) every 5 to 15 min as needed.

iv—Epinephrine 1:10,000: 3 to 10 ml (0.3 to 1 mg).

Pediatric

sc—Epinephrine aqueous suspension 1:200 (Sus-Phrine): initially, 0.005 ml/kg. The maximum single dose should not exceed 0.15 ml.

sc—Epinephrine 1:1000: 0.01 ml/kg (maximum dose: 0.5 ml). May repeat dose every 15 min for 2 doses, then every 4 hr as needed.

iv—Epinephrine 1:10,000: 0.05 to 0.1 ml/kg.

NOTE: Do not use if discolored (red or brown) or if sediment is present.

Nurse and patient considerations

* Be extremely cautious with dosage calculations and administration.
* Isoproterenol and epinephrine should not be administered simultaneously, since both drugs are potent cardiac stimulants. They may be given alternately, however.
* Palpitation, tachycardia, headache, tremor, weakness, and dizziness are common side effects. Serious arrhythmias, ventricular fibrillation, anginal pain, nausea, respiratory difficulty, and cerebral hemorrhage may also occur. Vital signs should be monitored during and after the administration of epinephrine.
* Dosage should be adjusted carefully in elderly patients; in patients with coronary insufficiency, diabetes, hyperthyroidism, and hypertension; and in psychoneurotic individuals. All patients are particularly sensitive to sympathomimetic amines.

Drug interactions

Tricyclic antidepressants, such as doxepin (Sinequan), nortriptyline (Aventyl), amitriptyline hydrochloride (Elavil), protryptyline hydrochloride (Vivactil), imipramine (Tofranil), and desipramine (Norpramin), strongly potentiate the actions of epinephrine. If they must be used concurrently, start with significantly lower doses of epinephrine.

Use epinephrine with caution in patients receiving pro-pranolol. Vagal reflex has resulted in marked bradycardia.

Epinephrine causes hyperglycemia. Diabetic persons may require increased doses of insulin or oral hypoglycemic agents.

Epinephrine may produce arrhythmias in patients anesthetized with cyclopropane.

Isoproterenol hydrochloride AHFS 12:12
(Isuprel)
CATEGORY Bronchodilator

Action and use

Isoproterenol is a beta-receptor stimulant that relaxes smooth muscle, particularly the bronchial and gastrointestinal musculature. It relieves bronchoconstriction in the smaller bronchi caused by drugs and bronchial asthma. Isoproterenol is used as a bronchodilator to treat bronchospasm associated with acute and chronic bronchial asthma, pulmonary emphysema, bronchitis, bronchiectasis, and laryngospasm caused by anesthesia. For its use as a cardiovascular agent, see Isoproterenol (Chapter 2, p. 141).

Administration and dosage
Adult and pediatric

INHALATION
1. Mistometer: 15 ml of isoproterenol 1:4000 solution, 2.8 mg/ml, 300 single inhalations per vial, each measured dose containing 125 μg of isoproterenol.
    Acute bronchial asthma: 5 to 6 inhalations daily as necessary.
    Bronchospasm in chronic obstructive lung disease: 6 to 8 inhalations daily, no more often than every 3 hr.
    Use of the Mistometer
    1. Hold the Mistometer in an inverted position.
    2. Close teeth and lips around the open end of the mouthpiece.
    3. Expel as much air from the lungs as possible.
    4. Press down on the sprayer while inhaling deeply. Hold the breath for several seconds before exhaling.
    5. Wait at least 1 min to determine the effect before starting a second treatment.

2. Hand-bulb nebulizer: 1:100 and 1:200 solutions. Do not use if there is a precipitate or brownish discoloration.

   Acute bronchial asthma: 5 to 6 treatments daily consisting of 3 to 7 deep inhalations of the 1:100 isoproterenol solution or 5 to 15 deep inhalations of the 1:200 isoproterenol solution.

   Bronchospasm in chronic obstructive lung disease: 6 to 8 treatments daily consisting of 3 to 7 deep inhalations of the 1:100 isoproterenol solution or 5 to 15 deep inhalations of the 1:200 isoproterenol solution. Repeat each treatment no more often than every 3 hr.

NOTE: 5 to 7 inhalations from a hand-bulb nebulizer using a 1:100 isoproterenol solution is equivalent to 1 inhalation of the Mistometer.

3. Intermittent positive pressure breathing (IPPB): 0.5 ml of isoproterenol 1:200 or 0.25 ml of isoproterenol 1:100 diluted with 2 to 2.5 ml of water or saline solution to provide concentrations of 1:800 and 1:1000, respectively. Administer usually over 15 to 20 min, up to 5 times daily as needed.

PO—Elixir contains 2.5 mg of isoproterenol/tbsp. (15 ml). The solution also contains 6 mg phenobarbital, 12 mg ephedrine sulfate, 45 mg of theophylline, 150 mg of potassium iodide, and 19% ethanol/tbsp (15 ml). Doses should be individualized for patients' needs, but an initial dosage is 2 tbsp 3 to 4 times daily.

NOTE: Patients using both the PO and inhalation forms of therapy may develop a tolerance to isoproterenol if the recommended dosages are exceeded frequently. Prolonged abuse has resulted in severe paradoxic airway resistance. If this should occur, isoproterenol therapy should be withdrawn immediately. Isoproterenol may also cause sputum and saliva to turn pink.

Nurse and patient considerations

* Administration of isoproterenol is contraindicated in patients with tachycardia caused by digitalis intoxication.
* Isoproterenol and epinephrine should not be administered simultaneously, since both drugs are direct cardiac stimulants. They may be given alternately, however.

* Dosage should be adjusted carefully in patients with coronary insufficiency, diabetes and hyperthyroidism and in patients sensitive to sympathomimetic amines.
* If the cardiac rate increases sharply, patients with angina pectoris may experience anginal pain until the cardiac rate decreases.
* Palpitation, tachycardia, headache, and flushing of the skin are common side effects. Serious arrhythmias, anginal pain, nausea, tremor, dizziness, weakness, and sweating occasionally occur.
* Patients should be advised that with prolonged use, isoproterenol may cause a pink discoloration of the sputum and saliva. It is, however, of no clinical significance.
* Although there have been no teratogenic effects reported, safe use in pregnant or lactating women has not been established.

Drug interactions

The beta-adrenergic stimulant effects of isoproterenol are blocked by propranolol, a beta-adrenergic blocker.

Isoproterenol may produce arrhythmias in patients anesthetized with cyclopropane.

Pseudoephedrine hydrochloride
(Sudafed)

AHFS 12:12
CATEGORY Vasoconstrictor

Action and use

Pseudoephedrine is a sympathomimetic agent that stimulates the alpha-adrenergic receptors and releases catecholamines within the upper respiratory tract to cause vasocontriction. The reduced blood flow to the area results in shrinkage of swollen nasal mucous membranes, allowing the airways to reopen and sinus secretions to drain. It also has some beta-adrenergic activity that may cause minor bronchodilatation. Pseudoephedrine may be used alone as a nasal decongestant, but it is also used in combination with antihistamine, analgesic, expectorant, and antitussive agents to provide symptomatic relief to patients with allergies or viral infections.

Characteristics

Onset: 30 min. Duration: 4 to 6 hr. Metabolism: liver to inactive metabolite. Excretion: 55% to 75% unchanged in urine. Dialysis: unknown.

Administration and dosage
Adult

PO—30 to 60 mg every 4 hr to a maximum dosage of 240 mg daily.

Pediatric
Ages 2 to 5

PO—15 mg every 4 hr to a maximum dosage of 60 mg daily.

Ages 6 to 12

PO—30 mg every 4 hr to a maximum dosage of 120 mg daily.

Nurse and patient considerations

* CNS stimulation manifested by nervousness, insomnia, irritability, dizziness, and headache may occur. Nausea and vomiting may result from large doses.
* Patients known to have hypertension, hyperthyroidism, diabetes mellitus, prostatic hypertrophy, elevated intraocular pressure, or cardiac arrhythmias may be particularly sensitive to adverse reactions and must be monitored closely.
* The effect of pseudoephedrine on the human fetus is unknown; therefore use in pregnant women must be determined on the basis of risk versus benefit. Infants are particularly susceptible to the pharmacologic actions of pseudoephedrine. The drug may enter breast milk and therefore should not be given to lactating women.

Drug interactions

Administration of pseudoephedrine in conjunction with other sympathomimetic agents may enhance cardiovascular and CNS side effects. Use with caution.

Use with extreme caution in patients receiving MAO inhibitors (pargyline [Eutonyl, Eutron] and tranylcypromine sulfate [Parnate]) because severe, prolonged hypertension may result.

Terbutaline
(Brethine, Bricanyl)

AHFS 12:12
CATEGORY Beta stimulant

Action and use

Terbutaline selectively stimulates beta$_2$ receptors, causing dilatation of bronchial, vascular, and uterine smooth muscle. In higher doses there is also stimulation of the beta$_1$ receptors of the heart. This selective activity makes terbutaline a useful agent in the treatment of bronchial asthma and reversible bronchospasm that may occur in bronchitis and emphysema. Because of its ability to relax uterine musculature, it may also be used in cases of premature labor or threatened abortion.

Characteristics

Onset: 1 to 2 hr. Peak blood levels: 2 to 3 hr. Duration: 4 to 8 hr. Metabolism: liver. Excretion: 60% unchanged in urine, 3% in feces.

Administration and dosage
Adults

Guidelines for use in premature labor:
1. Initiate a control IV of dextrose 5%, Ringer's lactate, or saline solution and administer 400 to 500 ml in 15 to 20 min before initiation of the medication. Then decrease to 100 to 125 ml/hr.
2. Add 20 mg of terbutaline to 1000 ml of dextrose 5%.
3. Administer a loading dose of 250 µg IV over 1 to 2 min.
4. Start the infusion at a rate of 10 µg IV (30 ml/hr) Table 6-1).
5. Increase the infusion rate by 3.5 µg/min (10 ml/hr) every 10 min until labor has stopped or a maximum dose of 26 µg/min (80 ml/hr) has been attained.
6. Maintain the effective dose for 1 hr or more, then begin decreasing the rate by 2 µg/min (6 ml/hr) every 30 min until the lowest effective dose is reached. Maintain the total IV fluid intake at 125 ml/hr.

Table 6-1. Terbutaline administration in premature labor*

ml/hr	15	20	30	40	50	60	70	80	90
µg/min	5	6.6	10	13	16	20	23	26	30

*Administer 20 mg/1000 ml or 20 µg/ml.

7. When the lowest effective IV dose is reached, begin PO terbutaline, 2.5 mg every 4 hr.
8. If labor has stopped, discontinue the IV infusion 24 hr after PO administration was initiated if the uterus is not irritable.
9. Continue the PO regimen (2.5 mg every 4 hr or 5 mg every 8 hr) until 36 weeks' gestation.
10. If labor begins again, restart the IV infusion as above.

Guidelines for treatment of pulmonary disease:
PO—5 mg 3 times daily while the patient is awake. Total daily dosage should not exceed 15 ml.
SC—250 µg. The dose may be repeated if significant clinical improvement is not seen within 15 to 30 min. No more than 500 µg should be administered in a 4 hr period.

Pediatric (12 to 15 years of age)

PO—2.5 mg 3 times daily.
NOTE: There are no dosage recommendations as yet for children under 12 years of age.

Nurse and patient considerations

* When terbutaline is used for premature labor, a sometimes significant drop in blood pressure (due to vasodilatory effects) can be observed at the time of the loading dose and when the infusion is started. Blood pressure and pulse monitoring should be done before and every 5 min after the loading dose has been administered and the infusion started until the patient is stable. Use continuous fetal monitoring. If the maternal pulse exceeds 120 beats/min and does not decrease with an increase in fluids or when the patient is rolled on her left side, or if there is any evidence of a decrease in uterine perfusion, discontinue the infusion.

* Most side effects are dose related. These inlcude tachycardia, tremor, nervousness, palpitations, and dizziness. Headache, nausea, vomiting, restlessness, drowsiness, sweating, and tinnitus also have been reported.
* Patients known to have hypertension, hyperthyroidism, diabetes mellitus, or cardiac disease with arrhythmias may be particularly sensitive to adverse reactions and must be observed closely.

Drug interactions

Propranolol (Inderal) may inhibit the pharmacologic effects of terbutaline.

Administration of terbutaline in conjunction with other sympathomimetic agents may enhance cardiovascular side effects. Therefore use terbutaline with caution.

Concurrent administration of corticosteroids (betamethasone, dexamethasone, others) with IV terbutaline may result in pulmonary edema. This adverse interaction is infrequently reported, but there is a higher incidence in patients with multiple pregnancy, occult cardiac disease, and fluid overload. Persistent tachycardia may be a sign of impending pulmonary edema. Observe patients closely, monitoring fluid input and output, breath sounds, and heart rate, as well as the patient's anxiety level and state of well-being.

Theophylline derivatives
GENERAL INFORMATION

The parent compound of the theophylline derivatives is theophylline. Because of the relative insolubility of theophylline, several synthetic salts have been developed in an attempt to increase water solubility and reduce gastrointestinal irritation (see Table 6-2). Regardless of the salt, all the theophylline derivatives have the same mechanism of action, side effects, metabolic pathways, and clinical indications as the theophylline base.

The mechanisms of action of theophylline have not been fully elucidated. Theophylline appears to work by three broad mechanisms: (1) translocation of intracellular calcium, (2) inhibition of the enzyme phosphodiesterase, allowing an accumulation of cyclic AMP, and (3) blockade of receptors of adenosine. Other pharmacologic actions are being studied, including potentiation of inhibitors of prosta-

Table 6-2. Theophylline content of theophylline salts

Salt	Percent pure theophylline	equivalent dosage (mg)
Theophylline NF	100	100
Theophylline mono-hydrate NF	91	110
Aminophylline USP	80	125
Oxtriphylline	65	154
Theophylline sodium glycinate	50	200
Theophylline sodium salicylate	48	209

glandin synthesis and reduction of the uptake and metabolism of catecholamines in nonneuronal tissues.

As indicated by diverse mechanisms of action, theophylline has extensive pharmacologic activity in the renal, cardiovascular, gastrointestinal, smooth muscle, skeletal muscle, and central nervous systems.

Therapeutically, theophylline is used as a bronchodilator in bronchial asthma, status asthmaticus, and reversible bronchospasm associated with chronic bronchitis, emphysema, and other obstructive pulmonary diseases. It is also used investigationally in infants to stimulate respirations to prevent apneic episodes.

Characteristics

Under the acidic conditions of the stomach, the theophylline salts release free theophylline. Absorption: (PO) uncoated tablets, capsules—1 to 2 hrs; solutions or microcrystalline tablets—1 hr. Half-life: significant interpatient variation due to different rates of metabolism; normal adults—3 to 20 hr; children—1.5 to 9.5 hr; premature infants—15 to 58 hr; cigarette smoking reduces half-life by up to 40%. Protein binding: adults and children—56%; premature infants—36%. Metabolism: liver to 1,3-dimethyluric acid, 1-methyluric acid, and 3-methylxanthine (25%); 3-methylxanthine has about 50% of the activity of theophylline. Excretion: renal, 10% unchanged, remainder as metabolites. Therapeutic levels: bronchodilatation—10 to 20 μg/ml; apnea—7 to 14 μg/ml. Toxic levels: > 20 μg/ml. Dialysis: yes, hemoperfusion; no, H, P. Breast milk: yes, 70% of plasma concentrations.

Administration and dosage

Because of the low therapeutic index of the theophyllines and the great interpatient variation in rates of metabolism, it is essential that dosages are individually determined and that each patient be monitored closely for response and tolerance with theophylline plasma levels.

The dosages of theophylline preparations are expressed in terms of the theophylline base. See Table 6-2 for the theophylline content of the theophylline salts available, and see Table 6-3 for a representative list of products available and their theophylline equivalence. See monographs on aminophylline (p. 279), dyphylline (p. 284), and oxtriphylline (p. 285).

For bronchodilator therapy:

Adult

PO—9 to 20 mg theophylline/kg daily in 4 divided doses. Use an approximation of the patient's lean body weight.

Pediatric

PO—16 to 25 mg theophylline/kg in 4 divided doses.

For apnea:

Pediatric

See Aminophylline (p. 279).

NOTE: Theophylline products may be taken with food, milk, or antacids to reduce local gastrointestinal irritation.

Nurse and patient considerations

* All theophylline products, regardless of the dosage form used, cause CNS stimulation and gastrointestinal irritation. The GI irritation is both locally and centrally mediated, causing nausea, vomiting, epigastric pain, abdominal cramps, and anorexia. The CNS side effects include headache, irritability, restlessness, insomnia, dizziness, and seizure activity. All these side effects are dosage dependent and may diminish with a reduction in dosage.
* Theophylline products should be administered cautiously to patients who have congestive heart failure, chronic obstructive pulmonary disease, cor pulmonale, or renal or hepatic disease. These patients metabolize theophylline much more slowly and may

develop toxicities more easily. Theophylline should also be used with caution in patients with angina pectoris, peptic ulcer disease, hyperthyroidism, glaucoma, and diabetes mellitus.

* *Abnormalities of laboratory tests:* theophylline may cause a false-positive elevation of serum and urinary uric acid when the colorimetric method is used. When the uricase method is used, there is no interference with test results. The following drugs may falsely elevate theophylline plasma levels when measured by spectrophotometric methods: furosemide, sulfathiazole, phenylbutazone, probenecid, and theobromine.

* Theophylline products have been used in pregnancy without evidence of teratogenicity or adverse effects to the fetus. Theophylline is secreted into the breast milk in sufficient quantities to occasionally produce irritability in infants. Attempt to schedule dosages when they will not conflict with nursing schedules.

Drug interactions

Erythromycin, clindamycin, lincomycin, troleandomycin, thiabendazole, influenza vaccine, cimetidine, and allopurinol significantly reduce hepatic metabolism of theophylline, causing an increase in serum levels with potential for toxicity. Patients at greater risk include those receiving large doses of theophylline and/or those with diseases that impair theophylline elimination. This potential drug interaction may be managed by (1) using alternative drugs, (2) keeping the theophylline dose constant, but monitoring the patient and serum levels for signs of toxicity, and (3) reducing the dose of theophylline by about 25% when the drug is started and observing the patient for signs of inadequate therapeutic response and toxicity.

Cigarette smoke induces hepatic metabolism of theophylline, requiring a 50% to 100% increase in the dosage for therapeutic response.

Phenytoin may significantly increase theophylline metabolism by induction of hepatic microsomal enzymes. The theophylline dose may have to be increased 50% to 100% to maintain the same therapeutic response.

Table 6-3. Xanthine-derivative products

Product name	Aminophylline	Oxtriphylline	Theophylline	Theophylline Na Glycinate	Dyphylline	Dosage forms	Equivalent to X mg theophylline
Accurbron			X			50 mg/5 ml liquid	50 mg
Aminophylline	X					100,200 mg tablets	79,158 mg
	X					125,250,500 mg suppository	99,198,395 mg
	X					250 mg/10 ml IV	198 mg
	X					500 mg/20 ml IV	395 mg
	X					500 mg/2 ml IM	395 mg
Airet LA					X	400 mg tablets, long-acting	—
Aminodur Dura-tabs	X					300 mg tablets, sustained release (8-12 hr)	236 mg
Bronkodyl			X			100,200 mg capsules	100,200 mg
			X			300 mg caps, sustained release	300 mg
			X			26.6 mg/5 ml elixir	26.6 mg

Continued.

Table 6-3. Xanthine-derivative products—cont'd

Product name	Xanthine derivative					Dosage forms	Equivalent to X mg theophylline
	Aminophylline	Oxtriphylline	Theophylline	Theophylline Na Glycinate	Dyphylline		
Choledyl		X				100,200 mg tablets	64,128 mg
		X				50 mg/5 ml pediatric syrup	32 mg
		X				100 mg/5 ml elixir	64 mg
Choledyl SA		X				400,600 mg tablets, sustained action	256,384 mg
Dilor					X	200,400 mg tablets	—
					X	53.5 mg/5 ml elixir	—
					X	250 mg/ml injection	—
Droxine					X	100 mg/5 ml liquid	—
Elixicon			X			100 mg/5 ml suspension	100 mg
Elixophyllin			X			100,200 mg capsules	100,200 mg
			X			125,250 mg capsules, timed release	125,250 mg
Lufyllin					X	33.3 mg/5 ml elixir	—
					X	250 mg/ml injection	—

					Dosage form	Strength
Lufyllin 200				X	200 mg tablets	—
Lufyllin 400				X	400 mg tablets	—
Neothylline				X	200,400 mg tablets	—
				X	53.3 mg/5 ml elixir	—
				X	250 mg/ml injection	—
Quibron T Dividose			X		300 mg tablets	300 mg
Quibron T/SR			X		300 mg tablets, sustained release	300 mg
Slo-Phyllin			X		100,200 mg tablets	100,200 mg
Slo-Phyllin 80			X		26.6 mg/5 ml syrup	26.6 mg
Slo-Phyllin Gyrocaps			X		60,125,250 mg capsules, timed release	60,125,250 mg
Somophyllin		X			105 mg/5 ml liquid	90 mg
		X			300 mg/5 ml rectal solution	255 mg
Somophyllin-CRT			X		50,100,250 mg capsules, controlled release	50,100,250 mg
Somophyllin-T			X		100,200,250 mg capsules	100,200,250 mg
Synophylate			X		330 mg tablets	165 mg
			X		110 mg/5 ml elixir	110 mg
Theolair	X				125,250 mg tablets	125,250 mg
	X				26.6 mg/5 ml liquid	26.6 mg
Theolair SR	X				250,500 mg tablets, sustained release	250,500 mg

Continued.

Table 6-3. Xanthine-derivative products—cont'd

| Product name | Xanthine derivative | | | | | Dosage forms | Equivalent to X mg theophylline |
	Aminophylline	Oxtriphylline	Theophylline	Theophylline Na Glucinate	Dyphylline		
Theophyl		X				100 mg tablets (chewable)	100 mg
Theophyl-225		X				225 mg tablets	225 mg
		X				37.5 mg/5 ml elixir	37.5 mg
Theophyl SR		X				65,130,260 mg capsules, sustained release	65,130,260 mg
Theophylline		X				26.5 mg/5 ml elixir	26.6 mg
Theovent		X				125,250 mg capsules, long-acting	125,250 mg

Aminophylline, USP
AHFS 86:00

Actions and use
CATEGORY Bronchodilator, diuretic, myocardial stimulant

Aminophylline is used in the treatment of pulmonary emphysema, congestive heart failure, bronchial or cardiac asthma, status asthmaticus, Cheyne-Stokes respiration, and bronchitis. It is a direct myocardial stimulant, bronchodilator, and weak diuretic. It increases the depth and rate of respiration, cardiac output, and renal blood flow and diminishes bronchospasm.

Administration and dosage
Adult

PO 1. Initial: 3 mg/kg every 6 hr.
   2. Maintenance: readjust dosage every few days up to 6 mg/kg every 6 hr as indicated by serum levels and clinical response.

IM—Painful, with erratic absorption. Not recommended.

IV—Infusion: the usual initial loading dose is 5.6 mg/kg administered no faster than 25 to 50 mg/min.* The maintenance dose is adjusted according to the following schedule:

Young patients	— 0.9 mg/kg/hr*
Middle-aged patients	— 0.7 mg/kg/hr*
Patients with congestive heart failure or liver disease	— 0.45 mg/kg/hr*

For maintenance infusion rate adjustment see Table 6-4.
See NOTE below on converting a patient from IV to PO therapy.

RECTAL SUPPOSITORY—125 to 500 mg every 6 to 12 hr. This may be quite irritating to rectal tissues.

RETENTION ENEMA—500 to 700 mg in 20 to 30 ml of tap water 2 to 3 times daily.

Pediatric (greater than 1 year of age)

PO—Non–status asthmaticus: initially, 5 mg/kg every 6 hr. Readjust dosage every few days to 8 mg/kg every 6 hr as indicated by serum levels and clinical response.

---

*Dosage must be calculated on an estimated lean body weight.

Table 6-4. Aminophylline infusion*

mg/500 ml	500		1000		1500		2000	
Final volume	520		540		560		580	
mg/ml	0.96		1.85		2.68		3.45	
50 kg μgtts/min	mg/kg/hr	mg/hr	mg/kg/hr	mg/hr	mg/kg/hr	mg/hr	mg/kg/hr	mg/hr
10	0.2	9.6	0.4	18.5	0.5	26.8	0.7	34.5
20	0.4	19.2	0.7	37	1.1	53.6	1.4	69
30	0.6	28.8	1.1	55.5	1.6	80.4	2	103.5
40	0.8	38.4	1.5	74	2.1	107.2	2.8	138
50	1.0	48	1.8	92.5	2.7	134	3.5	172.5
60	1.1	57.6	2.2	111	3.2	160.8	4.1	207
60 kg μgtts/min	mg/kg/hr	mg/hr	mg/kg/hr	mg/hr	mg/kg/hr	mg/hr	mg/kg/hr	mg/hr
10	0.2	9.6	0.3	18.5	0.5	26.8	0.6	34.5
20	0.3	19.2	0.6	37	0.9	53.6	1.2	69
30	0.5	28.8	0.9	55.5	1.3	80.4	1.7	103.5
40	0.6	38.4	1.3	74	1.8	107.2	2.3	138
50	0.8	48	1.5	92.5	2.2	134	2.9	172.5
60	1.0	57.6	1.9	111	2.7	160.8	3.5	207

70 kg μgtts/min	mg/kg/hr	mg/hr	mg/kg/hr	mg/hr	mg/kg/hr	mg/hr	mg/kg/hr	mg/hr
10	0.2	9.6	0.3	18.5	0.4	26.8	0.5	34.5
20	0.3	19.2	0.5	37	0.8	53.6	1.	69
30	0.4	28.8	0.8	55.5	1.1	80.4	1.5	103.5
40	0.5	38.4	1.0	74	1.6	107.2	2	138.5
50	0.7	48	1.3	92.5	1.9	134	2.5	172.5
60	0.8	57.6	1.6	111	2.3	160.8	3	207

80 kg μgtts/min	mg/kg/hr	mg/hr	mg/kg/hr	mg/hr	mg/kg/hr	mg/hr	mg/kg/hr	mg/hr
10	0.1	9.6	0.2	18.5	0.3	26.8	0.4	34.5
20	0.2	19.2	0.5	37	0.7	53.6	0.9	69
30	0.4	28.8	0.7	55.5	1.0	80.4	1.3	103.5
40	0.5	38.4	0.9	74	1.3	107.2	1.7	138.5
50	0.6	48	1.2	92.5	1.7	134	2.2	172.5
60	0.7	57.6	1.4	111	2	160.8	2.6	207

*Using a microdrip administrations set—60 gtts/ml.

Continued.

Table 6-4. Aminophylline infusion—cont'd

mg/500 ml	500		1000		1500		2000	
Final volume	520		540		560		580	
mg/ml	0.96		1.85		2.68		3.45	
90 kg μgtts/min	mg/kg/hr	mg/hr	mg/kg/hr	mg/hr	mg/kg/hr	mg/hr	mg/kg/hr	mg/hr
10	0.1	9.6	0.2	18.5	0.3	26.8	0.4	34.5
20	0.2	19.2	0.4	37	0.6	53.6	0.8	69
30	0.3	28.8	0.6	55.5	0.9	80.4	1.2	103.5
40	0.4	38.4	0.8	74	1.1	107.2	1.5	138
50	0.5	48	1.0	92.5	1.5	134	1.9	172.5
60	0.6	57.6	1.2	111	1.8	160.8	2.3	207
100 kg μgtts/min	mg/kg/hr	mg/hr	mg/kg/hr	mg/hr	mg/kg/hr	mg/hr	mg/kg/hr	mg/hr
10	0.1	9.6	0.2	18.5	0.3	26.8	0.3	34.5
20	0.2	19.2	0.4	37	0.5	53.6	0.7	69
30	0.3	28.8	0.5	55.5	0.8	80.4	1	103.5
40	0.4	38.4	0.7	74	1	107.2	1.4	138
50	0.5	48	0.9	92.5	1.3	134	1.7	172.5
60	0.6	57.6	1.1	111	1.6	160.8	2	207

IV 1. Infusion: the usual initial loading dose is 5.6 mg/kg administered at a rate no faster than 25 to 50 mg/min.
2. Maintenance: 1.1 mg/kg/hr by continuous infusion or 5 mg/kg every 6 hr by intermittent bolus administered at a rate of 25 to 50 mg/min.

For apnea:

Up to 2 weeks of age

1. Loading dose: 6 mg/kg IV.
2. Maintenance dose: 1.1 mg/kg every 8 hr, IV or PO.

Two to 4 weeks of age

1. Loading dose: 6 mg/kg IV or PO. If oral, divide into 2 doses and administer 2 hr apart. Start the maintenance dose 8 hr later.
2. Maintenance dose: 1.7 to 2.5 mg/kg every 8 hr IV or PO.

Over 4 weeks of age

1. Loading dose: as above.
2. Maintenance dose: 3.0 to 4.2 mg/kg every 8 hr, IV or PO.

NOTE: When converting from IV to PO aminophylline therapy, the PO dose will be the same as the IV dose if similar plasma concentrations are desired. Multiply the hourly IV dose times the number of hours in the dosage interval (usually 6) to obtain the PO aminophylline dose. When converting from IV aminophylline to PO theophylline, oxtriphylline, or another salt, a dosage adjustment must be made because of actual theophylline content. See Table 6-2.

Aminophylline therapy is now quite easily monitored by serum levels. The normal therapeutic range is 7 to 20 µg/ml. Anorexia, nausea, and vomiting may occur at serum levels of 15 to 30 µg/ml. See also General information on theophylline derivatives (p. 271).

Nurse and patient considerations

* Common side effects particularly associated with rapid IV injection of aminophylline may produce nausea, headache, flushing, palpitation, dizziness, arrhythmias, tachycardia, hypotension, or precordial pain. PO administration is also irritating to the stomach and may result in erratic absorption.

* Since aminophylline is frequently administered via continuous infusion, a question arises as to what may be compatible with it. Consult a pharmacist, since the lists of compatibilities and incompatibilities are long and aminophylline is fairly unstable as a result of a high pH.
* The bronchodilatory effects of aminophylline are usually not influenced by beta-blocking agents (propranolol); therefore this drug may be useful in patients who develop bronchospasm while taking beta-blocking agents.

See General information on theophylline derivatives (p. 271).

Drug interactions

Aminophylline may increase the renal excretion of lithium carbonate. Patients may require increased dosages of lithium if they are on concomitant aminophylline and lithium carbonate therapy.

Aminophylline and propranolol may be mutually antagonistic in their actions. Patients must be observed for inhibition of either drug.

See General information on theophylline derivatives (p. 271).

Dyphylline
(Dilor, Lufyllin, Neothylline)

AHFS 86:00
CATEGORY
Bronchodilator

Action and use

Dyphylline is a xanthine derivative, structurally and pharmacologically similar to theophylline, but, contrary to popular belief, it is not a salt of theophylline and does not metabolize to theophylline. It is used as a bronchodilator to relieve acute bronchial asthma and for reversible bronchospasm associated with chronic bronchitis and emphysema.

Characteristics

Absorption: well absorbed, intact (PO). Half-life: adults, 2 hr. Metabolism: minimal. Excretion: renal, 85% unchanged.

Administration and dosage
Adult

PO—15 mg/kg every 6 hr, 3 to 4 times daily.
NOTE: See General information on theophylline derivatives
(p. 271).

Nurse and patient considerations

✳ See General information on theophylline derivatives
(p. 271).

Drug interactions

See General information on theophylline derivatives (p.
271).

Oxtriphylline
(Choledyl)

AHFS 86:00
CATEGORY Bronchodilator

Action and use

Oxtriphylline is a theophylline derivative about 65% as
potent as theophylline. When compared with theophylline or
aminophylline, it is theoretically less irritating to the gastric
mucosa, and because it is more stable and soluble, it is more
readily absorbed from the gastrointestinal tract. Oxtriphylline is used in long-term therapy to reduce bronchospasm in
patients with acute bronchial asthma, chronic bronchitis,
and emphysema.

Administration and dosage
Adult

TABLETS—200 mg 4 times daily. (Some patients may require
1200 mg daily for adequate therapy.)
ELIXIR—200 mg (10 ml) 4 times daily.

Pediatric (ages 2 to 12)

ELIXIR—100 mg (5 ml)/27 kg 4 times daily.

Nurse and patient considerations

✳ CNS stimulation manifested by nervousness, insomnia, irritability, nausea, and vomiting may
occur, particularly with children and with larger
doses.

* See General information on theophylline derivatives (p. 271).

Drug interactions

Administration of oxtriphylline in conjunction with other theophylline derivatives or with sympathomimetic agents may enhance cardiovascular and CNS adverse effects. Use with caution in drug combinations.

See General information on theophylline derivatives (p. 271).

CHAPTER SEVEN

Antihistaminic agents

Cyproheptadine
*   hydrochloride*
Diphenhydramine
Hydroxyzine
Meclizine hydrochloride

Cyproheptadine hydrochloride
(Periactin)

AHFS 4:00
CATEGORY Antihistamine, antipruritic

Action and use

Cyproheptadine has both anticholinergic and sedative effects. Its exact mechanism of action is unknown, but it is a potent blocking agent against histamine and 5-hydroxytryptamine. Cyproheptadine is effective in various allergic diseases such as seasonal allergic rhinitis, conjunctivitis, pruritis, urticaria, and angioedema secondary to reactions to food, airborne allergens, and minor drug or serum reactions. It has also been used as an appetite stimulant in children.

Administration and dosage
Adult

PO—Up to 20 mg/day in divided doses. The initial dosage recommended is 4 mg 3 times daily. A few patients may require as much as 32 mg daily for symptomatic relief.

Pediatric
Ages 2 to 6

PO—2 mg 2 to 3 times daily. Do not exceed 12 mg/day.

Ages 7 to 14

PO—4 mg 2 to 3 times daily. Do not exceed 16 mg/day.

Nurse and patient considerations

* The most frequent adverse effects are sedation and sleepiness. This usually passes with continued use of the drug.
* Less frequent effects include dry mouth, anorexia, nausea, dizziness, confusion, and ataxia.
* Cyproheptadine is not recommended for use in pregnant women and is excreted in breast milk of nursing mothers.

Drug interactions

There are no specific drug interactions with cyproheptadine except for additive sedative and anticholinergic activity when used in combination with CNS depressants and anticholinergic agents.

Diphenhydramine
(Benadryl)

AHFS 4:00, 48:00
CATEGORY Antihistamine

Action and use

Diphenhydramine blocks histamine activity by preventing the access of histamine to its receptor sites. It is used prophylactically and therapeutically against milk, local allergic reactions such as insect bites, and mild drug and blood transfusion reactions characterized by angioedema, urticaria, and pruritus.

It also has anticholinergic, antispasmodic, antitussive, antiemetic, and sedative effects. As an antiemetic, it may be effective in the treatment of motion sickness.

It is also effective in treating extrapyramidal reactions induced by other drugs, such as phenothiazines, and as a bedtime sedative for relief of simple insomnia.

Characteristics

Peak blood levels: 1 hr (PO). Duration: 4 to 6 hr. Metabolism: liver. Excretion: as metabolites within 24 hr. Therapeutic level: 0.1 mg/100 ml to 0.5 mg/100 ml. Fatal level: 1 mg/100 ml. Dialysis: yes, H.

Administration and dosage
Adult

PO—25 to 50 mg 3 to 4 times daily.
IM—10 to 50 mg, not to exceed 400 mg daily.
IV—As for IM administration.

Pediatric
Infants and children under 10 kg

PO—½ to 1 tsp (6 to 12 mg) 3 to 4 times daily.

Children over 10 kg

PO—1 to 2 tsp (12 to 24 mg) 3 to 4 times daily, not to exceed 300 mg.

IM—5 mg/kg/24 hrs in 4 divided doses, not to exceed 300 mg.

IV—As for IM administration.

NOTE: Diphenhydramine must not be used in patients with narrow-angle glaucoma, asthmatic attacks, prostatic hypertrophy, or bladder-neck obstruction.

Nurse and patient considerations

* Patients may become drowsy and should be warned against engaging in activities requiring mental alertness.
* Patients may complain of drowsiness, confusion, blurring of vision, difficulty in urination, dry mouth, nasal stuffiness, and constipation.
* Antihistamines should be used with caution in patients with chronic pulmonary disease, since these agents may thicken bronchial secretions and cause tightness of the chest and wheezing.
* The anticholinergic properties of diphenhydramine may inhibit lactation in nursing mothers.

Drug interactions

Diphenhydramine may have additive CNS depressant effects with alcohol, sedatives, hypnotics, tranquilizers, and narcotics.

Hydroxyzine
(Atarax, Vistaril)

AHFS 28:16.08
CATEGORY Tranquilizer

Action and use

Hydroxyzine is a CNS depressant, anticholinergic, antiemetic, and antispasmodic as well as an antihistaminic agent. It is used as a mild tranquilizer in emotional and psychiatric states characterized by anxiety, tension, and agitation.

Hydroxyzine may also be effective as a preoperative or

postoperative sedative to control emesis, diminish anxiety, and reduce the amount of narcotics needed for analgesia.

Hydroxyzine may also be used as an antipruritic agent to relieve the itching associated with allergic conditions.

Administration and dosage
Adult

PO—Tranquilizer: 25 to 100 mg 3 to 4 times daily.
IM   1. Tranquilizer: 50 to 100 mg every 4 to 6 hr.
    2. Preoperative and postoperative: 25 to 100 mg.
    3. Antiemetic: 25 to 100 mg.

Pediatric
Under 6 years of age

PO—50 mg daily in divided doses.
IM   1. Preoperative and postoperative: 0.2 mg/kg.
    2. Antiemetic: 0.2 mg/kg.

Over 6 years of age

PO—50 to 100 mg daily in divided doses.
IM—As for children under 6 years of age.
NOTE: When hydroxyzine is used preoperatively, narcotic requirements may be reduced up to half the normal dosage.

Nurse and patient considerations

* Drowsiness may occur, especially during the first few days of therapy, and patients must be warned about performing hazardous tasks while taking hydroxyzine.
* Dryness of the mouth and nasal stuffiness are common complaints.
* Safe use of hydroxyzine in pregnancy has not been proved, and its use is not recommended in early pregnancy.

Drug interactions

Hydroxyzine may potentiate the action of other CNS depressants including narcotics, analgesics, barbiturates or other sedatives, anesthetics, tranquilizers, and alcohol.

Meclizine hydrochloride
(Antivert, Bonine)

AHFS 56:20
CATEGORY Antihistamine, antinauseant

Action and use

Meclizine, a long-acting antihistaminic agent, is effective in controlling nausea, vomiting, and dizziness, especially when associated with motion sickness or with diseases affecting the vestibular system. Its mechanism of action is unknown.

Characteristics

Duration: 12 to 24 hr.

Administration and dosage

PO 1. Motion sickness: initially, 25 to 50 mg 1 hr prior to embarkation. The dosage may be repeated every 24 hr for the duration of the journey.
2. Vertigo: 25 to 100 mg daily in divided doses, depending on clinical response.

NOTE: Meclizine is not recommended for the nausea and vomiting of pregnancy. Teratogenic effects have been observed in laboratory animals. Safe use has not been established in pediatric patients.

Nurse and patient considerations

* A common side effect of meclizine is drowsiness. Patients must be warned against performing hazardous tasks at this time.
* Other side effects include blurred vision, dry mouth, constipation, and fatigue.

Drug interactions

Meclizine may display additive anticholinergic side effects (dry mouth, constipation, blurred vision) when administered with other antihistamines, phenothiazines, trihexyphenidyl (Artane), benztropine (Cogentin), and other agents with anticholinergic activity.

CHAPTER EIGHT

Analgesic agents

GENERAL INFORMATION ON ANALGESIA

Pain is an unpleasant subjective experience symptomatic of some underlying disorder. The "pain experience" includes, in addition to the sensation of pain, all the associated emotional sensations for a particular person under particular circumstances. Pain perception and response are influenced by such psychosocial factors as past experience, attention, and emotion. The intensity, duration, and location of harmful stimuli also influence pain perception and response. Whether it originates from physiologic or psychologic causes, it is still pain. Physiologically, it may serve as a key to pathology, that is, angina pectoris in coronary insufficiency, the pain of gout or rheumatoid arthritis. Pain also serves as a sign for other problems such as tense musculature, insomnia, stress, or high anxiety.

When the source of pain is not immediately obvious (that is, trauma), the diagnosis usually requires a detailed history and physical examination to determine the etiology. The region of pain can usually be localized (skin, skeletal muscle, or internal viscera), but the onset, course, and present status must also be identified. The patient should be asked what aggravates or relieves the pain, the effect of emotional disturbances, movement of the part, and other activities that may be associated with the intensity, quality, and distribution of pain.

If the diagnosis indicates that the source of pain has an emotional overlay without demonstrable physiologic changes, treatment of the psychologic dysfunction should be the primary approach to therapy.

When pain is related to a pathologic condition, factors to be considered when initiating therapy should include the cause, the site, the severity, and the probable duration of the pain. In selecting the type of analgesic to be used, the quality and intensity of pain are the most important factors. Mild analgesics (aspirin) are frequently and effectively used for pain originating in the integumental or musculoskeletal system. Those drugs that act centrally (morphine) are most effective for visceral pain.

Once a drug is selected, the optimal dose can be defined as the minimal dose repeated frequently enough to produce the desired therapeutic effect and yet be free of side effects that may further debilitate the patient or complicate therapy. Implicit in the selection of the optimal dose is the continued observation of the patient for proper evaluation of analgesia and the development of side effects. Analgesics must be administered on a regular basis for effective control of pain. It is essential, especially for patients with chronic and terminal pain, that the interval between doses is based on the half-life and duration of the analgesic, rather than on an arbitrary schedule. When a patient knows that he or she will not be expected to suffer until some appointed hour for the next dose, a cycle of anxiety, anticipation, and fear that may compound the pain will not develop. The evaluation of effective therapy may require the help of family members who may notice more subtle changes in patient behavior.

Tolerance to narcotic analgesics may develop relatively rapidly. Many patients and physicians fear that the use of pain-relieving drugs even for a short time must inevitably lead to a further problem of addiction. The number of people who become addicted after prolonged legitimate clinical use is small. When drugs are properly used in hospitals, few of the conditions predisposing to addiction exist. A critical factor predisposing to addiction is self-administration for immediate and continuing reward. A multifaceted approach frequently provides significant pain relief that is relatively uncomplicated by problems in drug dependence. Consequently, full and adequate doses of analgesic drugs should seldom be withheld simply because of fear of initiating drug dependence.

Nurse and patient considerations

Psychologic support and reassurance are quite important to a patient's sense of well-being. Patients are quick to sense an attitude of defeat or a lack of interest and may be easily demoralized by it. Feelings of isolation and anxiety may increase the patient's response to pain and decrease the effectiveness of analgesia. Therefore supportive, concerned communication is an effective tool in pain relief. Combine the analgesic with verbal assurance that it will be effective. Explain that the analgesic will help relieve pain and always indicate to the patient that you understand there is pain, that you have time to listen and to help.

Inform the patient of what may be expected—the quantity and duration of pain, how frequently the analgesic may be administered, by what routes, if and when it may be requested, and how long it will take for the effects to be noticeable.

Timing is of primary concern in planning analgesic care. Anticipate the need for pain medication, and do not force undue waiting, as the therapeutic effects will then take longer; the patient's anxiety, fear, and anticipation will increase before the next encounter. While visiting with the patient, evaluate the effectiveness of the analgesic being administered.

Assess the need for the analgesic at the time of administration if the patient gives no indication of needing it. Be cautious of developing a judgmental attitude about personality characteristics associated with pain and the patient's pain threshold. Never assume that the pain is typically from one source. Encourage patients to describe pain in their own words and investigate all possible causes, such as the development of infection of a wound or bandage tightness.

Nausea and vomiting are occasionally associated with the initial doses of morphine or meperidine. Maintaining a horizontal position for 15 to 20 min after administration and the use of antiemetics such as prochlorperazine or hydroxyzine will often control this adverse effect.

Constipation can result from the use of analgesics. Preventive treatment consists of bulk diet, adequate fluid intake, mobility, and the use of stool softeners.

Depression of the cough reflex by potent analgesics poses a serious threat to postoperative patients. It is essential that these patients deep-breathe, cough, and expectorate mucus to prevent postoperative pulmonary complications.

Measures to increase the effectiveness of analgesics include repositioning, hygiene, and general comfort measures. Reduce unpleasant environmental stimuli and avoid painful activities such as deep breathing and ambulation until the effects of analgesics are apparent. Periodic rest and sleep are essential in helping the patient tolerate pain.

Acetaminophen
(Tylenol, Datril)

AHFS 28:08
CATEGORY Antipyretic analgesic

Action and use

Acetaminophen is a nonnarcotic, synthetic analgesic used in the treatment of mild to moderate pain. Its analgesic and antipyretic effectiveness is similar to that of aspirin in equal doses. Acetaminophen has no antiinflammatory activity and is therefore ineffective (other than as an analgesic) in the symptomatic relief of rheumatoid arthritis.

Characteristics

Peak plasma levels: 10 to 60 min. Duration: 3 to 4 hr. Protein binding: 25%. Plasma half-life: 1.5 to 3 hr. Metabolism; hepatic. Excretion: urine 3% active, more than 80% metabolites. Therapeutic serum levels: 3 mg/100 ml. Dialysis: yes, H; no, P.

Administration and dosage
Adult

PO—300 to 600 mg every 4 to 6 hr. Daily dosage should not exceed 2.6 g.

Pediatric
Under 1 year of age

PO—60 mg every 4 to 6 hr.

Ages 1 to 3

PO—60 to 120 mg every 4 to 6 hr.

Ages 3 to 6

PO—120 mg every 4 to 6 hr.

Ages 6 to 12

PO—240 mg every 4 to 6 hr.
RECTAL—As for PO.

Nurse and patient considerations

∗ During the past decade acetominophen has often been recommended as the drug of choice for the relief of mild pain and fever. Its acquisition does not require a prescription, and its use has climbed steadily. Unfortunately overdosage due to acute and chronic ingestion has risen dramatically in the last few years. Severe, life-threatening hepatotoxicity has been reported in patients who either ingest 5 to 8 g daily for several weeks or attempt suicide by consuming large quantities at one time.

* Early indications of toxicity include anorexia, nausea, and vomiting—symptoms that are often attributed to other causes. A few days later the patient develops jaundice, and the SGOT and SGPT levels and prothrombin time rise dramatically. As more cases of toxicity are being recognized, the treatment modalities are becoming more refined. If acetaminophen toxicity is suspected, consult the manufacturer, a university drug information center, or a poison control center for the most current recommendations for therapy.

* Blood dyscrasias, including thrombocytopenia, leukopenia, pancytopenia, and agranulocytosis are rare side effects that may result from prolonged administration of large doses. Hemolytic anemia may be precipitated in those patients with a deficiency of glucose-6-phosphate dehydrogenase enzyme.

* See General information on analgesia (p. 292).

Drug interactions

There are no clinically significant drug interactions reported involving acetaminophen.

Alphaprodine hydrochloride
(Nisentil)

AHFS 28:08; C-II
CATEGORY Analgesic,
central narcotic

Action and use

Alphaprodine is a synthetically produced narcotic analgesic that is chemically related to meperidine. It is recommended for the relief of moderate to severe pain, but because of its short duration of action it is particularly well suited for use as an analgesic in minor surgical, dental and obstetric procedures. For urgent situations IV injection will provide more prompt relief than any other analgesic.

Characteristics

Onset: 1 to 2 min (IV), 5 to 10 min (SC). Duration: ½ to 1 hr (IV), 2 hr (SC). Metabolism: liver. Excretion: primarily in urine as free drug and inactive metabolites.

Administration and dosage
Adult

sc—Usual range: 0.4 to 1.2 mg/kg. The initial dose should not exceed 60 mg.

obstetrics—40 to 60 mg after cervical dilatation has begun. Repeat as needed.

preoperatively for major surgery—20 to 40 mg.

iv—Usual range: 0.4 to 0.6 mg/kg. The initial dose should not exceed 30 mg.

urologic procedures (e.g., cystoscopy)—20 to 30 mg. Preoperatively for major surgery: 10 to 20 mg.

NOTE: Doses of alphaprodine should be reduced 25% to 50% when phenothiazines or other tranquilizers are to be administered concomitantly.

NOTE: The total dose administered by any route should not exceed 240 mg/24 hr.

Pediatric

NOTE: Use of alphaprodine is recommended in children only for dental analgesia.

Submucosal—0.3 to 0.6 mg/kg. Routine reversal with naloxone should be performed following each procedure.

Nurse and patient considerations

* Alphaprodine must be used with extreme caution in patients with chronic, severe respiratory disease. Normal therapeutic doses have occasionally produced respiratory depression (see Antidote).
* If alphaprodine is used as a postoperative analgesic, the patient must be encouraged to cough and deep-breathe, to ambulate with caution or assistance, and to change positions every 2 hr to prevent respiratory pooling. Additional forms of comfort and support should be offered.
* Repeated use may lead to tolerance, dependence, and addiction. Therefore evaluate the *patient's* response to the analgesic and suggest a change to milder analgesics if indicated.
* See General information on analgesia (p. 292).

Antidote

Administer Naloxone (Narcan) 0.4 mg (1 ml) IV, IM, or SC. If the desired degree of counteraction and improvement in respiratory function is not obtained immediately, the dose may be repeated at 2 - to 3- min intervals (see Naloxone, p. 612).

Drug interactions

The depressant effects of alphaprodine are additive with those of general anesthetics, phenothiazines, tranquilizers, sedative-hypnotics, tricyclic antidepressants, antihistamines, and other CNS depressants, including alcohol. Respiratory depression, hypotension, and profound sedation or coma may result from these interactions unless the dose of alphaprodine has been reduced appropriately (usually by one third to half the normal dose).

Aspirin
(A.S.A., Aspergum)

AHFS 28:08
CATEGORY Analgesic, antipyretic, anti-inflammatory agent

Action and use

The pharmacologic activity of aspirin is rather extensive and quite dose dependent. It appears that the primary mechanism of action is inhibition of cyclooxygenase, a prostaglandin-synthetase enzyme necessary for production of the prostaglandins that mediate inflammation and certain types of pain.

Analgesia: aspirin is the most popular and effective agent for relief of mild to moderate pain. Relief comes from a combination of peripheral and central nervous system effects. The analgesic potency of 325 mg of aspirin is approximately equivalent to 32 mg of codeine.

Antipyresis: aspirin lowers elevated body temperature by action within the hypothalamus and by producing vasodilatation peripherally to allow heat dissipation.

The exact mechanism of aspirin's antiinflammatory effect is unknown but is thought to involve inhibition of prostaglandin synthesis and other inflammatory and immunologic processes.

Diminished platelet adhesiveness may result from minimal doses of 300 to 600 mg/day. Aspirin blocks the adhesion of platelets to connective tissue and collagen fibers by several mechanisms, thus prolonging the bleeding time for several days. In doses greater than 6 g/day, aspirin reduces the plasma prothrombin level by decreasing blood clotting factor VII plasma levels.

Small doses (1 to 2 g daily) inhibit tubular secretion of uric acid and may elevate serum uric acid levels. Doses greater than 5 g daily promote urinary excretion of uric acid, resulting in lower serum uptake levels.

Characteristics

Onset: 15 to 30 min. Peak activity: 1 to 2 hr. Duration: 4 to 6 hr. Protein binding: 50% to 80%. Plasma half-life: 5 to 9 hr. Metabolism: liver, plasma, and erythrocytes. Excretion: urine—time-dose dependent. Therapeutic blood levels: 20 mg/100 ml to 30 mg/100 ml. Toxic blood levels: 40 mg/100 ml to 50 mg/100 ml. Fatal levels: 90 mg/100 ml to 120 mg/100 ml. Dialysis: yes, H, P. Breast milk: Yes.

Administration and dosage
Adult

PO

1. Analgesia and antipyresis: 300 mg to 1 g every 3 to 6 hr.
2. Rheumatoid disorders: 2.4 to 3.6 g (8 to 12 325 mg tablets) in 4 to 6 daily divided doses. Doses may be increased if needed. Gastrointestinal side effects can usually be reduced by administering the dose with food, milk, antacids, or large amounts of water.

RECTAL—Analgesia and antipyresis: as for PO administration.

Pediatric

PO

1. Analgesia and antipyresis: 65 mg/kg/day divided into 4 to 6 doses. Daily dosage should not exceed 3.6 g.
2. Rheumatoid disorders: as tolerated, to 3.6 g in 4 to 6 daily divided doses.

RECTAL—Analgesia and antipyresis: as for PO administration.

Nurse and patient considerations

＊ In normal therapeutic doses aspirin may produce gastrointestinal discomfort, nausea, vomiting, gastric hemorrhage, peptic ulcer, and occult blood loss. Extreme caution should be used with administration to those patients with a history of peptic ulcer, liver disease, or coagulation disorders.

* In patients receiving higher dosages, salicylism (salicylate intoxication) may result. Symptomatology includes tinnitus, fever, sweating, dizziness, mental confusion, lethargy, dimness of vision, nausea, vomiting, and impaired hearing. This condition is reversible on reduction of dosage.

* "Analgesic nephropathy," resulting in papillary necrosis, chronic interstitial nephritis, and possible pyelonephritis, occurs with increasing frequency in patients who ingest large doses of combination products containing aspirin, phenacetin, and caffeine.

* Aspirin in various dosages will alter blood test results. Test results that may be elevated by aspirin either by interference with testing procedure or by pharmacologic effects include amylase, glucose, and red cell T_3 uptake. Test results decreased by aspirin include cholesterol, glucose, potassium, PBI, and platelets.

* Urine tests altered by aspirin include ketones, PSP, protein, steroids, and VMA. Ingestion of 8 to 18 of the 325 mg tablets of aspirin daily may result in false-positive Clinitest and false-negative Tes-Tape urine glucose determinations.

* Aspirin crosses the placental barrier and is excreted in breast milk. It may be used moderately during pregnancy, but is not recommended in the last month of pregnancy.

* See General information on analgesia (p. 292).

Drug interactions

Coagulation studies must be watched closely when anticoagulants (heparin, warfarin) are administered with aspirin. Aspirin inhibits platelet adhesiveness as well as potentially displacing oral anticoagulants from protein binding, especially in large doses. Aspirin has also been shown to reduce plasma prothrombin levels.

Aspirin displaces oral hypoglycemics (Diabinese, Orinase) from protein-binding sites, potentially producing hypoglycemia. This displacement has occurred at aspirin serum levels or less than 10 mg/100 ml.

Although often clinically indicated for concomitant use,

aspirin and corticosteroids may produce gastrointestinal ulceration. Corticosteroids also tend to enhance salicylate elimination, and larger than usual doses of salicylates may be required in patients receiving both drugs. If the corticosteroids are withdrawn, reductions in salicylate dosage may be required to avoid toxicity.

Salicylates may displace phenytoin (Dilantin) from protein-binding sites, increasing active serum levels and, potentially, the toxicity of phenytoin.

Aspirin may enhance the pharmacologic and adverse effects of methotrexate by displacement of methotrexate from protein-binding sites, as well as by blocking the renal tubular secretion of methotrexate.

Low doses of aspirin block the excretion of uric acid by sulfinpyrazone (Anturane) and probenecid (Benemid), while sulfinpyrazone and probenecid may inhibit the excretion of uric acid by large doses (5 g) of aspirin.

When possible, patients should avoid aspirin within 8 to 10 hr of heavy alcohol use. Aspirin and ethanol disrupt the gastric mucosal barrier, and the minor amount of bleeding secondary to aspirin use is doubled with the concomitant administration of ethanol. If aspirin therapy is absolutely necessary, an enteric-coated preparation may be preferable.

Butorphanol tartrate
(Stadol)

AHFS 28:08
CATEGORY Analgesic

Action and use

Butorphanol tartrate is a synthetic narcotic agonist-antagonist that is structurally related to morphine and naloxone but has pharmacologic properties similar to pentazocine and nalbuphine. Analgesic activity is thought to be mediated through opiate receptors in the limbic system. Narcotic antagonistic effects may be caused by competitive inhibition at the opiate receptor. A parenteral dose of 2 to 3 mg of butorphanol produces analgesia approximately equal to 10 mg of morphine or 80 mg of meperidine. The narcotic antagonist properties are about one fortieth of those of naloxone and 30 times the antagonist activity of pentazocine. In subjects who are dependent on 60 mg of morphine/day, butorphanol neither supresses nor precipitates a withdrawal syndrome.

The respiratory depressant properties of 2 mg of butorphanol are equivalent to 10 mg of morphine. However, unlike morphine, the depth of respiratory depression plateaus at doses greater than 2 mg. In contrast to nalbuphine, which also shows a plateau effect, the duration of respiratory depression induced by butorphanol becomes more prolonged as the dosage is increased. Like pentazocine, butorphanol produces an increase in the pulmonary artery pressure and cardiac index of the heart, while systemic arterial pressure is slightly decreased.

Butorphanol is recommended for the relief of moderate to severe acute and chronic pain associated with cancer, orthopedic disorders, burns, renal colic, preoperative analgesia, and obstetric and surgical analgesia.

Characteristics

Onset: less than 30 min (IM), less than 15 min (IV). Duration: 2 to 4 hr. Metabolism: liver to glucuronides.

Administration and dosage
Adult

IM—Initially, 2 mg every 3 to 4 hr. Dosage range is 1 to 4 mg, depending on the severity of pain.

IV—Initially, 1 mg every 3 to 4 hr. Dosage range is 0.5 to 2 mg, depending on the severity of pain.

Pediatric

Butorphanol is currently not recommended for use in children under 18 years of age.

NOTE: Butorphanol increases the work load of the heart and is therefore not recommended for patients with pain of cardiac origin unless a patient reacts adversely to morphine or meperidine.

Nurse and patient considerations

* The possibility that butorphanol may cause respiratory depression should be considered in the treatment of patients with bronchial asthma, obstructive respiratory diseases, cyanosis, or other respiratory depression from any cause.
* The respiratory depressant effects of butorphanol and its potential for elevating cerebrospinal fluid pressure may be markedly exaggerated in the presence of head injury, other intracranial lesions, or a preexisting increase in intracranial pressure. The use of butorphanol can produce effects such as mio-

sis that may obscure the clinical course of patients with head injuries.
* The most commonly reported adverse reactions are sedation, nausea, a clammy and sweaty sensation, and dizziness.
* Butorphanol has weak narcotic antagonist activity. It is not potent enough to antagonize the respiratory depression produced by morphine; however, when given to patients who have been receiving opiates on a regular basis, it may precipitate withdrawal symptoms.
* Safety of butorphanol during pregnancy or lactation has not been established.
* See General information on analgesia (p. 292).

Antidote

Naloxone (Narcan) is a specific antidote for butorphanol. The usual adult dose is 0.4 mg (1 ml) administered IV, IM, or SC. If the desired degree of counteraction and improvement in respiratory function is not obtained immediately, the dose may be repeated at 2 to 3 min intervals (see Naloxone, p. 612).

Drug interactions

The depressant effects of butorphanol are additive with those of general anesthetics, phenothiazines, tranquilizers, sedative-hypnotics, tricyclic antidepressants, antihistamines, and other CNS depressants, including alcohol. Respiratory depression, hypotension, and profound sedation or coma may result from this interaction unless the dose of butorphanol has been reduced appropriately (usually by one third to half the normal dose).

Codeine
(Codeine)

AHFS 28:08; C-II
CATEGORY Analgesic, narcotic

Action and use

Codeine has properties similar to morphine. Its analgesic and respiratory depressant effects are equivalent on an equianalgesic basis (120 mg codeine = 10 mg morphine parenterally). A particular advantage of codeine is its effectiveness on PO administration. It is approximately two-thirds as

effective orally as parenterally. Codeine is an effective antitussive agent as well as an analgesic in mild to moderate
pain.

Characteristics

Onset: 15 to 30 min. Duration: 4 to 6 hr. Metabolism:
liver, primarily inactive, 10% to morphine. Excretion: urine,
primarily inactive, less than 16% active. Therapeutic level:
2.5 mg/100 ml. Fatal level: 0.2 mg/100 ml. Dialysis:
unknown.

Administration and dosage
Adult

PO   1. Analgesia: 15 to 60 mg every 4 hr.
      2. Antitussive: 8 to 20 mg every 4 hr as needed.
SC—Analgesia: 15 to 60 mg every 4 hr.
IM—Analgesia: as for SC administration. Do not inject IM to
     anticoagulated patients or those suspected of suffering
     a myocardial infarction. Use with caution in debilitated
     patients and those with chronic obstructive pulmonary
     disease.

Pediatric

PO   1. Analgesia: 3 mg/kg/24 hr in 6 divided doses.
      2. Antitussive: 1 to 1.5 mg/kg/24 hr in 4 to 6 divided
        doses.
SC—Analgesia: as for PO administration.

Nurse and patient considerations

* Adverse reactions occur infrequently with codeine
  when it is used in normal doses. Reactions that may
  occur are listed in the morphine monograph.
* Additional supportive antitussive actions include
  maintaining high humidity, avoiding smoking, limiting talking. Deep-breathing exercises should be
  encouraged.
* Codeine appears in the milk of lactating women.
* See General information on analgesia (p. 292).

Antidote

Administer 0.4 mg (1 ml) of naloxone (Narcan) IV, IM,
or SC to reverse respiratory depression. The dose may be
repeated in 2 to 3 min (see Naloxone, p. 612).

Administer 5 mg of nalorphine (Nalline) IV every 3 to 5 min to 15 mg until the respiratory rate increases and the sensorium clears.

Drug interactions

See Drug interactions for morphine (p. 318).

Diflunisal
(Dolobid)

Action and use

Diflunisal is a synthetically produced derivative of the salicylate family but is not metabolized to salicylic acid. It has analgesic and antiinflammatory properties but only minimal (clinically insignificant) antipyretic activity. Its mechanisms of action are not known, but diflunisal is a prostaglandin-synthetase inhibitor.

Diflunisal is used as an analgesic in mild to moderate pain and as an antiinflammatory agent in osteoarthritis. Diflunisal, 500 mg, is comparable in analgesic potency to 650 mg of aspirin, 650 mg of acetaminophen, and 100 mg of propoxyphene napsylate with 650 mg of acetaminophen but has a considerably longer duration of action. Diflunisal, 500 to 750 mg daily, is equivalent to aspirin, 2 to 3 g daily, in the treatment of osteoarthritis. No evidence of habituation, tolerance, or addiction has been reported.

Characteristics

Peak plasma levels: 2 to 3 hr. Activity: nonlinear, concentration dependent; a doubling of the dose produces a greater than doubling of drug accumulation. Half-life: 8 to 12 hr. Protein binding: 99%. Metabolism: liver. Excretion: 90% in urine as inactive metabolites. Dialysis: no, H. Breast milk: yes.

Administration and dosage

NOTE: Do not administer to patients with hypersensitivity to aspirin or to those who have developed bronchospasm, urticaria, or rhinitis secondary to other nonsteroidal antiinflammatory agent therapy.

Adult

PO 1. Mild to moderate pain: 1000 mg followed by 500 mg every 12 hr. Dosage may be adjusted based on the age of the patient, pain severity, and patient's response. Dosage may range from 250 mg every 12 hr to 500 mg every 8 hr. Tablets may be administered with water, milk, or food. Do not crush tablets.

2. Osteoarthritis: 50 to 1000 mg daily in 2 divided doses. Dosage may be adjusted to patient response. Maintenance doses higher than 1500 mg are not recommended. Tablets may be administered with water, milk, or food. Do not crush tablets.

Pediatric

Not recommended for children under 12 years of age.

Nurse and patient considerations

* In normal therapeutic doses, diflunisal may produce nausea, vomiting, dyspepsia, gastrointestinal pain, diarrhea, constipation, flatulence, gastric hemorrhage, peptic ulcer, and occult blood loss. Extreme caution should be used with administration to those patients with a history of peptic ulcer, liver disease, renal disease, or coagulation disorders.

* Other adverse effects reported include dizziness, tinnitus, somnolence or insomnia, rash, headache, tiredness and fatigue, and edema. Use with caution in patients with compromised cardiac function, hypertension, or other conditions predisposing to fluid retention.

* Diflunisal was maternotoxic, embryocidal, and teratogenic in laboratory animals. Use in pregnancy is suggested only if the benefits significantly outweigh the risks of therapy to the fetus. Therapy during the third trimester is not recommended, because of the potential for inducing closure of the patent ductus arteriosus in the fetus.

* See General information on analgesia (p. 292).

Drug interactions

Coagulation studies must be closely monitored when anticoagulants (heparin, warfarin) are administered concurrently with diflunisal. Diflunisal displaces warfarin from protein-binding sites and in higher doses inhibits platelet aggregation.

Diflunisal has been reported *not* to displace tolbutamide (Orinase) from protein-binding sites, but it is not known whether this will be true for the other oral hypoglycemic agents (chlorpropamide, tolinase, others).

Diflunisal significantly inhibits the excretion of hydrochlorothiazide, resulting in accumulation. Diflunisal decreases the hyperuricemic effect of hydrochlorothiazide and furosemide.

An occasional dose of antacids will not significantly affect absorption of diflunisal, but they will if administered on a continuous schedule.

Diflunisal significantly increases plasma levels of acetaminophen. There is generally no need for concomitant therapy.

Administration of diflunisal to patients receiving indomethacin significantly increases plasma levels of indomethacin. Concurrent use significantly enhances adverse effects of both drugs. Concurrent administration is not recommended with diflunisal and any other nonsteroidal antiinflammatory agent.

Ibuprofen
(Motrin)

AHFS 28:08
CATEGORY Antipyretic analgesic

Action and use

Ibuprofen is an analgesic, antipyretic agent that has antiinflammatory properties when used in higher dosages. It is an arylacetic-acid derivative similar in structure to fenoprofen, naproxen, and zomepirac. As with other agents of this class, its mechanism is postulated to be the inhibition of prostaglandin synthetases, a series of enzymes necessary for the formation of prostaglandins that mediate pain and inflammatory activity.

Ibuprofen is used in the chronic symptomatic treatment of rheumatoid arthritis and osteoarthritis, for relief of mild to moderate pain, and for the symptomatic treatment of primary dysmenorrhea. It may be considered an alternative to aspirin therapy in those patients who cannot tolerate the side effects of salicylates. Clinical studies indicate that the antiinflammatory and analgesic effects are similar to those of salicylates and less than indomethacin.

Characteristics

Peak serum levels: 1 to 2 hr. Protein binding: 99%. Plasma half-life: 1.8 to 2 hr. Excretion: 1% in urine unchanged,

45% to 79% as metabolites in 24 hr. Therapeutic level: unknown.

Administration and dosage

NOTE: Do not administer to patients with hypersensitivity to aspirin or to those who have developed bronchospasm, urticaria, or rhinitis secondary to other nonsteroidal antiinflammatory agent therapy.

Adult

PO 1. Rheumatoid arthritis and osteoarthritis: 300 to 600 mg 3 to 4 times daily. Maximum dosage is 2.4 g daily. Antiinflammatory effects usually require 1600 mg/day. Two weeks of therapy are necessary to assess treatment.
2. Mild to moderate pain: 400 mg every 4 to 6 hr as needed.
3. Primary dysmenorrhea: 400 mg every 4 hr as necessary.

Pediatric

For juvenile rheumatoid arthritis:

Under 20 kg

PO—Maximum daily dose: 400 mg.

Between 20 and 30 kg

PO—Maximum daily dose: 600 mg.

Between 30 and 40 kg

PO—Maximum daily dose: 800 mg.

Over 40 kg

PO—As for adult dosages.

Once control is achieved, the lowest effective dose must be maintained. Adequate dosages may need to be maintained for up to 2 weeks before a therapeutic response may be fully evaluated. Ibuprofen may be given with food or milk to minimize gastric irritation.

NOTE: Ibuprofen is contraindicated in patients who are allergic to aspirin.

Nurse and patient considerations

* Gastric irritation causing nausea, vomiting, heartburn, diarrhea, gas, and constipation are the most common side effects of ibuprofen. Gastrointestinal ulceration and perforation have been reported, and the drug should be used with caution in patients with a history of ulcer disease.

* Other adverse effects that have been attributed to this agent include dizziness, headache, tinnitus, drowsiness, mental confusion, vision disturbances, and various rashes.

* There are many other rare side effects that are caused by ibuprofen. These include blood dyscrasias such as anemia, thrombocytopenia, and agranulocytosis; various dermatoses such as urticaria, purpura, pruritus, and rashes; and hepatotoxicity and renal toxicity. All these adverse effects warrant cessation of therapy.

* Safe use during pregnancy has not been established, and the use of ibuprofen is not recommended in patients less than 14 years of age. In preliminary studies, ibuprofen has not been detected in the milk of lactating women.

* See General information on analgesia (p. 292).

Drug interactions

Possible reactions that may occur include displacement of oral anticoagulants (warfarin) from protein-binding sites, enhancing the effects of the anticoagulant and potentiation of the ulcerogenic effects of salicylates, phenylbutazone, indomethacin, and corticosteroids when administered concomitantly with ibuprofen.

Indomethacin
(Indocin)

AHFS 28:08
CATEGORY Antipyretic analgesic

Action and use

Indomethacin is a nonsteroidal, antiinflammatory, and antipyretic analgesic. Although the exact mechanism of action is unknown, it is thought that indomethacin inhibits the biosynthesis of prostaglandins, which appear to contribute to inflammation. Indomethacin relieves pain and stiffness and reduces swelling and tenderness of joints. It may be effective in the treatment of active rheumatoid arthritis, rheumatoid (ankylosing) spondylitis, and degenerative joint disease of the hip. Because of its high incidence of side effects with chronic administration, its use is not recommended unless aspirin therapy is ineffective or not tolerated. About 25% of patients using this agent show significant improvement; however, if the patient does not show symptomatic improvement with 75 to 100 mg/day after 2 to 3 weeks, alternative therapy is recommended.

Characteristics

Onset: 1 to 2 hr. Duration: 4 to 6 hr. Protein binding: 90%. Plasma half-life: 2 hr. Metabolism: liver and kidneys. Excretion: metabolites, 35% in feces, 65% in urine. Therapeutic level: 10 to 18 mg/ml. Dialysis: unknown. Breast milk: yes.

Administration and dosage
Adult

PO—Initially, 25 mg 3 to 4 times daily, increasing the dosage by increments of 25 mg daily to a maximum of 150 to 200 mg daily. After the acute phase of the disease subsides, the dosage should be reduced until discontinued. Indomethacin should be administered with food, immediately after meals, or with antacids to reduce gastric irritation.

Pediatric

Do not use in patients under 14 years of age.

Nurse and patient considerations

* CNS effects are frequent. Headaches occurring 1 hr after administration and with increased severity in the morning are most common (25% to 50%). Patients also complain of dizziness, lightheadedness, and mental confusion. Patients should avoid activities requiring mental alertness, coordination, or judgment during the initiation of therapy.
* Indomethacin may adversely influence patients with psychiatric disorders and epilepsy. Use with caution in these patients.
* Gastrointestinal complaints include anorexia, nausea, vomiting, abdominal pain, and diarrhea. Indo-

methacin may initiate or reactivate ulcers of the stomach, esophagus, duodenum or small intestine. This ulcerogenic property appears to be unrelated to dosage. These complications may be minimized by administration with food or antacids.

* There are many other rare side effects caused by indomethacin that suppress bone marrow function and produce ophthalmic disorders, various dermatoses, hepatotoxicity, and hypersensitivity and warrant cessation of the drug.

* See General information on analgesia (p. 292).

Drug interactions

Concurrent administration with salicylates, phenylbutazone, other nonsteroidal antiinflammatory agents, or corticosteroids may enhance the ulcerogenic properties of indomethacin.

Caution must be used in patients receiving anticoagulants because of possible indomethacin-induced bleeding and possible displacement of oral anticoagulants from protein-binding sites.

Probenecid blocks the renal tubular secretion of indomethacin, resulting in the accumulation and prolongation of the half-life of indomethacin.

Indomethacin tends to cause accumulation of lithium by reducing renal excretion. Patients already receiving lithium should be observed for symptoms of toxicity (nausea, drowsiness, tremor, lethargy, speech difficulty) over the next 2 weeks. Monitoring plama lithium levels when adding or deleting indomethacin may help avoid inadequate therapy or toxicity.

Indomethacin and possibly other prostaglandin inhibitors inhibit the antihypertensive activity of propranolol (Inderal) and pindolol (Visken), resulting in loss of hypertensive control. The dosage of the beta blocker may need to be increased if long-term concomitant therapy is planned.

Indomethacin may impair the antihypertensive, although not the diuretic effects, of thiazide diuretics. Long-term concomitant use of nonsteroidal antiinflammatory agents may require an increase in dosage of the thiazide to maintain the antihypertensive effect.

Indomethacin may reduce the diuretic and antihypertensive effects of furosemide and thiazide diuretics. Monitor patients closely when adding or deleting indomethacin therapy.

Concomitant administration of indomethacin and triamterene results in a very significant reduction in renal creatinine clearance. Until more information is available concerning this potential drug interaction, it is preferable to avoid concomitant use of these agents.

Meclofenamate sodium
(Meclomen)

AHFS 28:08
CATEGORY Antiinflammatory,
Antipyretic analgesic

Action and use

Meclofenamate sodium is a nonsteroidal, antiinflammatory, antipyretic agent that is an anthranilic acid derivative, structurally related to mefenamic acid. As with other agents of this class, its mechanism of action is postulated to be the inhibition of prostaglandin synthetases, a series of enzymes necessary for the formation of prostaglandins that mediate inflammatory activity. It may also act by competing with prostaglandins at the binding site.

The antiinflammatory and analgesic effects of meclofenamate sodium are used to treat acute and chronic symptoms of rheumatoid arthritis and osteoarthritis. It is recommended that, because of the high incidence of gastrointestinal effects, meclofenamate sodium be used only in patients with symptoms of active inflammatory disease who have not received adequate relief from supportive measures and salicylate therapy.

Characteristics

Peak serum levels: 30 to 60 min. Protein binding: 99.8%. Half-life: single dose—0.6 to 2 hr; multiple doses—3.3 hr. Metabolism: many metabolites, one (hydroxymethyl) is active. Excretion: 70% to 80% in urine, minimal active drug; 20% to 30% excreted in feces. Dialysis: no, H, P. Breast milk: unknown.

Administration and dosage

NOTE: Do not administer to patients with hypersensitivity to aspirin or to those who have developed bronchospasm, urticaria, or rhinitis secondary to other nonsteroidal antiinflammatory agent therapy.

Adult

PO—The usual initial dose is 200 to 300 mg daily in 3 to 4 divided doses. Subsequent doses are adjusted to the patient's disease, response to therapy, and tolerance of side effects. Maximum daily dose should not exceed 400 mg. Symptoms start resolving within a few days, but 2 to 3 weeks of therapy may be necessary for optimum effects. After therapeutic goals have been achieved, doses should be retitrated to maintain therapeutic activity at the lowest dose. The frequency of gastrointestinal complaints may be reduced by administering with food, milk, or antacids.

Pediatric:

Not recommended for use in children under 14 years of age.

Nurse and patient considerations

* The most frequent adverse effects associated with meclofenamate sodium therapy are gastrointestinal complaints. Frequency of adverse effects are diarrhea 10 to 33% (4% required discontinuation of therapy), nausea with and without vomiting (11%), abdominal pain (3% to 9%) and other gastrointestinal disorders (10%), including constipation, flatulence, anorexia, stomatitis, GI bleeding, and peptic ulcer. These complications may be minimized by administration with food or milk.
* Side effects associated with the central nervous system include dizziness, headache, vertigo, lack of concentration, and confusion. Patients should be cautioned not to perform tasks requiring mental alertness or coordination until stabilized on therapy.
* Hematologic effects including leukocytosis, thrombocytopenia, leukopenia, and decreased hemoglobin and hematocrit levels have rarely been reported. Patients receiving long-term therapy should be monitored periodically.
* Other side effects associated with meclofenamate sodium therapy include rash, pruritus, urticaria, tinnitus, paresthesias, depression, and edema. Use with caution in patients with heart disease or hypertension.
* Meclofenamate sodium is fetotoxic and teratogenic in laboratory animals. Therapy is therefore not recommended in pregnancy.
* See General information on analgesia (p. 292).

Drug interactions

Meclofenamate sodium enhances the activity of warfarin (Coumadin). When administered to patients receiving warfarin, the dose of warfarin should be reduced to prevent hemorrhage.

Salicylates displace significant quantities of meclofenamate sodium from protein-binding sites. This causes more rapid excretion of meclofenamate sodium, but probably also enhances toxicity. Concomitant use of salicylates and meclofenamate sodium is not recommended.

Concurrent administration with other drugs such as corticosteroids that might potentiate adverse gastrointestinal effects should be discouraged.

Meperidine hydrochloride
(Demerol)

AHFS 28:08; C-II
CATEGORY Analgesic,
central narcotic

Action and use

Meperidine, like other narcotic analgesics, exerts its primary pharmacologic activity on the central nervous system. Therapeutic doses of meperidine produce analgesia, sedation, euphoria, and respiratory depression. Meperidine is recommended for the relief of moderate to severe pain and for preoperative analgesia (parenteral form only). Meperidine may also be used with caution in patients with gallbladder disease or pancreatitis, since in equianalgesic doses it causes less spasm of Oddi's sphincter or the biliary tract than morphine.

Characteristics

Onset: 10 min (IM). Peak analgesia: 30 to 50 min (IV). Duration: 2 to 4 hr. Protein binding: 40%; half-life. 5½ hr. Metabolism: PO—extensive first-pass effect to normeperidine. Excretion: 5% unchanged in urine. Therapeutic level: 60 μg/100 ml to 65 μg/100 ml. Toxic level: 200 μg/100 ml. Fatal level: 0.5 mg/100 to 3 mg/100 ml. Dialysis: unknown.

Administration and dosage
Adult

PO—50 to 150 mg every 3 to 4 hr.
IM—50 to 150 mg every 3 to 4 hr. Inject deeply, since

meperidine irritates subcutaneous tissue. Do not inject IM to anticoagulated patients or to those suspected of suffering a myocardial infarction.

IV—50 to 100 mg every 3 to 4 hr. Doses should be diluted and administered slowly. Severe tachycardia and hypotension may result. Side effects may also be diminished by having the patient in a recumbent position.

Pediatric

PO—1 to 2 mg/kg every 3 to 4 hr as needed. Do not exceed 100 mg/dose.

IM—As for PO administration.

SC—As for PO administration.

NOTE: Doses of meperidine should be reduced 25% to 50% when phenothiazines or other tranquilizers are to be administered concomitantly.

Nurse and patient considerations

* Adverse reactions are much the same as for morphine—dizziness, nausea, vomiting, and postural hypotension.
* Meperidine must be used with extreme caution in patients with chronic severe respiratory disease. Normal therapeutic doses may decrease respiratory drive while increasing airway resistance.
* Meperidine may precipitate or aggravate seizures in patients prone to convulsive activity.
* If meperidine is used as a postoperative analgesic, the patient must be encouraged to cough and deep-breathe, to ambulate with caution or assistance, and to change positions every 2 hr to prevent respiratory pooling. Offer additional forms of comfort, support, and interest.
* Repeated use may lead to tolerance, dependence, and addiction. Therefore evaluate the *patient's* response to the analgesic and suggest a change to milder analgesics when indicated.
* Use meperidine with caution as an obstetric analgesic. Meperidine crosses the placental barrier and may produce respiratory depression in newborn infants. Meperidine is excreted in breast milk of lactating women.

See General information on analgesia (p. 292).

Antidote

Nalorphine (Nalline) may be used to counteract the symptoms (particularly respiratory depression and hypotension) of excessive dosage of morphine, codeine, and meperidine. Dosage in the treatment of respiratory depression is 5 to 10 mg IV, repeated every 10 to 15 min if respirations remain depressed, but with a total dose not to exceed 40 mg.

Naloxone (Narcan), 0.4 mg (1 ml), may be administered IV, IM, or SC. If the desired degree of counteraction and improvement in respiratory function is not obtained immediately, the dose may be repeated at 2 to 3 min intervals (see Naloxone, p. 612).

Drug interactions

The depressant effects of meperidine are additive with those of general anesthetics, phenothiazines, tranquilizers, sedative-hypnotics, tricyclic antidepressants, antihistamines, and other CNS depressants, including alcohol. Respiratory depression, hypotension, and profound sedation or coma may result from this interaction unless the dose of meperidine has been reduced appropriately (usually by one third to half the normal dose).

A major metabolite of meperidine in normeperidine. Enzyme-inducing agents such as phenobarbital and phenytoin enhance the metabolism of meperidine to normeperidine. Chlorpromazine (and possibly other phenothiazines) also enhances normeperidine production. Patients receiving long-term, large oral doses of meperidine, those with renal impairment, and those with a highly acidic urine are predisposed to accumulating normeperidine. Evidence of toxic levels of normeperidine are seizures, tremors, and excitation.

Morphine sulfate

Action and use

AHFS 28:08; C-II
CATEGORY Analgesic,
central narcotic

Morphine is recommended for the relief of severe pain as a preanesthetic medication, for acute vascular occlusion, and to produce sleep in selected cases. It may also be quite effective in low doses to reduce anxiety and diminish venous return in acute pulmonary edema. Morphine has a biphasic action on the CNS. It sedates the cerebrum and has a mixture of stimulation and sedation on the medulla. In the medulla it sedates the respiratory center, emetic center, and the cough reflex. It also stimulates the chemoreceptor trigger zone in the medulla, which is responsible for the nausea and emesis noted as a side effect. The stimulation of the chemoreceptor trigger zone occurs before the sedative action on the emetic center.

Characteristics

Onset: immediate. Peak analgesia: 50 to 90 min (SC), 30 to 60 min (IM), and 20 min (IV). Duration: 4 to 5 hr. Metabolism primarily liver. Excretion: 90% in urine primarily as metabolites in 24 hr, 7% to 10% in feces. Therapeutic level: 0.01 mg/100 ml. Fatal level: 0.05 mg/100 ml to 0.4 mg/100 ml. Dialysis: unknown.

Administration and dosage
Adult

PO—10 to 30 mg every 4 hr as needed. There is great patient variation based on type of pain, age of pain, previous administration of opiates, and tolerance to side effects.

IM or SC—2 to 20 mg (10 mg average) every 4 hr. Do not inject IM to anticoagulated patients or to those suspected of suffering a myocardial infarction.

IV—2.5 to 16 mg diluted to 5 ml of saline solution. Inject slowly, observing patient's response (hypotension, respiratory depression).

Pediatric

SC—0.1 to 0.2 mg/kg. Do not exceed 15 mg.

IV—0.05 mg/kg. Inject slowly, observing patient's response (hypotension, respiratory depression).

Nurse and patient considerations

* The major hazards of narcotic analgesics are respiratory depression and, to a lesser degree, circulatory depression, respiratory arrest, shock, and cardiac arrest. Morphine renders the respiratory centers less responsive to increases in alveolar and serum P_{co2}. This may occur before either reduction in the respiratory rate or tidal volume is noticeable. Check the respiratory rate and depth frequently. Return to normal should occur within 3 to 4 hr.

* The most frequently observed adverse reactions include lightheadedness, dizziness, sedation, nausea, vomiting, and sweating. These effects seem to

> be more prominent in ambulatory patients and in
> those who are not suffering severe pain.
> * Use extreme caution in administration to patients
>   with head injuries, increased cerebrospinal pres-
>   sure, or decreased respiratory reserve.
> * Morphine may also cause constipation and urinary
>   retention.
> * Morphine is excreted in small amounts in human
>   breast milk.
> * See General information on analgesia (p. 292).

Antidote

Nalorphine (Nalline) is used to counteract the symptoms (particularly respiratory depression and hypotension)
of excess dosage of morphine, codeine, and meperidine.
Dosage in the treatment of respiratory depression is 5 to 10
mg IV, repeated every 10 to 15 min if respirations remain
depressed, but with a total dose not to exceed 40 mg.

Naloxone (Narcan), 0.4 mg (1 ml), can be administered
IV, IM, or SC. If the desired degree of counteraction and
improvement in respiratory function is not obtained immediately, the dose may be repeated at 2 to 3 min intervals (see
Naloxone, p. 612).

Drug interactions

The depressant effects of morphine are additive with
those of general anesthetics, phenothiazines, tranquilizers,
sedative-hypnotics, tricyclic antidepressants, antihistamines, and other CNS depressants, including alcohol.
Respiratory depression, hypotension, and profound sedation
or coma may result from this interaction unless the dose of
morphine has been reduced appropriately (usually by one
third to half the normal dose).

Nalbuphine hydrochloride
(Nubain)

AHFS 28:08
CATEGORY Analgesic

Action and use

Nalbuphine is a synthetic narcotic agonist-antagonist
that is structurally related to morphine and naloxone but has
pharmacologic properties similar to pentazocine and butor-

phanol. Analgesic activity is thought to be mediated through opiate receptors in the limbic system. Narcotic antagonistic effects may be due to competitive inhibition at the opiate receptor. Analgesic potency, on a milligram for milligram basis, is equal to morphine and 3 to 4 times more potent than pentazocine. The narcotic antagonist properties are about one fourth those of nalorphine (Nalline), but 10 times that of pentazocine. When administered to patients addicted to low doses (60 mg/day) of morphine, it precipitates narcotic withdrawal syndrome.

Nalbuphine is a respiratory depressant similar to equianalgesic doses of morphine. However, unlike morphine, nalbuphine's respiratory effects plateau out at about 30 mg, with no additional depression. Unlike butorphanol, the duration of depression produced by nalbuphine is not increased by increasing dosage. In contrast to pentazocine and butorphanol, nalbuphine does not produce an increase in cardiac index, pulmonary artery pressure, or cardiac work, and systemic blood pressure is not significantly altered.

Nalbuphine is recommended for the relief of moderate to severe acute and chronic pain associated with cancer, orthopedic disorders, renal or biliary colic, migraine or vascular headaches, preoperative analgesia, and obstetric and surgical analgesia. The potential for abuse is probably similar to that of pentazocine.

Characteristics

Onset: 15 min (IM, SC); 2 to 3 min (IV). Peak activity: 30 min (IM, SC); 30 min (IV). Duration: 2.5 to 5 hr (IM, SC, IV). Protein binding: minor. Half-life: 5 hr. Metabolism: liver. Excretion: fecal via biliary secretion; only 7% as unchanged drug and metabolites in urine. Dialysis: unknown. Breast milk: unknown.

Administration and dosage
Adult

sc, im, iv—Usual dose, 10 mg/70 kg every 3 to 6 hr as necessary. Adjustment is required, based on type and severity of pain, age, and clinical status. For those patients with no narcotic tolerance, the maximum single dose is 20 mg and the maximum daily dose is 160 mg.

Pediatric

Nalbuphine is currently not recommended for patients under 18 years of age.

Nurse and patient considerations

* The possibility that nalbuphine may cause respiratory depression should be considered in treatment of patients with bronchial asthma, obstructive respiratory conditions, cyanosis, or other respiratory depression from any other cause.
* The respiratory depressant effects of nalbuphine and its potential for elevating cerebrospinal fluid pressure may be markedly exaggerated in the presence of head injury, other intracranial lesions, or a preexisting increase in intracranial pressure. The use of nalbuphine can produce effects such as miosis that may obscure the clinical course of patients with head injuries.
* The most commonly reported adverse reactions are sedation (36%), nausea (6%), a clammy and sweaty sensation (9%), dizziness (5%), dry mouth (4%), and headache (3%).
* Nalbuphine may cause spasm of the sphincter of Oddi. Use with caution in patients with suspected gallbladder disease.
* Repeated use may lead to tolerance, dependence, and addiction. Abrupt discontinuance following extended use of nalbuphine may result in withdrawal symptoms. Evaluate the *patient's* response to the analgesic and suggest a change to milder analgesics when indicated.
* No teratogenic effects have been reported with nalbuphine, but it does cross the placental barrier. It should be administered with caution during pregnancy. Nalbuphine can produce respiratory depression in the neonate. It should be used with caution, especially in women delivering preterm infants.
* See General information on analgesia (p. 292).

Antidote

Naloxone (Narcan) is a specific antidote for nalbuphine. The usual adult dose is 0.4 mg (1 ml) administered IV, IM, or SC. If the desired degree of counteraction and improvement in respiratory function is not obtained immediately, the dose may be repeated at 2-to 3 min intervals (See Naloxone, p. 612).

Drug interactions

The depressant effects of nalbuphine are additive with those of general anesthetics, phenothiazines, tranquilizers, sedative-hypnotics, tricyclic antidepressants, antihistamines, and other CNS depressants, including alcohol. Respiratory depression, hypotension, and profound sedation or coma may result from this interaction unless the dose of nalbuphine has been reduced appropriately (usually by one third to one half the normal dose).

Although nalbuphine has narcotic antagonist activity, nalbuphine will not antagonize a narcotic analgesic administered to non-narcotic-dependent patients.

Pentazocine
(Talwin)

AHFS 28:08, C-IV
CATEGORY Analgesic

Action and use

Pentazocine is a synthetic compound structurally related to morphine, with a pharmacologic activity similar to nalbuphine and butorphanol. It has both narcotic agonist and weak opioid-antagonistic properties. A parenteral dose of 45 to 50 mg of pentazocine is approximately equivalent to 10 mg of morphine. An oral dose of 50 mg of pentazocine is equivalent to 60 mg of codeine.

The respiratory depressant effects of 20 mg of pentazocine are approximately equivalent to the effects of morphine, 10 mg. Unlike morphine, however, increasing the dose of pentazocine beyond 30 mg does not produce proportionate increases in respiratory depression.

The cardiovascular responses to pentazocine differ somewhat from those of morphine or codeine. Pentazocine, in high doses, causes an increase in blood pressure and heart rate. In patients with coronary artery disease, pentazocine elevates mean aortic pressure, left ventricular end diastolic pressure and mean pulmonary artery pressure, and causes an increase in cardiac work. Pentazocine is indicated for the relief of moderate to severe pain.

Characteristics

Peak plasma levels: 15 to 60 min (IM), 1 to 3 hr (PO). Duration: 5 hr (PO). Half-life: 2 hr. Metabolism: extensive variation among individuals. Excretion: 60% in urine in 24 hr, primarily as metabolites. Therapeutic level: 0.05 mg/100 ml. Toxic level: 0.2 mg/100 ml to 0.5 mg/100 ml. Fatal level: 0.3 mg/100 ml to 2 mg/100 ml. Dialysis: unknown.

Administration and dosage
Adult

PO—50 to 100 mg every 3 to 4 hr.

IM—30 to 60 mg every 3 to 4 hr. Do not administer IM to anticoagulated patients or those suspected of having a myocardial infarction.

IV—30 to 60 mg every 3 to 4 hr.

NOTE: Pentazocine is not recommended in children under 12 years of age.

Nurse and patient considerations

* The possibility that pentazocine may cause respiratory depression should be considered in treatment of patients with bronchial asthma, obstructive respiratory conditions, cyanosis, or other respiratory depression from any cause.
* The respiratory depressant effects of pentazocine and its potential for elevating cerebrospinal fluid pressure may be markedly exaggerated in the presence of head injury, other intracranial lesions, or a preexisting increase in intracranial pressure.
* The most commonly reported adverse reactions are nausea, dizziness or lightheadedness, vomiting, and euphoria.
* Pentazocine has weak narcotic antagonist activity. It does not antagonize the respiratory depression produced by morphine; however, when given to patients who have been receiving opiates on a regular basis, it may precipitate withdrawal symptoms.
* Use extreme caution in administration to patients with head injuries, increased cerebrospinal pressure, or decreased respiratory reserve.
* Pentazocine, when used in higher doses (50 mg IM), may elevate serum amylase levels, resulting from spasm of Oddi's sphincter.
* Seizures have occurred in association with the use of pentazocine in patients prone to convulsions. No direct cause-and-effect relationship has been found, however.
* Repeated use may lead to tolerance, dependence, and addiction. Abrupt discontinuance following extended use of pentazocine may result in withdrawal symptoms. Evaluate the *patient's* response

> to the analgesic and suggest a change to milder
> analgesics when indicated.
> * No teratogenic effects have been reported with pen-
> tazocine, but it does cross the placental barrier. It
> should be administered with caution during preg-
> nancy and delivery because both elevation and
> depression in fetal heart rate have occurred.
> * See General information on analgesia (p. 292).

Antidote

Nalorphine (Nalline) is not effective in antagonizing
pentazocine-induced respiratory depression.

Naloxone (Narcan) is a specific antidote for pentazocine. The usual adult dose is 0.4 mg (1 ml) administered IV,
IM, or SC. If the desired degree of counteraction and
improvement in respiratory function is not obtained immediately, the dose may be repeated at 2 to 3 min intervals (see
Naloxone, p. 612).

Drug interactions

The depressant effects of pentazocine are additive with
those of general anesthetics, phenothiazines, tranquilizers,
sedative-hypnotics, tricyclic antidepressants, antihistamines, and other CNS depressants, including alcohol.

Smokers metabolize pentazocine significantly more
rapidly than nonsmokers. Larger doses may be necessary to
gain adequate therapeutic response.

Phenylbutazone
(Azolid, Butazolidin)

AHFS 28:08
CATEGORY Antiinflammatory,
antipyretic, analgesic

Action and use

Phenylbutazone is a nonsteroidal, antiinflammatory,
antipyretic analgesic used for the symptomatic relief of gout,
rheumatoid arthritis, osteoarthritis, and rheumatoid spondylitis. It does not alter the course of the disease process. As a
result of many serious adverse effects it should be used only
after other drugs have failed. If significant improvement is
not observed within 7 days, it should be discontinued.

Characteristics

Peak blood levels: 2 hr. Protein binding: 98%. Plasma
half-life: 50 to 100 hr. Metabolized to oxyphenbutazone and

other active products. Excretion: 15% as metabolites in urine. Therapeutic level: 5 mg/100 ml to 15 mg/100 ml. Dialysis: unknown.

Administration and dosage
Adult

PO—300 to 600 mg daily in divided doses. Gastrointestinal side effects may be diminished by administering the dose with food or milk.

NOTE: Use of phenylbutazone is not recommended in children under 14 years of age and in senile, elderly patients. With patients 60 years of age and over, every effort must be made to discontinue the drug as soon as possible, especially after 7 days, because of the exceedingly high risk of potentially fatal reactions in this group. With all patients the goal of therapy should be short-term relief of severe symptoms with the smallest possible dose for the shortest administration time and course possible.

Nurse and patient considerations

* Known factors that increase the incidence of adverse reactions are age (over 40), weight, dosage, duration of therapy, concurrent diseases, and concurrent administration of other drugs.
* Serious and fatal blood dyscrasias, including agranulocytosis, aplastic anemia, and hemolytic anemia, have been reported. It is crucial that biweekly blood counts with differential are completed.
* Many gastrointestinal side effects have been attributed to phenylbutazone. These include creation and reactivation of ulcers, occult bleeding, nausea, vomiting, and abdominal distention.
* Phenylbutazone causes significant sodium and chloride retention that may result in congestive heart failure, edema, or hypertension in susceptible individuals. Check for signs of fluid retention in ankles, feet, and sacrum.
* Other complications include hypersensitivity reactions, various dermatoses, potentially fatal hepatitis, renal impairment, and visual disturbances.
* Phenylbutazone inhibits the thyroid uptake of iodine and may result in hypothyroidism.
* Phenylbutazone is not recommended in pregnant or nursing mothers. Teratogenic effects have been

noted in animals, and the drug is found in breast milk.
* See General information on analgesia (p. 292).

Drug interaction

Phenylbutazone displaces warfarin (Coumadin) from protein-binding sites, enhancing the anticoagulant activity of warfarin.

Phenylbutazone inhibits the metabolism of tolbutamide (Orinase) and acetohexamide (Dymelor) and may also displace tolbutamide from protein-binding sites, thus enhancing the hypoglycemic effects of these agents.

Phenytoin (Dilantin) metabolism may be inhibited by phenylbutazone, leading to phenytoin toxicities.

Phenylbutazone inhibits excretion of uric acid by high (5 g daily) doses of salicylates.

Piroxicam
(Feldene)

AHFS Unlisted
CATEGORY Antiinflammatory, antipyretic analgesic

Action and use

Piroxicam is a nonsteroidal, antiinflammatory, antipyretic agent that is an enolic acid derivative. Its mechanism of action is not completely known, but it is postulated to be an inhibitor of prostaglandin synthetases, a series of enzymes necessary for the formation of prostaglandins that mediate inflammatory activity.

The antiinflammatory and analgesic effects of piroxicam are used to treat acute and chronic symptoms of osteo-arthritis and rhematoid arthritis. It should be used only in patients with symptoms of active inflammatory disease who have not received adequate relief from supportive measures and salicylate therapy. Its primary advantage over other nonsteroidal antiinflammatory agents is its long half-life. It only needs to be administered once daily.

Characteristics

Peak serum levels: 3 to 5 hr. Steady state: 7 to 12 days. Protein binding: extensive. Half-life: 50 hrs; range—30 to 86 hr. Metabolism: extensive. Excretion: two-thirds in urine (5% unchanged drug); one-third in feces. Dialysis: unknown. Breast milk: unknown.

Administration dosage

NOTE: Do not administer to patients with hypersensitivity to aspirin or to those who have developed bronchospasm, urticaria, or rhinitis secondary to other nonsteroidal antiinflammatory agent therapy.

Adult

PO 1. 20 mg 1 time daily. If gastrointestinal irritation develops, the dose may be administered in 2 equally divided doses or with antacids. Although patients will notice symptomatic relief within a few days, the extent of therapeutic activity should not be fully assessed until after at least 2 weeks of therapy.

   2. Patients with renal impairment should be observed for signs of excessive accumulation and toxicity.

Pediatric

Not recommended for use in children.

Nurse and patient considerations

* The most frequent adverse effects associated with piroxicam therapy are gastrointestinal complaints (20%). Epigastric distress and nausea (3% to 6%), peptic ulceration (1%), stomatitis, constipation, diarrhea, abdominal pain, flatulence, and indigestion were reported. Of those patients experiencing gastrointestinal effects, 5% discontinued therapy.

* Other side effects reported include rash, headache, dizziness, malaise, thrombocytopenia, decreased hemoglobin and hematocrit levels, tinnitus, and edema (2%). Use with caution in patients with heart disease or hypertension.

* No teratogenic effects have been reported in laboratory animals or humans, but gastrointestinal tract toxicity was increased in pregnant females in the last trimester of pregnancy compared with nonpregnant females and females in earlier trimesters of pregnancy. Piroxicam therapy is not recommended in pregnant or nursing women.

* See General information on analgesia (p. 292).

Drug interactions

Salicylates displace significant quantities of piroxicam from protein-binding sites. This causes more rapid excretion of piroxicam but may also enhance toxicity. Concomitant use of salicylates and piroxicam is not recommended.

Concurrent administration with other drugs such as corticosteroids that may potentiate adverse gastrointestinal effects should be discouraged.

Drug interactions with warfarin (Coumadin) have not been reported, but patients receiving concomitant therapy should be monitored closely for enhanced hypoprothrombinemic effects and hemorrhage.

Propoxyphene hydrochloride
(Darvon)

AHFS 28:08
CATEGORY Central Analgesic

Action and use

Propoxyphene is a synthetic analgesic that acts on the central system for pain relief. Propoxyphene has no antipyretic or antiinflammatory activity. It is used for the relief of mild to moderate pain. Clinical studies indicate that 65 mg of propoxyphene may have equivalent analgesic strength to 60 mg of codeine or 650 mg of aspirin. Greater pain relief may be attained when used in combination with aspirin, phenacetin, or acetaminophen.

Characteristics

Onset: 1 hr. Peak plasma levels: 2 hr. Biologic half-life: 3½ to 4 hr. Therapeutic serum levels: 0.05 to 0.2 µg/ml. Toxic serum levels: 1 to 10 µg/ml. Dialysis: minimally effective.

Administration and dosage

PO—65 mg every 4 to 6 hr.
NOTE: Propoxyphene is not recommended in children.

Nurse and patient considerations

* Side effects of propoxyphene include gastrointestinal disturbances, headache, dizziness, somnolence, and skin rashes.

* Tolerance and psychologic and physical dependence have been reported.
* Symptoms of acute overdose are similar to those of acute narcotic intoxication. These include coma, respiratory depression, pulmonary edema, circulatory collapse, and convulsions. Symptoms may be complicated by salicylism if combination products are consumed.
* See General information on analgesia (p. 292).

Antidote

Naloxone (Narcan), 0.4 mg (1 ml), may be administered IV, IM, or SC. If the desired degree of counteraction and improvement in respiratory function is not obtained immediately, the dose may be repeated at 2 to 3 min intervals (see Naloxone, p. 612).

For respiratory depression administer nalorphine (Nalline), 5 to 10 mg IV. Repeat the dose every 10 to 15 min if respirations remain depressed, but with a total dose not to exceed 40 mg.

Drug interactions

Orphenadrine (Norflex, Disipal) and propoxyphene may cause mental confusion, anxiety, and tremors if used together.

Patients receiving carbamazepine and propoxyphene concurrently should be monitored closely for signs of carbamazepine toxicity (dizziness, nausea, drowsiness, and headache). Propoxyphene inhibits metabolism of carbamazepine, causing a significant increase in serum levels. Carbamazepine dosages usually need to be reduced.

Zomepirac sodium
(Zomax)

AHFS 28:08
CATEGORY Antiinflammatory, antipyretic analgesic

Action and use

Zomepirac is a nonsteroidal, antiinflammatory, antipyretic agent that is a arylacetic acid derivative, structurally related to tolmetin and indomethacin. As with other agents of this class, its mechanism of action is postulated to be the inhibition of prostaglandin synthetases, a series of enzymes necessary for the formation of prostaglandins that mediate inflammatory activity.

Zomepirac was developed primarily for its analgesic properties. Whereas the other agents of this class have analgesic potency equivalent to aspirin, studies indicate that 50 mg of zomepirac is comparable in analgesic potency to 650 mg of aspirin, and 100 mg of zomepirac (PO) is more effective than 60 mg of codeine (PO) or 8 mg of morphine (IM). It is recommended for use in mild to moderately severe pain associated with dental surgery, orthopedic disorders, cancer, and osteoarthritis. Long-term studies show no evidence of tolerance or addiction to zomepirac.

Characteristics

Onset: 30 min. Peak serum levels: 1 to 2 hr. Duration: 4 to 6 hr. Protein binding: 98%. Kinetics change with multiple dosing. Half-life: single-dose—4 hr; multiple doses for 3 weeks—9 to 10 hr. Metabolism: liver, other; multiple metabolites. Excretion: 20% unchanged in urine; passive tubular reabsorption dependent on acidic media. Dialysis: no, H. Breast milk: unknown.

Administration and dosage

NOTE: Do not administer to patients with hypersensitivity to aspirin or to those who have developed bronchospasm, urticaria, or rhinitis secondary to other nonsteroidal antiinflammatory agent therapy.

Adult

PO 1. Mild pain: 50 mg every 4 to 6 hr.
 2. Moderately severe pain: 100 mg every 4 to 6 hr. Maximum daily dose should not exceed 600 mg. Dosages should be reduced in patients with impaired renal function.
 3. Antacids may be used if gastrointestinal symptoms occur.

Pediatric

Not recommended for use in children.

Nurse and patient considerations

* The most frequent adverse effects associated with zomepirac therapy are gastrointestinal complaints. Nausea is most common (6% on short-term therapy, 12% on long-term therapy). Abdominal pain, diarrhea, gastrointestinal distress, dyspepsia, constipation, flatulence, and vomiting have been reported with a frequency of 3% to 9%. Other gastrointestinal effects reported include gastritis, peptic ulcer, GI bleeding, and stomatitis. These complications may be minimized by administration with food or antacids.

* Other adverse effects reported with a frequency of 3% to 9% include dizziness, insomnia, edema, elevated blood pressure, rash, and asthenia. Use with caution in patients with heart disease or hypertension.
* Patients treated with zomepirac for longer than 2 months are at greater risk (6.8%) for developing urinary tract signs and symptoms of dysuria, cystitis, frequency, hematuria, pyuria, and urinary tract infections. The mechanism of this activity is unknown. It is recommended that patients who require zomepirac therapy for longer than 6 months have renal function monitored periodically.
* Two 2-year studies in laboratory animals reported an increased frequency in the development of adrenal medullary tumors. No potential for teratogenicity has been reported. Because of the possibility of tumorigenicity and long-term effects on the urinary system, zomepirac therapy is not recommended in children or pregnant or nursing patients.
* See General information on analgesia (p. 292).

Drug interactions

Although zomepirac does not displace warfarin from protein-binding sites and does not alter the prothrombin time, it should be used with caution in patients receiving anticoagulants because zomepirac does inhibit platelet adhesiveness and can induce gastrointestinal bleeding.

Salicylates displace significant quantities of zomepirac from protein-binding sites. This interaction may enhance therapeutic activity, but it probably induces greater toxicity as well. Therefore concomitant use of aspirin and zomepirac is not recommended.

Concurrent administration with other drugs such as corticosteroids that might potentiate adverse gastrointestinal effects should be discouraged.

Do not administer with sodium bicarbonate. Alkalinization of the urine significantly reduces renal reabsorption, decreasing the duration of therapeutic activity.

Table 8-1. Nonsteroidal antiinflammatory agents

Drug	Peak level (hr)	Protein binding (%)	Half-life (hr)	Excretion	Dosage[a]	Notes*
ANTHRANILIC ACID DERIVATIVES						
Mefenamic acid (Ponstel)	2-4	Unknown	2	Urine and feces as active drug and metabolites	PO Mild to moderate pain: 500 mg initially, followed by 250 mg every 6 hr. Maximum daily dose: 1 g.	1. Therapy should not exceed 7 days. 2. Use with caution in patients with a history of kidney or liver disease.

*Nurse and patient considerations

1. Do not administer to patients with hypersensitivity to aspirin or to those who have developed bronchospasm, urticaria, or rhinitis secondary to other nonsteroidal antiinflammatory agents.

2. Use extreme caution with patients who have a history of ulcer disease or GI bleeds. All these agents induce bleeding or exacerbate existing bleeds. All these agents are inhibitors of platelet aggregation to varying degrees.

3. All agents may be administered with antacids, food, or milk to reduce gastric irritation.

4. All agents produce varying degrees of peripheral edema. Use with caution in patients with heart disease or hypertension.

5. All agents may potentially induce renal papillary necrosis. Patients receiving long-term therapy should have renal function monitored periodically.

6. Concomitant administration of aspirin significantly reduces serum levels of these agents, while possibly potentiating toxicity. Do not administer concurrently with aspirin.

Continued.

Table 8-1. Nonsteroidal antiinflammatory agents—cont'd

Drug	Peak level (hr)	Protein binding (%)	Half-life (hr)	Excretion	Dosage[4]	Notes*
						3. Enhances anticoagulant effects of warfarin.
						4. False positive urine bilirubin test when the Diazo tablet test is used.
						5. See Meclofenamate sodium (p. 312).
Meclofenamate sodium (Meclomen) (See p. 312)						

ARYLACETIC ACID DERIVATIVES

| Fenoprofen (Nalfon) | 2 | 99 | 3 | 3% excreted unchanged in urine | PO | Analgesia: 200 mg every 4 to 6 hr as needed. Rheumatoid and osteoarthritis: initially, 600 mg 4 times daily; increase every few days by response and tolerance. Do not exceed 3.2 g/day. | 1. Use with caution in patients with renal disease. Patients may develop dysuria, cystitis, hematuria, allergic nephritis, and nephrotic syndrome.
2. Phenobarbital induces metabolism of fenoprofen.
3. Fenoprofen enhances anticoagulant effects of warfarin.
4. See Ibuprofen (p. 307). |

Continued.

Table 8-1. Nonsteroidal antiinflammatory agents—cont'd

Drug	Peak level (hr)	Protein binding (%)	Half-life (hr)	Excretion	Dosage[4]		Notes*
Ibuprofen (Motrin) (see p. 307) Indomethacin (Indocin) (see p. 309) Naproxen (Naprosyn)	2-4	99	13	10% excreted unchanged in urine	PO	Musculoskeletal and soft tissue inflammation: initially, 250 to 375 mg every 12 hr; do not exceed 1 g/day. Acute gout: initially, 750 mg followed by 250 mg every 8 hr.	1. Do not administer concurrently to patients receiving Naproxen sodium (Anaprox). 2. Use with caution in patients with renal disease.

					Dosage	
					Juvenile arthritis: 10 mg/kg in 2 divided doses. Mild to moderate pain and primary dysmenorrhea: initially, 500 mg, then 250 mg every 6 to 8 hr; do not exceed 1250 mg/day.	3. Naproxen enhances anticoagulant effects of warfarin. 4. Probenecid elevates serum levels and prolongs half-life of naproxen. 5. See Ibuprofen (p. 307).
		10% excreted unchanged in urine	13	PO	Mild to moderate pain and primary dysmenorrhea: initially, 550 mg followed by 275 mg every 6 to 8 hr; do not exceed 1375 mg/day.	1. Do not administer concurrently to patients receiving Naproxen (Naprosyn). 2. As for Naproxen, above.

ANTHRANILIC ACID DERIVATIVES

Naproxen sodium (Anaprox)	1-2	99				

Continued.

Table 8-1. Nonsteroidal antiinflammatory agents—cont'd

Drug	Peak level (hr)	Protein binding (%)	Half-life (hr)	Excretion	Dosage[4]	Notes*
					Musculoskeletal and soft tissue inflammation: initially, 275 mg every 12 hr; do not exceed 1100 mg/day. Acute gout: initially, 825 mg, followed by 275 mg every 8 hr.	
Sulindac (Clinoril)	Unknown	Sulindac, 93; sulfide metabolite, 98	Sulindac, 7.8; sulfide metabolite, 16.4	Active sulfide metabolite: 50% renal, 25% fecal excretion	PO Rheumatoid and osteoarthritis, ankylosing spondylitis: initially, 150 mg every 12 hr; do not exceed 400 mg/day.	1. Use with caution in patients with hepatic and renal disease. 2. Probenecid has only a slight effect

| Tolmetin sodium (Tolectin) | 0.5 to 1 | 99 | 1 | 20% excreted unchanged in urine; remainder as inactive | PO | Rheumatoid and osteoarthritis: initially, 400 mg 3 times/day; effective range is 600 to 1800 mg/day. Juvenile arthritis: start at 20 mg/kg/day in 3 to 4 divided doses; effective range is 15 to 30 mg/kg/day. | on sulfide levels, while plasma levels of sulindac are significantly increased. 3. See Indomethacin (p. 309). 1. Use with caution in patients with impaired renal function. 2. Do not use in acute gout attacks. It is not effective. Acute shoulder tendonitis, acute gouty arthritis: 200 mg every 12 hr; reduce dosage according to response. |

Continued.

Table 8-1. Nonsteroidal antiinflammatory agents—cont'd

Drug	Peak level (hr)	Protein binding (%)	Half-life (hr)	Excretion	Dosage[4]	Notes*
						3. Metabolites may give false-positive results for urine protein when the sulfosalicylate method is used. No interference is seen with Albustix or Uristix.
						4. See Indomethacin (p. 309).
Zomepirac sodium (Zomax) (see p. 328)						
ENOLIC ACID DERIVATIVES						
Piroxicam (Feldene) (see p. 324)						

CHAPTER NINE

Sedative-hypnotic agents

GENERAL INFORMATION ON SEDATIVE-HYPNOTICS

Sleep is a naturally occurring phenomenon that occupies about one third of an adult's life. What constitutes optimal or *sound* sleep has been frequently debated and is a highly individual matter, but *adequate* sleep is important. Natural sleep is a rhythmic progression through stages that provide physical rest and psychic equilibrium. Stages I and II are light sleep periods that allow easy arousal. Stage III is a transition from the lighter to the deeper state of sleep, stage IV. These first four stages of sleep are called nonrapid eye movement (NREM) sleep. Stage V is referred to as rapid eye movement (REM) sleep, during which rapid eye movements occur, muscle tension increases, and most dreaming occurs. All stages of sleep are irregularly interrupted by REM sleep, which is thought to provide a psychic release of anxiety and tension.

Unfortunately, many of the details of what constitutes *normal* sleep are unknown. Normal sleep patterns may be altered by anxiety, pain, environmental conditions, physical exhaustion, forced awakenings, and drugs.

The ideal sedative-hypnotic agent should induce and maintain sleep as naturally as possible, that is, rapid induction of stages I, II, and III without significantly diminishing the time of stages IV or V. Frequently the most commonly used sedative-hypnotics increase total sleeping time, especially in stages III and IV (NREM) sleep; however, they also decrease the number of REM periods and the total time in REM sleep. When REM sleep is decreased, there is a strong tendency to "make it up." Compensatory REM sleep seems to occur even when hypnotics are used for only 3 or 4 days.

After chronic administration of sedative-hypnotic agents, REM rebound may be severe, accompanied by restlessness and vivid nightmares. Depending on the frequency of hypnotic administration, normal sleep patterns may not be restored for weeks. It is suspected that the effects of REM rebound may enhance chronic use and dependence of these agents by the patient to avoid the unpleasant consequences of rebound.

A primary responsibility of patient care is to provide a resting and relaxing environment, and sleep is a major part of hospital therapy. Hypnotic agents should not be forced on patients ("a good patient is a quiet patient"), but patients should be aware that sleeping medication is available. Treatment should be continued only on an intermittent basis and the smallest dose suitable for obtaining the desired effects should be used.

Nurse and patient considerations

Individual responses vary. Discuss with the patient the quality and quantity of sleep to assess whether adjustments in dosage and/or medication are indicated.

Irritation to the gastric mucosa and aftertaste may be minimized by administration with fruit juice, milk, or a bedtime snack if dietary requirements allow this.

Safety measures, such as siderails and assistance with ambulation, should be implemented shortly after ingestion. Hypnotic doses often have a rapid onset of action, resulting in transient dizziness and excitation. This occurs most frequently when administered on an empty stomach or to an ambulating patient.

Patients may complain of "morning hangover," drowsiness, blurred vision, and transient hypotension on arising. Explain to the patient the need for arising first to a sitting position, equilibrating, and then standing. Again, assistance with ambulation may be required. If "hangover" becomes troublesome, there should be a reduction in dosage and/or change in medication.

These drugs are psychologically and/or physiologically habit-forming. Withdrawal after long-term use may produce symptoms of anxiety, insomnia, tremors, vivid dreams, agitation, and confusion. Use as many natural aids as possible (for example, a relaxing backrub, a warm cup of milk, a quiet and soothing environment, a clean body and bed) to help produce relaxation and sleep.

Therapeutic, toxic, and fatal blood levels listed in the characteristics section of each monograph are much lower when more than one CNS depressant (for example, alcohol, tranquilizers, antihistamines, anesthetics, narcotics) have been ingested.

GENERAL INFORMATION ON BARBITURATES

The barbiturates are a class of structurally related chemicals that may reversibly depress the activity of all excitable tissues. The central nervous system is particularly sensitive, but the degrees of depression (ranging from mild sedation to deep coma and death) depend on the dosage, route of administration, tolerance from previous use, degree of excitability of the central nervous system at the time of administration, and condition of the patient. Usual hypnotic doses produce mild respiratory depression similar to that of natural sleep; with large doses, the rate, depth, and volume of respiration are markedly diminished.

Barbiturate-induced sleep varies from normal sleep by decreased REM time. With chronic administration of hypnotic doses, the amount of REM sleep gradually returns to normal as tolerance develops to the REM suppressant effect. When barbiturate therapy is discontinued, a rebound increase in REM sleep occurs in spite of the tolerance. Irregularities in REM sleep cycles may take weeks to fully dissipate.

Barbiturates are recommended primarily for their sedative and hypnotic effects. Some of the intermediate (secobarbital, pentobarbital) and long-acting (phenobarbital) barbiturates are also used for their anticonvulsant activity. The ultrashort-acting (methohexital, thiopental) agents may be administered IV as general anesthetics.

Nurse and patient considerations

General adverse effects of barbiturates include drowsiness, lethargy, headache, muscle or joint pain, and mental depression. Barbiturate "hangover" frequently occurs after administration of hypnotic doses or with long-term anticonvulsant therapy. Patients may display dulled affect, subtle distortion of mood, and impaired coordination.

Elderly patients and those in severe pain may respond paradoxically to barbiturates with excitement, euphoria, restlessness, and confusion.

Hypersensitivity reactions to barbiturates are infrequent, but the sequelae are quite serious and potentially fatal. Barbiturate therapy should be discontinued immediately if the patient develops symptoms of hypersensitivity, including high fever, inflammation of mucous membrane, or any type of dermatitis.

Blood dyscrasias have been attributed to barbiturate administration. Blood counts should be repeated periodically during long-term therapy. The patient should be reminded to report symptoms, including sore throat, easy bruisability, fever, or petechiae.

Barbiturates readily cross the placental barrier, appearing in fetal circulation. They are also present in breast milk. Neonates and nursing infants whose mothers receive barbiturates must be observed for signs of toxicity.

See General information on sedative-hypnotics (p. 339).

Treatment of overdosage

General management should consist of symptomatic and supportive therapy, including gastric lavage, administration of IV fluids, and maintenance of blood pressure, body temperature, and adequate respiratory exchange.

Forced diuresis enhances excretion of all barbiturates, and alkalinization of the urine (pH = 7.5) further enhances the excretion of phenobarbital.

Barbiturate abuse

The habitual use of barbiturates may result in physical dependence. Rapid discontinuance of barbiturates after long-term use of high dosages may result in symptoms similar to alcohol withdrawal. They may vary from weakness and anxiety to delirium and grand mal seizures. Treatment consists of cautious and gradual withdrawal of barbiturates over a 2- to 4-week period.

Drug interactions

The CNS depressant effects of antihistamines, analgesics, anesthetics, tranquilizers, and sedative-hypnotics may be potentiated by the barbiturates.

Barbiturates, especially phenobarbital, may induce hepatic microsomal enzymes enhancing the metabolism of warfarin (Coumadin), digitoxin, corticosteroids (prednisone), propranolol (Inderal), doxycycline (Vibramycin), phenytoin (Dilantin), and chlorpromazine (Thorazine). If the barbiturate is discontinued, the patient must be observed closely for signs of secondary drug toxicity requiring reduction of dosage.

Disulfiram (Antabuse) and valproic acid (Depakene) inhibit metabolism of barbiturates, leading to potential barbiturate toxicity.

MAO inhibitors (isocarboxazid [Marplan], pargyline hydrochloride [Eutonyl], tranylcypromine sulfate [Parnate]) may inhibit the metabolism of barbiturates, resulting in prolonged barbiturate effects. Barbiturate dosage reduction may be required.

Barbiturates, especially phenobarbital, may induce

hepatic microsomal enzymes, enhancing the metabolism of the estrogens contained in oral contraceptives. Cases have been reported whereby patients have developed spotting and breakthrough bleeding, especially when using the oral contraceptives with lower estrogen content. If bleeding should occur, a change in oral contraceptives and the use of alternative forms of contraception should be considered.

Phenobarbital
(Luminal, Eskabarb)

AHFS 28:12, 28:24; C-IV
CATEGORY Sedative-hypnotic, anticonvulsant

Action and use

Phenobarbital is a long-acting barbiturate used as a daytime sedative and as an adjunct in the prophylactic management of epilepsy.

Characteristics

Onset: 2 to 3 hr (PO). Peak blood levels: 8 to 12 hr. Protein binding: 40% to 60%. Half-life: 2 to 6 days. Metabolism: hydroxylation in liver to inactive forms. Excretion: 10% to 25% unchanged in urine, 75% as inactive metabolites. Therapeutic level: 1 mg/100 ml to 2.5 mg/100 ml. Toxic level: 4 mg/100 ml to 6 mg/100 ml. Fatal levels: 8 mg/100 ml to 11 mg/100 ml. Dialysis: yes, H, P (only 25% as effective as hemodialysis).

Administration and dosage
Adult

PO 1. Sedation: 30 to 120 mg daily in 3 to 4 divided doses.
2. Hypnosis: 100 to 320 mg.
3. Anticonvulsant: 100 to 200 mg usually given at bedtime.

IM—As for PO administration.

IV—As for PO administration. Administer at a rate no greater than 60 mg/min. Monitor the respiratory rate and blood pressure closely and administer with extreme caution to patients with respiratory disease.

Pediatric

PO 1. Sedation: 2 to 3 mg/kg every 8 hr.
2. Hypnosis: 6 to 10 mg/kg.
3. Anticonvulsant—status epilepticus: initially, 5 to 8 mg/kg, then 3 to 4 mg/kg every 5 min until seizures stop.

4. Maintenance: 5 to 10 mg/kg/day divided into 4 doses.

IM—As for PO administration

IV—As for PO administration. Administer at a rate no greater than 60 mg/min. Monitor the respiratory rate and blood pressure closely.

Nurse and patient considerations

* See General information on barbiturates (p. 341).
* Phenobarbital may produce paradoxic excitement and hyperactivity in children.
* Alkalinization of the urine and forced diuresis significantly increase the excretion of phenobarbital.

Drug interactions

See General information on barbiturates (p. 341).

Secobarbital
(Seconal)

AHFS 28:24; C-III
CATEGORY Sedative-hypnotic

Action and use

Secobarbital is a short-acting barbiturate used as a sedative-hypnotic and as an anesthetic in the control of acute convulsive conditions such as status epilepticus, tetanus, and toxic reactions to strychnine.

Characteristics

Onset: 10 to 30 min (PO). Duration: 6 to 8 hr. Half-life: 20 to 28 hr. Metabolism: liver. Therapeutic level: 0.1 mg/100 ml to 0.5 mg/100 ml to 0.5 mg/100 ml. Toxic level: 1 mg/100 ml to 3 mg/100 ml. Fatal level: 3 mg/100 ml to 5 mg/100 ml. Dialysis; no, H, P; however, dialyzable as a poison.

Administration and dosage
Adult

PO—Hypnosis: 100 mg at bedtime.

Preoperatively: 200 to 300 mg 1 to 2 hr before surgery.

NOTE: When secobarbital sodium is being prepared for parenteral administration, use sterile water for injection as a diluent. Do not use if the solution is not absolutely clear within 5 min of reconstitution. As a result of instability, use within 30 min of opening the ampule.

IM—Doses exceeding 250 mg are not recommended. After deep IM injection the patient should be watched closely for 20 to 30 min to ensure that respiratory depression does not develop.

IV—Injections should not exceed 50 mg/15 sec intervals. Rapid administration may cause respiratory depression, apnea, laryngospasm, vasodilatation, and hypotension.

RECTAL—120 to 200 mg.

Pediatric

PO 1. Sedation: 2 mg/kg/day in 4 divided doses.
2. Hypnosis: 6 mg/kg.
3. Preoperatively: 50 to 100 mg 1 to 2 hr before surgery.

To 6 months of age

RECTAL—15 to 60 mg.

Ages 6 months to 3 years

RECTAL—60 mg.

Over 3 years of age

RECTAL—60 to 120 mg.

Nurse and patient considerations

* See General information on barbiturates (p. 341).

Drug interactions

See General information on barbiturates (p. 341).

Chloral hydrate
(Noctec, Somnos)

AHFS 28:24; C-IV
CATEGORY Sedative-hypnotic

Action and use

Chloral hydrate is rapidly metabolized to trichlorethanol, which is believed to cause the CNS depression seen with this product. Chloral hydrate is used as a nocturnal sedative and does not have any specific restrictions as to the type of patient, other than those who should not receive any CNS depressant. Suppression of REM sleep occur at doses greater than 800 to 1000 mg.

Characteristics

Onset: 15 to 30 min. Duration: 5 to 8 hr. Half-life (trichloroethanol): 8 hr. Metabolism: chloral hydrate is rapidly metabolized by alcohol dehydrogenase to trichloroethanol, which is subsequently conjugated and excreted in the feces and urine. Therapeutic level: 1 mg/100 ml. Toxic level: 10 mg/100 ml. Fatal level: 10 mg/100 ml to 25 mg/100 ml. Dialysis: yes, H.

Administration and dosage
Adult

PO—500 mg to a maximum of 2 g.

Pediatric

PO 1. Sedative: 8 mg/kg 3 times daily (maximum dose: 1500 mg daily).
    2. Hypnosis: 50 mg/kg to a single maximum dose of 1 g.

NOTE: Chloral hydrate should be administered well diluted with milk, water, or fruit juices to minimize irritation and mask an aftertaste.

Nurse and patient considerations

* The habitual use of chloral hydrate may result in physical dependence and addiction similar to that of alcohol. Sudden withdrawal may result in delirium.
* Allergic reactions, although rare, include erythema, urticaria, and dermatitis. The eruption usually begins on the face or back and spreads to the neck, chest, and arms. The dermatitis may occur soon after administration or as long as 10 days after administration.
* Large doses may produce false-positive results with Clinitest tablets.
* Chloral hydrate passes the placental barrier and is excreted in breast milk.
* See General information on sedative-hypnotics (p. 339).

Drug interactions

Trichloroacetic acid, a major metabolite of chloral hydrate, displaces warfarin from protein-binding sites, thereby increasing anticoagulant activity and lengthening the prothrombin time. This reaction is potentially more significant in patients stabilized on warfarin therapy when chloral hydrate therapy is being initiated.

Ethanol may significantly potentiate the sedative action of chloral hydrate.

Chloral hydrate may be potentiated by other CNS depressants such as phenothiazines, narcotics, barbiturates, antihistamines, and antidepressants.

Ethchlorvynol
(Placidyl)

AHFS 28:24; C-IV
CATEGORY Sedative-hypnotic

Action and use

Ethchlorvynol is a nonbarbiturate CNS depressant with a rapid onset and short duration of action. It is used as a hypnotic agent in the short-term management of insomnia.

Characteristics

Onset: 15 to 30 min. Peak plasma levels: 1 to 1½ hr. Duration: 5 hr. Protein binding: minimal. Half-life: biphasic-distribution phase—5 to 6 hr; elimination phase—70 hr. Metabolism: liver, possibly kidneys, activity of metabolites unknown. Excretion: negligible amounts in urine unchanged. Therapeutic level: 0.2 mg/100 ml to 1.5 mg/100 ml. Toxic level: 2 mg/100 ml. Fatal level: 10 mg/100 ml to 15 mg/100 ml. Dialysis: yes, H,P.

Administration and dosage
Adult

PO—500 mg to 1 g at bedtime. Ethchlorvynol should be administered with food or milk to help prevent aftertaste, transient giddiness, dizziness, and ataxia.

NOTE: Ethchlorvynol is not recommended in children.

Nurse and patient considerations

* Chronic use of ethchlorvynol may result in physical and psychologic dependence. Sudden discontinuance may result in withdrawal symptoms similar to delirium tremens.
* Mild "hangover" effects from the drug are relatively common.

> * Due to rapid onset of action (15 to 20 min), side effects (dizziness, giddiness, ataxia) are likely to occur before the induction of sleep. Safety measures such as maintenance of bedrest, siderails, and observation should be implemented during this period.
> * Ethchlorvynol administration is not recommended during the first and second trimesters of pregnancy.
> * See General information on sedative-hypnotics (p. 339).

Drug interactions

Ethchlorvynol may enhance the metabolism of oral anticoagulants, such as warfarin (Coumadin), resulting in a decreased prothrombin time. Use particular caution when discontinuing ethchlorvynol with patients receiving oral anticoagulants.

Transient delirium has been reported with the combination of amitriptyline (Elavil) and ethchlorvynol.

Ethchlorvynol may be potentiated by other CNS depressants such as alcohol, phenothiazines, narcotics, barbiturates, and antihistamines.

Flurazepam
(Dalmane)

AHFS 28:24; C-IV
CATEGORY Hypnotic

Action and use

Flurazepam is a benzodiazepine derivative used specifically for inducing and maintaining sleep. It may be effective in those patients who have difficulty falling asleep, those patients with frequent awakenings and/or early morning awakenings, and in those patients with acute or chronic medical situations where restful sleep is essential. Laboratory data indicate that doses of 30 mg or less generally do not alter REM sleep, or cause rebound on withdrawal of the drug. Doses of 60 mg do inhibit REM sleep, but again, there appears to be no rebound on discontinuance of therapy. A disadvantage of flurazepam therapy is that, because of its long half-life, there is occasional "hangover" with notable impairment of performance the next day.

Characteristics

Onset: 20 to 45 min. Duration: 6 to 8 hr. Half-life: active metabolites—50 to 100 hr. Metabolism: liver. Excretion: renal. Dialysis: unknown.

Administration and dosage
Adult

PO—15 to 30 mg at bedtime. It is recommended that elderly and debilitated patients start with 15 mg at bedtime to determine response.

Pediatric

The use of flurazepam is not recommended in patients under 15 years of age.

Nurse and patient considerations

* See General information on benzodiazepines (p. 358).
* Overdosage may be manifested by somnolence, confusion, coma, and respiratory depression. Treatment consists of general physiologic and supportive measures including maintenance of an airway and administration of oxygen. Methylphenidate (Ritalin) or caffeine may be used for severe CNS or respiratory depression. Do not use barbiturates in patients who develop excitation after ingestion of flurazepam.
* See General information on sedative-hypnotics (p. 339).

Drug interactions

See General information on benzodiazepines (p. 358).

Glutethimide
(Doriden)

AHFS 28:24; C-III
CATEGORY Sedative-hypnotic

Action and use

Glutethimide is a nonbarbiturate hypnotic used for insomnia of short-term duration. Its mechanism of CNS depression is unknown, but is thought to be similar to that of the barbiturates. It, too, suppresses REM sleep but will not diminish the number of nocturnal awakenings or prolong the total sleeping time. It also appears to lose its effectiveness after a few weeks of continual administration.

Characteristics

Onset: 30 min. Duration: 4 to 8 hr. Protein binding: 50%. Half-life: 10 hr. Metabolism: almost complete. Excretion: urine and feces, inactive. Dialysis: no, H, P.

Administration and dosage

PO   1. Daytime sedation: 125 to 250 mg 3 times daily after meals.
      2. Hypnosis: 500 mg at bedtime.

NOTE: Total daily dosages above 1 g are not recommended. Glutethimide is not recommended in children under 12 years of age.

Nurse and patient considerations

* Chronic use of glutethimide may result in physical and psychologic dependence. Sudden discontinuance may result in withdrawal symptoms that include nausea, abdominal discomfort, tremors, and delirium.
* General adverse effects include nausea, vomiting, headache, dizziness, confusion, and generalized skin rash. Anticholinergic effects of blurred vision, constipation, dry mouth, and tenacious secretions are also occasionally seen.
* Glutethimide must be used with caution in pregnancy. Newborn infants of mothers dependent on glutethimide may also exhibit withdrawal symptoms.
* See General information on sedative-hypnotics (p. 339).

Drug interactions

Glutethimide enhances the metabolism of warfarin (Coumadin) by induction of hepatic microsomal enzymes. Use particular caution when discontinuing glutethimide in patients stabilized on oral anticoagulants.

Patients receiving tricyclic antidepressants and glutethimide concurrently may display additive anticholinergic effects.

Glutethimide may be potentiated by other CNS depressants such as alcohol, phenothiazines, narcotics, barbiturates, and antihistamines.

Methaqualone
(Quaalude, Sopor)

AHFS 28:24; C-II
CATEGORY Sedative-hypnotic

Action and use

Methaqualone is a CNS depressant that acts on the cortex, midbrain, and spinal cord. In addition to its sedative-hypnotic activity, methaqualone has mild antitussive and anticonvulsant activity. The primary use of methaqualone is to produce sleep in simple insomnia. There is disagreement in the literature as to whether methaqualone suppresses REM sleep. In low doses it may be used as a daytime sedative.

Characteristics

Onset: 15 to 30 min. Duration: 6 to 8 hr. Half-life: 2½ hr. Metabolism: liver microsomal enzymes to 9 metabolites. Excretion: primary urine, inactive. Therapeutic level: 0.5 mg/100 ml. Toxic level: 1 mg/100 ml to 3 mg/100 ml. Fatal levels: 2 mg/100 ml to 3 mg/100 ml. Dialysis: yes, H, P.

Administration and dosage
Adult

PO—150 to 300 mg at bedtime for insomnia; 75 mg 3 to 4 times daily as a sedative.

NOTE: Methaqualone is not recommended for continuous use for periods exceeding 3 months. It is also not recommended for use in pediatric patients.

Nurse and patient considerations

* Psychologic and physiologic dependence have been observed with methaqualone. It has also been a popular agent of abuse with the drug culture. Severe grand mal seizures may occur after withdrawal from high doses. Use of succinylcholine accompanied by assisted respiration has been proposed for prolonged convulsions.
* Patients frequently complain of "hangover," fatigue, dizziness, and headache after ingestion of hypnotic doses.
* Patients may occasionally experience transient numbness and tingling in extremities, restlessness, and anxiety before falling asleep after ingestion of hypnotic doses.

> * Methaqualone administration is not recommended
> in pregnant women or those who may become preg-
> nant. Teratogenic effects have been noted in off-
> spring of laboratory animals.
> * See General information on sedative-hypnotics (p.
> 339).

Drug interactions

One case has been reported of a patient who developed
apnea after receiving diazepam (Valium), 10 mg IV, to treat
an overdose of diphenhydramine and methaqualone combination (Mandrax).

The CNS depressant activity of methaqualone is
enhanced by barbiturates, reserpine, phenothiazines, narcotics, antihistamines, and alcohol.

Paraldehyde
(Paral)

AHFS 28:24; C-IV
CATEGORY Sedative-hypnotic

Action and use

The mechanism of action of paraldehyde is unknown,
although it does depress many levels of the central nervous
system. Its sedative-hypnotic properties may be effective in
suppressing the withdrawal symptoms of alcohol, narcotics,
and barbiturates. It may also be used to control seizures arising from tetanus, poisons, and status epilepticus.

Characteristics

Onset: 10 to 15 min (PO). Peak activity: 30 to 60 min.
Duration: 8 hr. Half-life: 7½ hr. Metabolism: 70% to 80%
metabolized in liver. Excretion: 11% to 28% exhaled, up to
2.5% in urine. Therapeutic level: 5 mg/100 ml to 8 mg/100
ml. Toxic level: 20 mg/100 ml to 40 mg/100 ml. Fatal level:
50 mg/100 ml. Dialysis: unknown.

Administration and dosage
Adult

PO—10 to 30 ml well diluted in milk or iced fruit juice to
disguise the odor and taste and to minimize gastrointestinal irritation.

IM—5 to 10 ml undiluted deep into the buttocks with no
more than 5 ml/injection site. Use caution; permanent
sciatic nerve injury, sterile abscesses, and skin sloughing have been reported.

IV—5 to 10 ml diluted with several volumes of 0.9% sodium chloride and injected slowly with caution.

RECTAL—5 to 10 ml diluted in 200 ml of 0.9% sodium chloride or 120 ml of olive oil to minimize mucosal irritation.

Pediatric

PO—0.15 ml/kg well diluted in milk or iced fruit juice to disguise the odor and taste and to minimize gastrointestinal irritation.

IM—0.15 ml/kg undiluted. Use caution; permanent sciatic nerve injury, sterile abscesses, and skin sloughing have been reported.

IV—0.15 ml/kg mixed with several volumes of 0.9% sodium chloride and injected slowly with caution.

RECTAL—0.3 ml/kg diluted with at least 2 volumes of olive or cottonseed oil to prevent rectal irritation.

NOTE: Paraldehyde should not be stored or administered in plastic containers such as syringes and cups, because of the instability with various plastics.

Preparations with a brownish color or a sharp odor of acetic acid (vinegar) should not be used. The unused contents of any container should be discarded within 24 hr after being opened. Paraldehyde is inactivated by light.

Nurse and patient considerations

* Paraldehyde must be used with caution in patients with hepatic disease. The drug is metabolized more slowly, and the hypnotic effects may be prolonged.
* Paraldehyde by-products are excreted through the lungs, giving the breath a characteristic odor.
* The most frequent adverse effects associated with normal doses are gastric irritation and erythematous skin rash.
* Acetaldehyde, a metabolic by-product, may produce false-positive serum and urine ketone values when Acetest tablets are used.
* Paraldehyde readily diffuses across the placenta and appears in fetal circulation in quantities sufficient to induce respiratory depression in newborn infants.
* See General information on sedative-hypnotics (p. 339).

Drug interactions

Disulfiram may slow the metabolism of paraldehyde, resulting in more prolonged blood levels of paraldehyde and acetaldehyde.

Paraldehyde may be potentiated by other CNS depressants such as alcohol, phenothiazines, narcotics, barbiturates, and antihistamines.

Temazepam
(Restoril)

AHFS 28:24;C-IV
CATEGORY Sedative-hypnotic

Action and use

Temazepam is an intermediate-acting benzodiazepine derivative used specifically for inducing and maintaining sleep. It may be effective in those patients who have difficulty falling asleep and those patients with frequent nocturnal awakenings and/or early morning awakenings. Laboratory data indicate essentially no change in REM sleep. Minor sleep disturbances (rebound insomnia) may occur, primarily during the first night, after discontinuation of therapy. There is no evidence of tolerance developing after 1 month of therapy. Temazepam has the specific advantage when compared with flurazepam (Dalmane) that, due to its intermediate half-life, there is minimal impairment of performance the next day.

Characteristics

Onset: 20 to 40 min. Peak plasma levels: 2.5 hr. Duration: 6 to 8 hr. Protein binding: 96%. Half-life: biphasic— short half-life, 0.4 to 0.6 hr; terminal half-life, 9.5 to 12.4 hr. Metabolism: liver, to inactive metabolites. Excretion: completely metabolized, inactive, 80% to 90% via urine. Dialysis: unknown. Breast milk: unknown.

Administration and dosage
Adult

PO—15 to 30 mg at bedtime. It is recommended that elderly and debilitated patients start with 15 mg at bedtime to determine response. Patients having difficulty falling asleep should ingest the medication 1 to 2 hr before bedtime. Do not allow the patient to attempt any hazardous tasks before retiring.

Pediatric

The use of temazepam is not recommended in patients under 18 years of age.

Nurse and patient considerations

* See General information on benzodiazepines (p. 358).
* The most common adverse effects were drowsiness, dizziness, and lethargy. Other side effects include confusion, euphoria, weakness, anorexia, and diarrhea. Rare adverse effects include hallucinations, paradoxic agitation, wakefulness, and hyperactivity.
* Overdosage may be manifested by somnolence, confusion, coma, and respiratory depression. Treatment consists of general physiologic and supportive measures including use of pressor agents for hypotension, maintenance of an airway, and administration of oxygen. Do not use barbiturates in patients who develop excitation after ingestion of temazepam.
* Temazepam is contraindicated for use in pregnant women. Patients should be warned to discontinue use before becoming pregnant or discontinue use immediately if pregnancy is suspected.
* See General information on sedative-hypnotics (p. 339).

Drug interactions

See General information on benzodiazepines (p. 358).

Triazolam
(Halcion)

AHFS 28:24; C-IV
CATEGORY Sedative-Hypnotic

Action and use

Triazolam is a short-acting benzodiazepine derivative used specifically for inducing and maintaining sleep. It may be effective in those patients who have difficulty falling asleep and those with frequent nocturnal awakenings and/or early morning awakenings. Laboratory data indicate essentially no changes in the distribution of time spent in various stages of sleep; however, after 2 weeks of consecutive nightly administration, tolerance or adaptation develops, leading to an increased frequency of wakefulness during the last third of the night. There is usually a rebound increase in total wake time the first few nights after discontinuation of therapy. This rebound insomnia can be minimized by tapering rather than abruptly discontinuing therapy. Triazolam has the advantages when compared with flurazepam (Dalmane) or temazepam (Restoril) of relatively rapid onset of activity, and, because of its short half-life, no impairment of performance the next day.

Characteristics

Onset: 10 to 20 min. Peak plasma levels: 1.3 hr. Duration: 6 to 7 hr. Half-life: 1.7 to 3 hr. Metabolism: liver, to an active metabolite. Excretion: 80% as inactive metabolites in urine. Dialysis: unknown. Breast milk: unknown.

Administration and dosage
Adult

PO—0.25 to 0.5 mg at bedtime. It is recommended that elderly and debilitated patients start with 0.125 to 0.25 mg at bedtime to determine response.

Pediatric

The use of triazolam is not recommended in patients under 18 years of age.

Nurse and patient considerations

* See General information on benzodiazepines (p. 358).
* The most common side effects observed are extensions of pharmacologic activity and include drowsiness (14%), dizziness (7%), and light-headedness (5%). Other side effects include nausea, headache, confusion, euphoria, tachycardia, and brief memory impairment. Rare adverse effects include nightmares, taste alterations, insomnia, tinnitus, and paresthesias.
* Overdosage may be manifested by somnolence, confusion, impaired coordination, slurred speech and ultimately coma. Treatment consists of general physiologic and supportive measures, including the use of levarterenol, dopamine, or metaraminol for

hypotension, maintenance of an airway, and administration of oxygen.
* Triazolam is contraindicated for use in pregnant women. Patients should be warned to discontinue use before becoming pregnant or discontinue use immediately if pregnancy is suspected.
* See General information on sedative-hypnotics (p. 339).

Drug interactions

See General information on benzodiazepines (p. 358).

CHAPTER TEN

Tranquilizing agents

Benzodiazepines
GENERAL INFORMATION

The benzodiazepines are a group of structurally related chemicals that selectively act on polysynaptic neuronal pathways throughout the central nervous system. They act primarily as presynaptic inhibitors by simulating the effects of gamma aminobutyric acid (GABA). Although the benzodiazepines have similar activities as CNS depressants, individual derivatives act more selectively at specific sites, allowing them to be subclassified into three categories based on their predominant clinical use. Individual benzodiazepines are used as anticonvulsants, hypnotics, or antianxiety agents.

The three agents approved for use as anticonvulsants are diazepam, clonazepam, and clorazepate. Clonazepam is useful in the oral treatment of absence seizures in children. Diazepam must be administered intravenously to control seizures but is the drug of choice for treatment of status epilepticus. Clorazepate is used with other antiepileptic agents to control partial seizures. The anticonvulsant properties of the benzodiazepines are derived from their ability to suppress the spread of seizure activity produced by epileptogenic foci in the cortex, thalamus, and limbic systems. They do not abolish the abnormal discharge of the focus. See Clonazepam (p. 412) and Diazepam (p. 367).

Those benzodiazepine derivatives approved as hypnotics are flurazepam, triazolam, and temazepam. As hypnotic agents, they decrease the time needed to fall asleep, and diminish the number of awakenings and the amount of time lapsed during these awakenings. They have multiple effects on different stages of sleep, but studies show that benzodiazepines increase total sleep time and impart a sense of deep or refreshing sleep. Tolerance to some of these effects may develop after a few weeks of therapy, and there is a rebound in increased total wake time after withdrawal of triazolam and temazepam as there is with barbiturates. See Flurazepam (p. 348), Triazolam (p. 355), and Temazepam (p. 354).

Table 10-1 provides a list of benzodiazepine derivatives approved to treat anxiety. Those patients with relatively acute anxiety reactions or those patients with modifiable primary illnesses or anxiety neuroses respond most readily to benzodiazepine therapy. Since all the benzodiazepines have qualitatively similar mechanisms of action, selection of the appropriate derivative is partially dependent on the individual metabolic characteristics of each of the agents. Those with similar characteristics may be selected based on dosage forms available and price. In patients with reduced hepatic function or in the elderly, alprazolam, lorazepam, or oxazepam may be most appropriate, since they have a relatively short duration of action and have no active metabolites. Oxazepam has been most thoroughly investigated. The other benzodiazepines all have active metabolites that significantly prolong the duration of action and may accumulate to the point of excessive side effects with chronic administration. The primary active ingredient of both prazepam and clorazepate is desmethyldiazepam; therefore similar activity and patient response should be expected. Halazepam and diazepam are therapeutically active, but their major metabolite is again desmethyldiazepam, so similar response should be expected with chronic administration. Oxazepam, chlordiazepoxide, diazepam; and clorazepate are all approved for use in treating the anxiety associated with alcohol withdrawal. Oxazepam is the drug of choice because it has no active metabolites. Its use is somewhat limited, however, in those patients that cannot tolerate oral administration because of nausea and vomiting. Chlordiazepoxide or diazepam may be administered intramuscularly for this indication.

Nurse and patient considerations

The more common side effects of benzodiazepines are extensions of their pharmacologic properties. Drowsiness, fatigue, lethargy, and ataxia are relatively common, dose-related, adverse effects of this class of agents.

Paradoxic reactions occasionally occur within the first few weeks of therapy. These reactions are manifested by increased anxiety, hyperexcitation, hallucinations, acute range, and insomnia.   *Text continued on p. 365.*

AHFS 28:16.08

Table 10-1. Benzodiazepine derivatives

Name	Peak serum level (hr)	Half-life (hr)	Dosages	Notes
Alprazolam (Xanax)	1-2	12-15	PO Initially, 0.25 to 0.5 mg 3 times daily. Elderly or debilitated patients should start at 0.25 mg 2 to 3 times daily. Maximum dose: 4 mg daily in divided doses.	Use for anxiety disorders, for the short-term relief of the symptoms of anxiety, and for anxiety associated with depression.
Clonazepam (Clonopin)	See p. 412			
Clorazepate (Tranxene)	—	30-100	PO For anxiety: 10 mg 3 times daily. Range—15 to 60 mg daily. Elderly or debilitated patients should start at 7.5 to 15 mg daily. For partial seizures: Adults—Initially 7.5 mg 3 times daily. Increase	After patients are stabilized on a certain total daily dose, consideration may be given to switching to the long-acting tablets for once-daily administration.

dose by 7.5 mg/week.
Do not exceed 90 mg/
day.
Children (9 to 12 yr)—
Initially 7.5 mg 2
times daily. Increase
by 7.5 mg/week. Do
not exceed 60 mg/day.
Alcohol withdrawal:
Day 1—Initially 30 mg,
followed by 30 to 60
mg in divided doses.
Day 2—45 to 90 mg in
divided doses.
Day 3—22.5 to 45 mg in
divided doses.
Day 4—15 to 30 mg in
divided doses.
Continue to reduce to
7.5 to 15 mg/day, then
discontinue when no
longer needed.

Chlordiazepoxide
  (Librium, A-poxide)
  See p. 365
Diazepam (valium)   See p. 367

Continued.

Table 10-1. Benzodiazepine derivatives—cont'd

Name	Peak serum level (hr)	Half-life (hr)	Dosages	Notes
Flurazepam (Dalmane)	See p. 348			
Halazepam (Paxipam)	1-3	14; 50-100	PO Anxiety: Initially, 20 to 40 mg 3 to 4 times daily. Optimal dosage is usually 80 to 160 mg daily. Elderly or debilitated patients should start at 20 mg 1 or 2 times daily.	
Lorazepam (Ativan)	2	10-15	PO Anxiety: 2 to 3 mg 2 to 3 times daily. Elderly or debilitated patients should start at 1 to 2 mg daily in divided doses. IM Preoperative medication: 0.05 mg/kg to a maximum of 4 mg at least 2 hr before the procedure.	

			IV Anxiety and sedation: 0.044 mg/kg or a maximum of 2 mg.	Just before administration, dilute with an equal volume of parenteral fluid. Administer at a rate of 2 mg/min. Use with caution in patients with respiratory disease.
Oxazepam (Serax)	2-4	5-20	PO Anxiety: Mild to moderate—10 to 15 mg 3 or 4 times daily. Severe—15 to 30 mg 3 or 4 times daily. Elderly or debilitated patients—start with 10 mg 3 times daily. Alcohol withdrawal: Initially, 15 to 30 mg 3 or 4 times daily.	
Prazepam (Verstran)	6	30-100	PO Anxiety: Initially, 20 mg at bed time. Adjust as needed. Range—20 to 60 mg daily in divided doses.	

Continued.

Table 10-1. Benzodiazepine derivatives—cont'd

AHFS 28:16.08

Name	Peak serum level (hr)	Half-life (hr)	Dosages	Notes
Temazepam (Restoril)	See p. 354			Elderly and debilitated patients should start with 10 to 15 mg daily.
Triazolam (Halcion)	See p. 355			

Physical and psychologic dependence are relatively rare but may occur on discontinuance after prolonged therapy with high dosages. Abrupt withdrawal may result in seizure activity and symptoms similar to barbiturate withdrawal. The symptoms may not appear for more than a week after discontinuance as a result of the long half-lives and conversion to active metabolites.

Benzodiazepines should be administered with caution to patients with a history of blood dycrasias or hepatic or renal damage. Cases of agranulocytosis, jaundice, and elevated SGOT, SGPT, bilirubin, and alkaline phosphatase levels have been reported.

Benzodiazepines should not be administered during the first trimester of pregnancy. Congenital malformations have been reported.

Chronic administration during pregnancy may cause physical dependence with withdrawal symptoms in the infant after delivery.

Benzodiazepines and their metabolites are secreted in breast milk in sufficient quantities to produce drowsiness and feeding difficulties in infants.

Drug interactions

Benzodiazepines may be potentiated by other CNS depressants such as phenothiazines, narcotics, barbiturates, antihistamines, and antidepressants.

Cimetidine inhibits the metabolism of most benzodiazepines, significantly prolonging the duration of action. Cimetidine does not affect lorazepam or oxazepam, because of different metabolic pathways.

Smoking tends to enhance the metabolism of the benzodiazepines. Larger dosages may be necessary to maintain sedative effects in patients who smoke.

Chlordiazepoxide
(Librium)

AHFS 28:16.08; C-IV
CATEGORY Tranquilizer

Action and use

Chlordiazepoxide is a benzodiazepine derivative used in mild to moderate states of anxiety and tension. It is also used as a tranquilizer for acute alcohol withdrawal syndrome.

Characteristics

Onset: 30 to 60 min (PO), 15 to 30 min (IM), 3 to 15 min (IV). Peak blood level: 2 to 4 hr (PO). Half-life: 24 to 30 hr.

Metabolism: liver, to two active metabolites. Excretion: urine and feces. Therapeutic level: 0.1 mg/100 ml to 0.3 mg/100 ml. Toxic level: 0.5 mg/100 ml. Fatal level: 2 mg/100 ml to 3 mg/100 ml. Dialysis: no, H, P.

Administration and dosage
Adult

PO
1. Mild to moderate anxiety and tension: 5 to 10 mg 3 to 4 times daily.
2. Severe anxiety and tension: 20 to 25 mg 3 to 4 times daily.
3. Alcohol withdrawal syndrome: 50 to 100 mg initially, then 25 to 50 mg 3 to 4 times daily as needed.

IM—As for PO administration. IM administration appears to provide longer onset of activity and lower blood levels than PO administration. It may be more beneficial to administer dosage PO if the patient's clinical status will allow it. Add 2 ml of Special Intramuscular Diluent to the contents of the 5 ml dry-filled amber ampule to make 100 mg of IM chlordiazepoxide. Agitate gently to prevent formation of bubbles and inject deeply and slowly into a large skeletal muscle.

IV—As for PO administration. Add 5 ml of sterile water for injection or saline solution to the contents of the 5 ml dry-filled amber ampule to make 100 mg of the chlordiazepoxide for IV use. Administer at a rate no faster than 100 mg/min. Solutions prepared for IV administration are not recommended for IM use because of pain on injection.

NOTE: Total doses of greater than 300 mg/24 hr are not recommended.

Pediatric

NOTE: Not recommended in children under 6 years of age.
PO—Initially, 5 mg 2 to 4 times daily.
IM—0.5 mg/kg/24 hr in 3 or 4 divided doses. See IM administration instructions for adult dosages.

Nurse and patient considerations

* Acute overdosage or cumulative effects from chronic ingestion may be manifested by somnolence, confusion, coma, and respiratory depression. Treatment consists of general physiologic supportive measures including maintenance of an airway and

administration of oxygen. Methylphenidate (Ritalin) or caffeine may be effective against severe respiratory depression. Do not use barbiturates in patients who develop excitation after ingestion of chlordiazepoxide.

* Hypotension and tachycardia may occur, particularly on parenteral administration. Severe hypotensive effects may be reversed with levarterenol (Levophed), dopamine (Intropin), or metaraminol (Aramine).

* Use with caution in pregnant women. Fetal blood levels are similar to that of maternal circulation. Safe use in pregnancy has not been established.

* See General information on benzodiazepines (p. 358).

Drug interactions

See General information on benzodiazepines (p. 358).

Rare cases have been reported where chlordiazepoxide has inhibited the metabolism of phenytoin (Dilantin), resulting in increased serum levels of phenytoin.

Diazepam
(Valium)

AHFS 28:16.08; C-IV
CATEGORY Tranquilizer, anticonvulsant

Action and use

Diazepam is a benzodiazepine derivative used in mild to moderate states of anxiety and tension. It may also be used as a tranquilizer for acute alcohol withdrawal syndrome.

Diazepam has beneficial tranquilizing and amnesic effects when administered parenterally for the relief of anxiety and tension before endoscopy, surgical procedures, and cardioversion of atrial fibrillation. Diazepam displays some mild muscle relaxant properties, as do other CNS depressants.

Diazepam is often effective in controlling various types of partial and generalized seizures and in controlling tonic-clonic status epilepticus.

Characteristics

Onset: immediate (IV), 15 to 30 min (IM), 30 to 60 min (PO). Peak plasma levels: 1 to 3 hr (PO). Protein binding:

highly bound. Half-life: 1 to 2 days (parent compound and active metabolites). Metabolism: liver, active. Excretion: metabolites in urine and feces. Therapeutic level: 0.1 mg/100 ml to 0.25 mg/100 ml. Toxic level: 0.5 mg/100 ml to 2 mg/100 ml. Fatal level: 2 mg/100 ml. Dialysis: no, H.

Administration and dosage
Adult
PO—2 to 10 mg 2 to 4 times daily.

IM—Should be discouraged; it is painful, with erratic absorption.

IV—2 to 40 mg depending on use and should be added in small increments. Inject slowly, monitoring the patient's response. Take at least 1 min for each 5 mg (1 ml) given. A fine, white precipitate will develop when diazepam is added to other solutions, including dextrose 5% and saline solution. Administer as close to the venipuncture site as possible.

Pediatric
PO—0.12 to 0.8 mg/kg/24 hr divided into 3 to 4 doses.

IV—0.1 to 0.3 mg/kg repeated in 2 to 4 hr as needed.

NOTE: Diazepam is not recommended in infants less than 30 days of age. However, if seizure activity cannot be arrested with maximum doses of phenobarbital, 0.1 to 0.8 mg/kg/24 hr may be used. Sodium benzoate, a preservative in parenteral solutions of diazepam, has been associated with clinically significant displacement of bilirubin from protein-binding sites.

Nurse and patient considerations
* See General information on benzodiazepines (p. 358).
* Overdosage may be manifested by somnolescence, confusion, coma, and respiratory depression. Treatment consists of general physiologic supportive measures including maintenance of an airway and administration of oxygen. Methylphenidate (Ritalin) or caffeine may be effective against severe CNS or respiratory depression. Do not use barbiturates in patients who develop excitation after ingestion of diazepam.
* Hypotension may occur, particularly with parenteral administration. Severe hypotensive effects may be reversed with levarterenol (Levophed) or metaraminol (Aramine).

✻ Use with caution in pregnant women. Fetal blood levels are similar to those in maternal circulation. Small amounts are found in breast milk.

Drug interactions

When diazepam is used with a narcotic analgesic, the dosage of the narcotic should be reduced by at least one third and administered in small increments.

Rare cases have been reported where diazepam has inhibited the metabolism of phenytoin (Dilantin), resulting in increased serum levels of phenytoin and potential toxicity.

Rifampin may significantly decrease serum levels of diazepam. Dosage adjustment for anticonvulsant therapy may be necessary.

Cimetidine inhibits the metabolism of diazepam, enhancing its sedative effects. A decrease in dosage of diazepam may be necessary.

Isoniazid may inhibit the metabolism of diazepam, causing moderately prolonged activity. Observe patients for altered response to diazepam when isoniazid therapy is started or stopped.

See General information on benzodiazepines (p. 358).

Haloperidol
(Haldol)

AHFS 28:16.08
CATEGORY Tranquilizer

Action and use

Haloperidol is a butyrophenone derivative structurally unrelated but with pharmacologic properties similar to the piperazine group of phenothiazine tranquilizers. Haloperidol may be effective in the control of agitated states associated with psychotic behavior such as schizophrenia and manic phases of bipolar or major affective disorders. The butyrophenones offer an excellent alternative therapy for patients who are phenothiazine resistant or allergic to or suffer intolerable adverse effects from the phenothiazines or thioxanthines. The exact mechanism of action is unknown.

Characteristics

Peak plasma levels: 10 to 15 min (IM), 2 to 6 hr (PO). Duration: up to 72 hr. Metabolism: concentration in liver. Excretion: urine and feces.

Administration and dosage

NOTE: Dosage must be carefully adjusted according to individual requirements and tolerance. Geriatric or debilitated patients frequently require lower initial doses to achieve the same therapeutic effect. Haloperidol is not approved for use in children.

PO   1. Initial: moderate symptoms, 0.5 to 2 mg 2 to 3 times daily; severe symptoms, 3 to 5 mg 2 to 3 times daily. Dosages up to 100 mg daily may be required in severely disturbed individuals.

2. Maintenance: after achieving a desired therapeutic response, dosage should be gradually reduced to the lowest effective maintenance level.

IM—2 to 5 mg for immediate control of the acutely agitated patient. Depending on the patient's response, doses may be repeated every hour, but may need to be repeated only every 4 to 8 hr.

Nurse and patient considerations

* Extrapyramidal symptoms (akathisia or parkinsonian manifestations of marked drowsiness and lethargy, drooling and hypersalivation, fixed stare, and muscular rigidity) are the most common side effects of haloperidol. These symptoms often occur during the first few days of therapy and may require reduction in dosage, initiation of antiparkinsonian drug therapy (benztropine, [Cogentin] 2 to 4 mg) or complete discontinuance of haloperidol therapy. Antiparkinsonian drugs should be continued after haloperidol has been discontinued because the slow elimination of haloperidol may cause a recurrence of the extrapyramidal symptoms.

* Tardive dyskinesia, manifested by recurrent protrusion of the tongue, puffing of the cheeks, puckering of the mouth, and chewing movements, may develop with long-term treatment with haloperidol. There appears to be a higher incidence in elderly female patients on high-dose therapy. This syndrome is irreversible in some patients, but may be prevented if the drug is discontinued at the first sign of fine tremorlike movements of the tongue.

* Haloperidol should be administered with caution in patients prone to seizures, since haloperidol may

lower the convulsive threshold. Dosages of anticonvulsant therapy may require readjustment.

* Hypotension occurs infrequently but may be observed on IM injection or overdosage. It may be treated with IV fluids, plasma, albumin, or vasopressors such as norepinephrine or phenylephrine. *Do not use epinephrine,* since haloperidol blocks its vasopressor effects, resulting in further lowering of blood pressure.

* Other general adverse effects of haloperidol include mild and transient leukopenia and leukocytosis, impaired liver function and/or jaundice, skin rashes and alopecia, anorexia, dry mouth, constipation, nausea and vomiting, blurred vision, urinary retention, bronchospasm, drowsiness, euphoria, and agitation.

* Haloperidol therapy is not recommended in pregnant women. Teratogenic effects have been reported; however, a causal relationship has not been established. Haloperidol also appears in the milk of lactating mothers.

Drug interactions

Haloperidol may reverse the hypotensive effects of guanethidine.

Haloperidol may have additive CNS depressant effects with ethanol, barbiturates, sedatives, antihistamines, anesthetics, analgesics, and tranquilizers.

Loxapine succinate
(Loxitane)

AHFS 28:16.08
CATEGORY Tranquilizer

Action and use

Loxapine succinate represents the first of a new class of tricyclic neuroleptic agents called the dibenzoxazepine derivatives. They are chemically unrelated to the phenothiazines, butyrophenones, and thioxanthines. Loxapine is used to control the symptoms of schizophrenia such as disorientation, perceptual distortion, hallucination, emotional withdrawal, conceptual disorganization, and hostility. The exact mechanism of action is unknown. Clinical studies indicate that loxapine offers no greater effectiveness than chlorpromazine, thiothixene, or trifluoperazine, but it may be of value in chronic, long-term schizophrenic patients who have not benefited from or are allergic to other antipsychotic medication. It does not have any antidepressant activity.

Characteristics

Onset of sedation: 20 to 30 min. Peak serum levels: 1 to 2 hr. Peak sedation: 1.5 to 3 hr. Duration of sedation: 12 hr. Half-life: biphasic—first phase, 5 hr; second phase, 19 hr. Metabolism: liver, extensive; 2 major, active metabolites. Excretion: 50% in urine and feces in 24 hr as metabolites. Dialysis: no, H. Breast milk: unknown.

Administration and dosage
Adult

PO 1. Weeks to months of therapy may be necessary to produce maximum clinical improvement.
    2. Initially, 10 mg 2 times daily. Increase dosage over the next 7 to 10 days as required and tolerated to a maximum of 250 mg daily in divided doses.
    3. The usual maintenance dose is 60 to 100 mg daily in 2 to 4 divided doses.
    4. The oral loxapine concentrate may be mixed with orange or grapefruit juice. Measure the concentrated liquid only with the calibrated dropper provided.

IM 1. Use for prompt control of the symptomatic patient.
    2. Administer 12.5 to 50 mg every 4 to 6 hr as needed. Adjust to individual requirements.
    3. Patients should be converted to the oral liquid or capsules as soon as possible.

Pediatric

Use of loxapine is not recommended in patients under 16 years of age.

NOTE: Signs of overdosage range from mild CNS depression to profound hypotension, tachycardia, arrhythmias, respiratory depression, unconsciousness, and seizure activity. Treatment is primarily supportive. Early gastric lavage may be helpful. Do not use emetics or CNS stimulants. Severe hypotension may be controlled with infusions of levarterenol (Levophed) or phenylephrine (Neo-Synephrine). Do *not* use epinephrine, because of partial alpha-adrenergic receptor blockade by loxapine. Profound hypotension may result. Severe extrapyramidal symptoms may be treated with diphenhydramine (Benadryl), 2.5 to 5 mg/kg with a maximum single IV dose of 50 mg over 2 min.

Nurse and patient considerations

* Transient initial drowsiness is the most commonly reported side effect. Tolerance usually develops with continued therapy.

* Some of the most troublesome side effects noted with loxapine are "extrapyramidal" effects. These include the parkinsonian symptoms of tremor, muscular rigidity, masklike facies, shuffling gait, and loss or weakness of motor function; dystonias and dyskinesias, which are spasmodic movements of the body and limbs (dystonias) and coordinated, involuntary rhythmic movements (dyskinesias); and akathisias, which consist of involuntary motor restlessness, constant pacing, and inability to sit still and are often accompanied by fidgeting, with lip and limb movements. These extrapyramidal symptoms may require control by antiparkinsonian agents (benztropine or trihexyphenidyl).

* Tardive dyskinesia is a drug-induced neurologic disorder manifested by facial grimaces and involuntary movement of the lips, tongue, and jaw, producing smacking and frequent, recurrent protrusions of the tongue. This adverse drug effect is usually irreversible and appears after several years of antipsychotic therapy. It may also appear after discontinuation of therapy. The incidence appears to be higher in patients taking both antiparkinsonian and antipsychotic agents concomitantly. It has been reported that fine movements of the tongue may be an early sign of tardive dyskinesia. If the medication is stopped, the syndrome may not develop.

* Side effects associated with anticholinergic activity include blurred vision, nasal stuffiness, constipation, and dry mouth. Use with caution in patients with inadequately treated narrow-angle glaucoma, prostatic hypertrophy, or urinary retention.

* Use with extreme caution in patients with a history of seizure disorders. Normal therapeutic doses of loxapine have been reported to induce seizure activity in predisposed patients.

* Cardiovascular side effects include tachycardia, hypotension, hypertension, syncope, and minor electrocardiographic changes. Use with caution in patients with cardiac disease.

* Other adverse effects reported with loxapine therapy include dermatitis, photosensitivity, edema of the face, nausea, weight gain, headache, and paresthesias.
* Although loxapine differs structurally and to some degree pharmacologically from the phenothiazines, it does contain a piperazine side chain similar to certain phenothiazines. Similar adverse reactions should be anticipated. Grouped into classes, the potential adverse reactions include liver dysfunction and jaundice, hematologic dyscrasias, hypotensive effects, allergic reactions, endocrine disorders, skin pigmentation, and ocular changes.
* Laboratory studies have given no indication of fetotoxic or teratogenic effects when loxapine is administered to pregnant animals. However, loxapine should not be administered to pregnant patients unless therapeutic benefits significantly outweigh possible adverse effects to the fetus.

Drug interactions

Loxapine may be expected to have additive CNS depressant effects with ethanol, sedatives, antihistamines, anesthetics, analgesics, and tranquilizers.

Loxapine may display additive anticholinergic effects (dry mouth, constipation, urinary retention, acute glaucoma, blurred vision) when administered with antihistamines (Benadryl), phenothiazines, trihexiphenidyl (Artane), benzotropine (Cogentin), meperidine (Demerol), and other agents with anticholinergic activity. Usually, however, the side effects are not serious enough to require discontinuance of therapy.

Do not administer epinephrine to patients receiving loxapine. Due to the alpha-adrenergic blocking activity of loxapine, a paradoxic hypotension may result after use of epinephrine.

Meprobamate
(Equanil, Miltown)

AHFS 28:16.08; C-IV
CATEGORY Tranquilizer

Action and use

Meprobamate is a minor tranquilizer used effectively as an antianxiety agent and mild skeletal muscle relaxant. It acts on multiple sites within the central nervous system, producing mild sedation and relaxation. Meprobamate is indicated for the relief of anxiety and tension in anxious, tense patients. Meprobamate is of little value in the treatment of psychoses.

Characteristics

Onset: 30 min. Peak activity: 2 to 3 hr. Plasma half-life: 10 hr. Metabolism: microsomal enzymes in the liver; may produce enzyme induction. Excretion: 10% unchanged in urine. Therapeutic level: 0.5 mg/100 ml to 2 mg/100 ml. Toxic level: 5 mg/100 ml to 20 mg/100 ml (lower with ethanol). Fatal dose: 12 to 40 g. Dialysis: yes, H, P.

Administration and dosage
Adult

PO—400 mg 3 to 4 times daily. Smaller doses may suffice for elderly and debilitated patients. Maximum daily doses should not exceed 2400 mg.

Pediatric

PO—The usual dosage in children 6 to 12 years of age is 100 to 200 mg 2 or 3 times daily. Meprobamate is not recommended for children under 6 years of age.

Nurse and patient considerations

* Psychologic and physiologic dependence and abuse have occurred. Symptoms of the chronic use of high doses include ataxia, slurred speech, and dizziness. Withdrawal reactions such as vomiting, tremors, confusion, hallucinosis, and grand mal seizures may develop within 12 to 48 hr after abrupt discontinuance. Symptoms usually abate within the next 12 to 48 hr. Withdrawal from high and prolonged dosage should gradually be completed over 1 to 2 weeks. Alternatively, a patient may be stabilized on short-acting barbiturates and then gradually tapered from the barbiturate.
* Meprobamate may precipitate seizures in patients prone to convulsive episodes.
* Adverse reactions to meprobamate are generally mild and include dizziness, slurred speech, headache, paradoxic excitement, various arrhythmias, hypotension, dermatologic and allergic reactions, blood dyscrasias, and exacerbation of intermittent porphyria.

* Meprobamate may interfere with urinary steroid determinations as a result of interference with the testing procedure.
* Meprobamate readily crosses the placental barrier and is found in breast milk in concentrations 2 to 4 times that of the mother's blood level. Neonates and nursing infants whose mothers receive meprobamate must be observed for signs of toxicity.

Drug interactions

The CNS depressant effects of antihistamines, analgesics, anesthetics, other tranquilizers, and sedative-hypnotics may be potentiated by meprobamate.

Meprobamate may induce hepatic microsomal enzymes, enhancing the metabolism of warfarin (Coumadin), digitoxin, corticosteroids (for example, prednisone), doxycycline (Vibramycin), phenytoin (Dilantin), and chlorpromazine (Thorazine). If meprobamate is discontinued, the patient must be observed closely for signs of secondary drug toxicity requiring reduction of dosage.

Molindone hydrochloride (Moban hydrochloride)

AHFS 28:16.08
CATEGORY Tranquilizer

Action and use

Molindone hydrochloride represents the first of a new class of neuroleptic agents called the dihydroindolone derivatives. Although not structurally related to the butyrophenones, thioxanthenes, or phenothiazines, molindone has pharmacologic properties similar to these agents. Molindone is used to control the symptoms of schizophrenia such as grandiosity, tension, disorientation, perceptual distortion, and withdrawal. The exact mechanism of activity is unknown.

Characteristics

Peak plasma levels: 1 hr. Duration: 36 hr. Plasma half-life: 1½ hr. Metabolism: liver. Excretion: 3% unchanged in urine, small amount via lungs as CO_2, remainder in urine and feces as inactive metabolites. Therapeutic level: unknown. Dialysis: no, H, P.

Administration and dosage

NOTE: Dosage must be carefully adjusted to individual requirements and tolerance. Geriatric or debilitated patients frequently require lower initial doses to achieve the same therapeutic effect. Molindone is not recommended for use in children under 12 years of age.

PO
1. Initial: mild, 5 to 15 mg 3 to 4 times daily; moderate, 10 to 25 mg 3 to 4 times daily; severe, daily dosages as high as 225 mg may be required.
2. Maintenance: once the patient is stabilized, a single daiy dose is adequate.

Weeks or months of therapy with molindone may be necessary to produce maximum clinical improvement.

Nurse and patient considerations

* Transient initial drowsiness is the most frequently reported side effect.
* Extrapyramidal symptoms (akathisia or parkinsonian reactions characterized by muscle rigidity, recurring drowsiness and lethargy, drooling and hypersalivation, fixed stare, reduction of voluntary movement, and tremor) are frequently noted, particularly with increasing doses. These extrapyramidal symptoms may require control by antiparkinsonian drugs (benztropine or trihexyphenidyl).
* Other adverse effects noted with molindone include restlessness, depression, dizziness, blurred vision, hyperactivity, nausea, vomiting, euphoria, dry mouth, and tachycardia.
* Although molindone differs structurally and to some degree pharmacologically from the phenothiazines, similar adverse reactions should be anticipated. Grouping these potential adverse reactions into classes, they include liver dysfunction and jaundice, hematologic dyscrasias, hypotensive effects, allergic reactions, endocrine disorders, skin pigmentation, and ocular changes. Many of these reactions have not yet been reported, but as molindone gains more widespread use, the possibility of the development of these effects increases.
* Molindone is not recommended for use in pregnant or nursing women. No teratogenetic abnormalities in animals have yet been observed. Data are not available on the content of molindone in breast milk.

Drug interactions

No drug interactions have as yet been reported; however, molindone may be expected to have additive CNS depressant effects with ethanol, sedatives, antihistamines, anesthetics, analgesics, and tranquilizers.

Phenothiazines
GENERAL INFORMATION

The phenothiazine derivatives are among the oldest and most popular antipsychotic agents used in medicine today. There are several classes of phenothiazine derivatives, all based on different structural substituents attached to the basic phenothiazine molecule. These subgroups (with examples) are: (1) ethylamino derivatives (promethazine—Phenergan), (2) propylamino derivatives (chlorpromazine—Thorazine, promazine—Sparine), (3) piperazine derivatives (trifluroperazine—Stelazine, fluphenazine—Prolixin), and (4) piperidine derivatives (thioridazine—Mellaril). See the individual monographs on these agents for particular advantages and disadvantages of these classes of phenothiazines.

Phenothiazines are major tranquilizers believed to act by blocking receptors in the brain to dopamine and norepinephrine. The exact mechanisms of action are unknown. Their actions on the central and autonomic nervous systems affect many different sites within the body, thus giving rise to the many varied actions and side effects of phenothiazines.

Administration and dosage

Dosages must be individualized according to the degree of mental and emotional disturbance. It will often take several weeks for a patient to show optimal improvement and to become stabilized on an adequate maintenance dosage. As a result of the cumulative effects of phenothiazines, patients must be periodically reevaluated to determine the lowest effective dosage necessary to control psychiatric symptoms.

After patients have become stabilized on the lowest effective maintenance dosage, phenothiazines can often be given in a single daily dose. Single daily dosages at bedtime offer the advantages of improved sleep, which masks minor side effects. Other patients, however, may experience fewer side effects when the doses are spread out. Consequently patients must be placed on an individualized dosage regimen that will provide optimal symptomatic improvement and compliance with the fewest adverse effects.

Nurse and patient considerations

Some of the most troublesome side effects noted with antipsychotic agents are extrapyramidal effects. These include the parkinsonian symptoms of tremor, muscular rigidity, masklike facies, shuffling gait, and loss or weakness of motor function; dystonias and dyskinesias, which are spasmodic movements of the body and limbs (dystonias) and coordinated, involuntary rhythmic movements (dyskinesias); and akathisias, which consist of involuntary motor restlessness, constant pacing, inability to sit still, and are often accompanied by fidgeting, with lip and limb movements.

Tardive dyskinesia is a drug-induced neurologic disorder manifested by facial grimaces and involuntary movement of the lips, tongue, and jaw, producing smacking and frequent, recurrent protrusions of the tongue. This adverse drug effect is usually irreversible and appears after several years of antipsychotic therapy. The incidence appears to be higher in patients taking both antiparkinsonian and antipsychotic agents concomitantly. It has been reported that fine movements of the tongue may be an early sign of tardive dyskinesia. If the medication is stopped, the syndrome may not develop.

Dry mouth and constipation are other frequent side effects that may caused decreased compliance. Sugarless hard candy or gum may help the dry mouth. The use of stool softeners such as docusate (Colace) and occasionally a potent laxative such as bisacodyl (Dulcolax) may be required for constipation.

Chronic drowsiness and fatigue may occur during initiation or adjustment in therapy. Tolerance will usually develop, but a single daily dose at bedtime may also be effective.

Phenothiazines lower the seizure threshold. Seizures may occur in those with and without a history of seizure activity. Adjustment of anticonvulsant therapy may be required, especially in those seizure-prone patients.

Hypersensitivity reactions include cholestatic jaundice (upper abdominal pain, yellow skin, rash, fever, eosinophilia, elevated liver function tests), blood dyscrasias, dermatoses, and photosensitivity. Most hypersensitivity reactions occur within the first few months of therapy.

Adverse effects, listed according to organ systems involved, include:

1. Hematologic: blood dyscrasias are rare, but the mortality rate can be high. Agranulocytosis occurs most frequently in women and after 4 to 10 weeks of therapy. Leukopenia frequently occurs after prolonged therapy with high dosages of phenothiazines and is usually an indication to stop therapy. Other blood dyscrasias include eosinophilia, hemolytic anemia, thrombocytopenia, and aplastic anemia. If signs of blood dyscrasias (sore throat, fever, weakness) occur, phenothiazine therapy should be discontinued until a complete blood count has eliminated the possibility of a blood dyscrasia.

2. Hepatic: a cholestatic jaundice may appear in 0.5% to 4% of those patients ingesting phenothiazines. It usually appears within 2 to 4 weeks after initiating therapy. Patients may complain of upper abdominal pain, yellow skin, rash, and fever, and display elevated levels in liver function tests (SGOT, SGPT, bilirubin, alkaline phosphatase).

3. Skin: photosensitivity may develop while a patient is on phenothiazine therapy. Patients should be warned to wear protective clothing and avoid direct sunlight. A contact dermatitis may develop in those patients who have contact with solutions of phenothiazine derivatives. These patients should avoid physical contact with these solutions. Skin pigmentation, usually yellowish brown but possibly changing to grayish purple, may result from long-term (3 years or more) administration of large doses of phenothiazines. The pigmentation is more frequent in women, is usually restricted to exposed areas of the body, and may fade on discontinuance of therapy.

4. Ophthalmic: long-term administration may lead to deposition of fine particulate matter in the lens and cornea. These eye lesions appear to be reversible on discontinuance of phenothiazine therapy.

5. Cardiovascular: hypotension, tachycardia, fainting, and dizziness may occur, especially after parenteral administration. ECG changes similar to those caused by hypokalemia or quinidine may also occur.

6. Endocrine: menstrual irregularities, delayed ovulation, galactorrhea, alterations in libido, glycosuria, hypoglycemia, weight gain, and high or prolonged glucose tolerance curves may occur.

7. Other: phenothiazines may produce a myriad of side effects other than those already listed. These include gastrointestinal effects, alterations in body temperature regulation, particularly hypothermia, and respiratory depression, especially in those with impaired pulmonary function.

Phenothiazines cross the placental barrier and may appear in the milk of nursing mothers. The effects of phenothiazine therapy on the human fetus is unknown. Therefore these derivatives should be used on a risk versus benefit basis in pregnant women or those women planning to become pregnant while on phenothiazine therapy.

Overdosage

Treatment of phenothiazine overdosage is essentially symptomatic. Establish and maintain an airway. Early gastric lavage may be helpful. Extrapyramidal effects may be treated with diphenhydramine (Benadryl) 2.5 to 5 mg/kg with a maximum single IV dose of 50 mg over 2 min. Hypotension may be treated with an infusion of levarterenol (Levophed) or phenylephrine (Neo-Synephrine). Epinephrine is not recommended. As a result of the alpha-adrenergic blocking activity of phenothiazines, a paradoxic hypotension may result after the use of epinephrine.

Drug interactions

Phenothiazines display enhanced CNS depressant activity with ethanol, barbiturates, narcotics, tranquilizers, antihistamines, sedative-hypnotics, and anesthetics. Because of enhanced activity the phenothiazines may allow a dosage reduction to about half the usual dosage of these other agents.

The absorption of orally administered phenothiazines may be diminished by antacids. Spacing the time intervals between administration of the two products will minimize the gastrointestinal mixing that leads to diminished absorption.

Barbiturates may increase the rate of metabolism by enzyme induction, potentially leading to decreased phenothiazine activity.

Although the mechanism is unknown, phenothiazines may produce hyperglycemia. Diabetic patients controlled on insulin or oral hypoglycemic agents may require readjustment of dosages to control the diabetes mellitus.

Although the cases are rare, there are reports of phenytoin (Dilantin) metabolism being inhibited by prochlorperazine and chlorpromazine. Caution is recommended, and the dosage of phenytoin may require adjustment to maintain antiarrhythmic or anticonvulsant control.

Phenothiazines may inhibit the antihypertensive effect of guanethidine by diminishing the uptake of guanethidine into the adrenergic neurons. Patients must be observed for loss of antihypertensive control. Remember that phenothiazines also cause hypotension and may enhance the drop in blood pressure.

Beta blockers may enhance the hypotensive effect of phenothiazines. Patients should be observed for hypotensive effects, especially during adjustment to either beta blockers or phenothiazine therapy.

Phenothiazine effects on the heart are in some respects similar to those of quinidine. Phenothiazine-induced ventricular tachycardia should not be treated with quinidine, but should be treated similar to quinidine toxicity.

Chlorpromazine
(Thorazine)

AHFS 28:16.08
CATEGORY Tranquilizer

Action and use

Chlorpromazine is a representative of the propylamino phenothiazine derivatives. It may be used in the treatment of psychomotor agitation associated with various types of acute and chronic psychoses, control of the manic phase of bipolar major affective disorders, moderate to severe agitation, hyperactivity or aggressiveness in disturbed children, and control of nausea and vomiting. Sedative effects are predominant (although tolerance soon develops) while the frequency of extrapyramidal symptoms are moderate.

Characteristics

Absorption: dependent on formulation of the product, decreased significantly by the presence of food and anticholinergic drugs, as well as great intersubject variation. Peak plasma levels: 2 to 3 hr. Protein binding: 90%. Half-life (plasma): less than 6 hr. Metabolism: liver to greater than 100 metabolites. Excretion: about 10% unchanged in urine, metabolites about equal in urine and feces. Some metabolites are detectable in the urine 6 months after discontinuance of therapy. Therapeutic level: plasma concentrations of free chlorpromazine do not correlate with the therapeutic responses. Dialysis: no, H, P.

Administration and dosage

For anxiety, tension, and agitation:

Adult

PO—Initially 10 to 50 mg 4 times daily. Increase daily dosages by 25 to 50 mg semiweekly until the patient becomes calm and cooperative.

IM—25 to 50 mg for prompt control of severe symptoms. This dosage may be repeated in 1 hr. Observe patient closely for hypotensive effects, especially on initial dosages. Gradually increase dosages over several days. As a result of irritation, inject deeply into the upper outer quadrant slowly. Rotate injection sites.

IV—Not recommended because of potential cardiovascular effects.

Pediatric

PO—2 mg/kg/24 hr divided into 4 to 6 doses.

NOTE: Maximum improvement may not be seen for several weeks. Daily dosages of 1 to 2 g may be required in some patients with severe symptomatology. After symptoms have been controlled for a few weeks, dosages should be slowly reduced to the lowest effective level.

For nausea and vomiting:

Adult

PO—10 to 25 mg every 4 to 6 hr as needed.

IM—25 mg. Observe closely for hypotension. If hypotension is not evident, subsequent dosages may be increased to 50 mg every 3 to 4 hr as needed.

IV—If symptoms persist, inject 25 to 50 mg in 500 ml of saline slowly. The patient should remain flat in bed, and the blood pressure be monitored closely.

RECTAL—50 to 100 mg suppository every 6 to 8 hr as needed.

Pediatric

PO—0.1 mg/kg every 4 to 6 hr.

IM—0.1 mg/kg every 6 to 8 hr.

RECTAL—0.2 mg/kg every 6 to 8 hr as needed.

NOTE: Not recommended in children under 6 months of age unless potentially lifesaving.

NOTE: Pain on IM injection may be minimized by diluting with 2% procaine or saline. Abrupt withdrawal after long-term use of high dosages of chlorpromazine may result in symptoms of physical dependence (gastritis, nausea, vomiting, dizziness, and tremulousness). Gradual dosage reduction or continuation of antiparkinsonian agents for several weeks may avoid these complications.

Nurse and patient considerations

✳ See General information on phenothiazines (p. 378).

Overdosage

See General information on phenothiazines (p. 378).

Drug interactions

See General information on phenothiazines (p. 378).

Prochlorperazine
(Compazine)

AHFS 56:20 and 28:16.08
CATEGORY Antiemetic, tranquilizer

Action and use

Prochlorperazine is a piperazine phenothiazine derivative. It is an antipsychotic agent effective in controlling the psychomotor agitation of schizophrenia; the manic phase of manic-depressive psychosis; and the anxiety, tension, and confusion associated with various neuroses. Its most frequent use, however, is in the prevention and control of severe nausea and vomiting.

Administration and dosage

For severe nausea and vomiting:

Adult

PO—5 to 10 mg 3 to 4 times daily or 15 mg (in sustained release form) on arising or 10 mg (in sustained release form) every 12 hr.

IM—Initially, 5 to 10 mg injected deeply into the upper outer quadrant of the buttock. Repeat every 3 to 4 hr as needed. Total IM dosage should not exceed 40 mg/day.

IV—Initially, 5 to 10 mg. Observe for hypotension. An infusion of 20 mg of prochlorperazine/L of solution may be used to control nausea during surgery.

RECTAL—25 mg 2 times daily.

Pediatric

NOTE: Prochlorperazine should be used with caution when administered to children. There has been some suspicion that centrally acting antiemetics may contribute, in combination with viral illnesses, to the development of Reye's syndrome, a potentially fatal acute childhood disease. Administration of antiemetics is not recommended until the cause of vomiting can be determined.

Under 10 kg or 2 years of age

PO or RECTAL—Not recommended

Between 10 and 14 kg

PO or RECTAL—2.5 mg 1 or 2 times daily, not to exceed 7.5 mg/day.

IM—One half the PO or rectal dosage. More than 1 dose is seldom necessary.

Between 15 and 18 kg

PO or RECTAL—2.5 mg 2 or 3 times daily, not to exceed 10 mg/day.

IM—As for children between 10 and 14 kg.

Between 19 and 40 kg

PO or RECTAL—2.5 to 5 mg 2 or 3 times daily, not to exceed 15 mg/day.

IM—As for children between 10 and 14 kg.

NOTE: Prochlorperazine is not recommended for use in pediatric surgery. Children seem more prone to develop extrapyramidal reactions, even with moderate doses.

Nurse and patient considerations

* See General information on phenothiazines (p. 378).
* Other measures that enhance antiemetic activity include frequent small feedings or dry carbohydrates when allowed by dietary restrictions and avoidance of high fat foods and antacids. Decrease noxious stimuli in the environment such as odors, smoke, unpleasant sounds, drainage, and waste products. Good oral hygiene for improved patient comfort is frequently overlooked after emesis.
* One must be aware of excessive vomiting and must observe patient for deficiencies in fluids, electro-

lytes, and nutrients. See Table 4-1, Indications of electrolyte imbalance (p. 237).

* Safe use during pregnancy has not been established.

Drug interactions

See General information on phenothiazines (p. 378).

Promethazine hydrochloride
(Phenergan)

AHFS 4:00 and 28:24
CATEGORY Antihistaminic, tranquilizer

Action and use

Promethazine hydrochloride is a representative of the ethylamino phenothiazine derivatives. Although promethazine is a phenothiazine and has the potential for many of the side effects of phenothiazines, it has no use as an antipsychotic agent. Ethylamino derivatives are used for their antihistaminic and sedative properties. Antihistaminic activity makes promethazine useful in the symptomatic treatment of seasonal allergies, mild hypersensitivity reactions of urticaria and angioedema, and for the prevention of allergic reactions to blood or plasma transfusions. The sedative effects may be useful for mild preoperative and postoperative apprehension. Antiemetic activity may be effective in preventing or treating motion sickness and postoperative nausea.

Administration and dosage

For allergy:

Adult

PO—12.5 to 25 mg 2 or 3 times daily.
RECTAL—25 mg suppositories. May be repeated within 2 hr if necessary.

Pediatric

PO—0.1 mg/kg every 6 hr and 0.5 mg/kg at bedtime as needed or 6.25 to 12.5 mg 3 times daily and 25 mg at bedtime as needed.

For motion sickness, prophylaxis:

Adult

PO—25 mg twice daily. The initial dose should be administered 30 to 60 min before departure.

Pediatric

PO—0.5 mg/kg every 12 hr as needed or 12.5 to 25 mg every 12 hr as needed.

For nausea and vomiting:

Adult

PO—25 mg every 4 to 6 hr as needed.
RECTAL—12.5 to 25 mg suppository every 4 to 6 hr as needed.

Pediatric

PO—12.5 to 25 mg every 4 to 6 hr as needed.
RECTAL—As for adult dosages or 0.25 to 0.5 mg/kg every 4 to 6 hr as needed.
IM—0.25 to 0.5 mg/kg every 4 to 6 hr as needed.

To relieve apprehension and induce sleep:

Adult

PO—25 to 50 mg.

Pediatric

PO—12.5 to 25 mg.
RECTAL—12.5 to 25 mg.
IM—0.5 to 1 mg/kg.

Nurse and patient considerations

* See General information on phenothiazines (p. 378).
* A paradoxic reaction manifested by hyperexcitability and nightmares has been reported in children receiving single PO doses of 75 to 125 mg.

Drug interactions

See General information on phenothiazines (p. 378).

Thioridazine
(Mellaril)

AHFS 28:16.08
CATEGORY Tranquilizer

Action and use

Thioridazine is a representative of the piperidine phenothiazine derivatives. It may be effective in reducing psychomotor excitement, agitation, and tension associated with various types of acute and chronic psychoses and neuroses. The piperidine group of phenothiazines display minimal antiemetic activity, prominent sedative effects, and have the lowest incidence of extrapyramidal side effects of any of the classes of phenothiazines.

Administration and dosage
Adult

For neurotic depressive reaction, psychoneuroses, senility:

PO—10 to 50 mg 3 to 4 times daily.

For psychotic manifestations:

PO—50 to 100 mg 3 times daily, with gradual increments to a maximum of 800 mg if required.

NOTE: Once effective control of symptoms is achieved, the dosage should be reduced gradually to determine the minimum maintenance dose.

Pediatric (2 to 12 years of age)

NOTE: Thioridazine is not intended for children under 2 years of age. Dosage range for children age 2 to 12 years: 0.5 to 3.0 mg/kg.

Children with moderate disorders

PO—10 mg 2 or 3 times daily is the usual starting dose.

Children with severe disorders

PO—25 mg 2 to 3 times daily is the usual starting dose. Dosage may be increased gradually until optimal therapeutic effect or maximal dosage has been attained.

Nurse and patient considerations

＊ See General information on phenothiazines (p. 378).

Drug interactions

See General information on phenothiazines (p. 378).

Thiothixene
(Navane)

AHFS 28:16.08
CATEGORY Tranquilizer

Action and use

Thiothixene is an antipsychotic agent used in the treatment of acute and chronic psychoses. Its mechanism of action is not known, but it produces pharmacologic responses similar to those of the piperazine phenothiazines (trifluoperazine [Stelazine]) and butyrophenones (haloperidol [Haldol]). Thiothixene also displays some mild cholinergic and alpha-adrenergic blocking activity. Thiothixene may be used successfully in patients who are withdrawn, apathetic schizophrenics, and suffering from delusions and hallucinations. It is less effective in those patients displaying severe psychomotor excitement.

Characteristics

Onset: 1 to 6 hr (IM), a few days to several weeks (PO). Metabolism: liver. Excretion: primarily in bile and feces as unchanged drug and metabolites. Therapeutic level: unknown. Dialysis: no, H, P.

Administration and dosage
Adult

For mild to moderate psychotic states:

PO—Initially, 2 mg 3 times daily, gradually increased up to 15 mg daily. Dosage in elderly patients should be one third to half the normal adult dosage.

For severe psychotic states:

PO—Initially, 5 mg 2 times daily, with subsequent increases as needed. The usual optimal dose is 15 to 30 mg daily, although 60 mg daily may be required in some patients with severe symptomatology. A single daily dosage is usually adequate for maintenance therapy.

IM—In acutely agitated states, 4 mg 2 to 4 times daily may be effective. Subsequent doses may require adjustment. The usual optimal daily IM dose is 16 to 20 mg, with a total daily IM dosage not to exceed 30 mg. PO therapy should replace parenteral administration as soon as possible.

NOTE: Use in children under 12 years of age is not recommended.

Nurse and patient considerations

* See General information on phenothiazines (p. 378).
* Safe use in pregnancy has not been established.

Drug interactions

See General information on phenothiazines (p. 378).

Trifluoperazine
(Stelazine)

AHFS 28:16.08
CATEGORY Tranquilizer

Action and use

Trifluoperazine is a piperazine phenothiazine derivative used to treat anxiety, tension, and agitation associated with various neurotic and psychotic disorders. There appear to be fewer symptoms of sedation, blurred vision, and hypotension than with other classes of phenothiazine derivatives, but the extrapyramidal symptoms occur more frequently than with other classes of phenothiazines.

Administration and dosage
Adult

PO—1 to 5 mg 2 times daily. Optimal therapeutic dosage levels should be reached within 2 to 3 weeks. Most patients respond well at 15 to 20 mg/day, but an occasional patient will require 40 mg or more daily.

IM—1 to 2 mg by deep injection every 4 to 6 hr as needed. The injection should be protected from light. Slight yellow discoloration should not alter potency, but if markedly discolored, the solution should be discarded.

NOTE: As a result of the cumulative effects of trifluoperazine, patients should be periodically reevaluated to determine whether a lower maintenance dose may be adequate or whether drug therapy may be discontinued.

Pediatric (hospitalized patients 6 to 12 years of age)

PO—1 mg 1 to 2 times daily. Most patients respond to less than 15 mg/day. Gradually increase dosages until symptoms are controlled or until side effects become unacceptable.

IM—1 mg 1 or 2 times daily. The injection should be protected from light. Slight yellow discoloration should not alter potency, but if markedly discolored, the solution should be discarded.

Nurse and patient considerations

* See General information on phenothiazines (p. 378).

Overdosage

See General information on phenothiazines (p. 378).

Drug interactions

See General information on phenothiazines (p. 378).

GENERAL INFORMATION ON TRICYCLIC ANTIDEPRESSANTS

Tricyclic antidepressants are a class of compounds that are believed to relieve depression primarily by inhibiting the pump mechanism responsible for the reuptake of norepinephrine and serotonin into adrenergic neurons. Investigators have proposed that this may potentiate or prolong sympathetic activity by accumulation of these amines in the synaptic cleft. The tricyclic antidepressants may be subdivided into the tertiary amines (amitriptyline, doxepin, imipramine, trimipramine) and the secondary amines (amoxapine, desipramine, nortriptyline, protriptyline). The important differences between these agents is their relative selectivity for the receptor sites of the neurotransmitters, norepinephrine and serotonin. Amitriptyline is the most specific in affecting serotonin activity, while desipramine is most specific in affecting norepinephrine activity. The other tricyclic compounds affect both types of receptor sites to varying degrees, increasing the concentrations of both of the neurotransmitters in the synaptic cleft.

Tricyclic antidepressants have been found to be more specifically effective in treating patients with endogenous (psychotic) depression. Combination therapy with phenothiazine derivatives may be beneficial in treating the depression of schizophrenia or moderate to severe anxiety and depression associated with psychosis or psychoneurosis. Lithium and the tricyclic antidepressants are occasionally used concomitantly in treating acute depressive episodes of manic-depressive illness. Tricyclic antidepressants must be used with caution in manic-depressive patients, however, because these agents may induce a rapid return to the manic state (the "switch effect"). Tricyclic antidepressants may also be used in conjunction with electroconvulsive therapy in treating depression. Although data are conflicting, the use of antidepressants may reduce the amount of electroconvulsive therapy required.

The tricyclic antidepressants are equally effective in treating depression, assuming that appropriate dosages are used for an adequate duration of time. Consequently, the selection of an antidepressant is based primarily on the secondary characteristics of each individual agent. Sedation is more notable with amitriptyline, doxepin, and trimipramine, while protriptyline has no sedative properties and may actually produce mild stimulation in some patients. All tricyclic compounds display anticholinergic activity, with amitriptyline displaying the most, and desipramine the least. This should be considered in patients with cardiac disease, prostatic hypertrophy, or glaucoma. If a patient is not adequately treated after a course of therapy with a tertiary amine, a trial with a secondary amine may be indicated before moving to other treatment modalities (See Table 10-2). Other factors to consider are that men tend to respond better to imipramine than women, and the elderly tend to respond better to amitriptyline than younger patients.

Administration and dosage

Dosage should be initiated at a low level and increased gradually, particularly in elderly or debilitated patients. Increases in dosage should be made in the evening, since increased sedation is often present.

Manifestations of depression may improve within a few days (that is, increase in appetite, sleep, and psychomotor activity). However, the depression still exists, and it usually takes several weeks of therapeutic doses of antidepressants and psychotherapy before improvement is noted. Suicide precautions should be maintained during this time.

After an optimal response has been obtained, dosage should be reduced to the minimum necessary to maintain relief of depression.

When high doses are abruptly discontinued after several months of therapy, withdrawal symptoms (abdominal cramping, nausea, vomiting, chills, insomnia, akathisia, headache, dizziness, and irritability) often occur. Tapering should be done over a 1- or 2-month period.

See Table 10-2 for generic and brand names and recommended dosages.

Nurse and patient considerations

The most common side effects are those associated with anticholinergic activity. These include dry mucous mem-

Table 10-2. Tricyclic antidepressants

AHFS 28:16.04

Generic name	Trade name	Initial dosage		Maintenance daily dosage (mg)	Maximum daily dosage (mg)
		PO	IM		
Tertiary Amines					
Amitriptyline hydrochloride	Elavil	25 mg 3 times daily	20-30 mg 4 times daily	150 to 250	300
Doxepin hydrochloride	Sinequan	25 mg 3 times daily	—	No less than 150	300
Imipramine hydrochloride	Presamine Tofranil	30 to 75 mg daily	Up to 100 mg	150 to 250	300
Trimipramine maleate	Surmontil	75 to 100 mg daily	—	50 to 150	200 (out-patients) 300 (in-patients)

Continued.

Table 10-2. Tricyclic antidepressants—cont'd

AHFS 28:16.04

Generic name	Trade name	Initial dosage PO	Initial dosage IM	Maintenance daily dosage (mg)	Maximum daily dosage (mg)
Amoxapine	Asendin	50 mg 3 times daily	—	200 to 300	400 (out-patients) 600 (in-patients)
Secondary Amines					
Desipramine hydrochloride	Norpramin Pertofrane	25 mg 3 times daily	—	75 to 200	300
Nortriptyline hydrochloride	Aventyl	25 mg 3 to 4 times daily	—	50 to 75	100
Protriptyline hydrochloride	Vivactil	5-10 mg 3 to 4 times daily	—	20 to 40	60

branes, metallic taste, constipation, mydriasis, and cycloplegia resulting in blurred vision, epigastric distress, and urinary retention. Sugarless hard candy or chewing gum may help the dry mouth. The use of stool softeners such as docusate (Colace) or the occasional use of a potent laxative such as bisacodyl (Dulcolax) may be required for constipation. Reduction in dosage of the antidepressant may relieve symptoms of urinary retention. Tolerance to these side effects tends to develop with continued therapy.

Extrapyramidal side effects are rare, but a fine rapid tremor of the hands may occur in about 10% of the patients receiving tricyclic therapy. Occasionally, patients have reported numbness and tingling of arms and legs. The tremor may be controlled with small doses of propranolol. If parkinsonian symptoms develop, the tricyclic antidepressant dosage must be reduced or discontinued. Antiparkinsonian medications will not control tricyclic antidepressant–induced symptoms.

Patients with cardiovascular disorders must be observed for development or aggravation of existing arrhythmias, congestive heart failure, sinus tachycardia, and hypotension. The tricyclic antidepressants inhibit the reuptake of norepinephrine in cardiac tissue and have direct, quinidine-like depressant effects on the myocardium. Orthostatic hypotension is commonly seen with therapeutic dosages. Tricyclic antidepressants may cause flattening or inversion of the T wave of an electrocardiogram in about 20% of patients without previous history of cardiovascular disease. Deaths from coronary occlusion, cardiac arrest, and ventricular fibrillation have been reported, as well as cases of severe arrhythmias.

High doses of tricyclic antidepressants lower the seizure threshold. Seizures may occur in those with and without a history of seizure activity. Adjustment of anticonvulsant therapy may be required, especially in those seizure-prone patients.

Safe use in pregnancy has not been established. Fetal malformation, urinary retention, lethargy, and withdrawal symptoms have been reported in neonates whose mothers ingested tricyclic antidepressants during pregnancy.

Overdosage

Toxicity caused by acute overdosage is characterized by hyperpyrexia, hypertension, hypotension, arrhythmias, seizures, and coma. Gastric lavage may be of value in acute overdosage. Vital signs and ECG should be monitored continuously. Sudden fatal arrhythmias have been reported late in the course.

Physostigmine salicylate (Antilirium) may reverse the anticholinergic manifestations of delirium, convulsions, coma, and arrhythmias. (See Physostigmine salicylate, p. 615, for use.)

Hypotensive activity may be reversed with fluids. If a pressor agent is required, levarterenol or dopamine may be titrated as needed. Initiate therapy with very low doses, as tricyclics increase the pressor response to levarterenol.

Convulsions may be treated with IV diazepam (Valium). Arrhythmias refractory to physostigmine may be treated with phenytoin (Dilantin). Propranolol (Inderal) may be effective in arrhythmias caused by adrenergic hyperactivity resulting from blockade of the reuptake of catecholamines. In patients with conduction defects, the doses of physostigmine, propranolol, and phenytoin should be reduced to prevent complete heart block.

Drug interactions

Severe reactions (convulsions, hyperpyrexia, and fatalities) have been observed with the concomitant administration of an MAO inhibitor (isocarboxazid [Marplan], pargyline hydrochloride [Eutonyl], tranylcypromine sulfate [Parnate]). It is recommended that 2 weeks lapse between discontinuing an MAO inhibitor and starting tricyclic antidepressants. If used concomitantly, start with very low doses of both classes of compounds.

The antihypertensive effects of quanethidine (Ismelin) and clonidine (Catapres) are blocked by the tricyclic antidepressants because of inhibition of uptake into the adrenergic neuron.

Tricyclic antidepressants may display additive anticholinergic effects (dry mouth, constipation, urinary retention, acute glaucoma, blurred vision) when administered with antihistamines (Benadryl), phenothiazines, trihexiphenidyl (Artane), benzotropine (Cogentin), meperidine (Demerol), and other agents with anticholinergic activity. Usually, however, the side effects are not serious enough to require discontinuance of therapy.

Methylphenidate (Ritalin) and thyroid hormones may increase serum levels of tricyclic antidepressants. This reaction has been advantageous in attempts to gain a faster onset of antidepressant activity. Beware, however, of an increased incidence of arrhythmias.

Barbiturates may stimulate the metabolism of tricyclic antidepressants and may decrease their blood levels. Barbiturates may also potentiate the adverse effects (respiratory depression) of toxic doses of tricyclic antidepressants.

Tricyclic antidepression may enhance meperidine-induced respiratory depression. This reaction may be particularly significant in those patients with lung disease.

Tricyclic antidepressants may cause a synergistic response in patients receiving infusions of pressor amines—levarterenol (Levophed), epinephrine, and phenylephrine (Neo-Synephrine).

The sedative properties of the tricyclic antidepressants will be enhanced by concomitant use of ethanol, barbiturates, narcotics, tranquilizers, antihistamines, sedative-hypnotics, and anesthetics.

Concomitant therapy with tricyclic antidepressants and phenothiazines may result in elevated serum levels of both drugs. Additive anticholinergic effects and sedative effects may require a reduction in dosage of one or both agents.

Maprotiline hydrochloride AHFS 28:16.04
(Ludiomil) CATEGORY Antidepressant

Action and use

Maprotiline hydrochloride represents the first of a new class of tetracyclic antidepressants. The mechanism of action is similar to the tricyclic antidepressants in that it blocks the reuptake of norepinephrine at the neuronal membrane, but it does not affect the reuptake of serotonin. The overall pharmacologic activity is similar to that of the tricyclic antidepressants, but the frequency and severity of anticholinergic effects, cardiac arrhythmias, and orthostatic hypotension are reported to be lower with maprotiline. There does appear to be a slightly higher incidence of seizure activity and delirium associated with maprotiline therapy.

Characteristics

Peak serum levels: 8 to 24 hr (average: 12 hr). Protein binding: 88%. Half-life: maprotiline, 27 to 58 hr (average: 51 hr). Metabolism: liver, extensive; desmethylmaprotiline is active. Excretion: 60% in urine as metabolites; 30% in feces, within 3 weeks. Dialysis: no, H. Breast milk: unknown.

Administration and dosage
Adult

PO   1. Dosage should be initiated at a low level and increases gradually, particularly in elderly or debilitated patients. Increases in dosage should be made in the evening, since increased sedation is often present.

2. Initially, 75 mg daily. Increase in increments of 25 to 50 mg daily as required and tolerated. The usual effective dose is 150 mg daily. Some severely ill patients require 225 mg daily. Do not exceed 300 mg daily.

3. After an optimal response has been obtained, dosage should be reduced to the minimum necessary to maintain relief of depression, usually 75 to 150 mg daily.

Pediatric

Safe use and effectiveness in patients under 18 years of age have not been determined.

Nurse and patient considerations

* Manifestations of depression may improve within a few days (that is, increase in appetite, sleep, and psychomotor activity). However, the depression still exists, and it usually takes 2 to 4 weeks of therapeutic doses of antidepressants and psychotherapy before improvement is noted. Suicide precautions should be maintained during this time.

* Maprotiline should be used with caution in patients with a history of seizure disorders or those who may be predisposed to seizure activity. Maprotiline is associated with a higher incidence of seizures than the tricyclic antidepressants.

* Laboratory studies have given no indication of fetotoxic or teratogenic effects when maprotiline is administered to pregnant animals. However, maprotiline should not be administered to pregnant patients unless therapeutic benefits significantly outweigh possible adverse effects to the fetus.

* Maprotiline shares the same adverse effects as those of the tricyclic antidepressants. See General information on tricyclic antidepressants (p. 391).

Drug interactions

See General information on tricyclic antidepressants (p. 391).

Trazodone Hydrochloride
(Desyrel)

AHFS 28:16.04
CATEGORY Antidepressant

Action and use

Trazodone hydrochloride represents the first of a new class of antidepressants called the triazolopyridine derivatives. They are chemically unrelated to tricyclic and tetracyclic antidepressants. As with other antidepressants, the mechanism of action is not fully elucidated, but it is known that trazodone selectively inhibits serotonin uptake at brain synapses and potentiates the behavioral changes induced by the serotonin precursor, 5-hydroxytryptophan.

Clinical studies have shown that trazodone is an effective antidepressant when compared with placebo and is at least as effective as imipramine and amitriptyline in treating various types of depression. It has a low incidence of anticholinergic side effects when compared with other antidepressants, making trazodone particularly valuable as an alternative treatment for patients whose antidepressant dosages are limited by anticholinergic side effects and in those patients with severe angle-closure glaucoma, prostatic hypertrophy, organic mental disorders, and cardiac rhythm disturbances.

Characteristics

Peak serum levels: 1 to 2 hr. Protein binding: 89% to 95%. Half-lives: biphasic—3 to 10 hours after dosing, 4.4 hr; 10 to 34 hr after dosing, 7 to 8 hr. Metabolism: extensive. Excretion: 70% to 75% excreted in urine within 72 hr, less than 1% as active drug; 25% to 30% in feces. Dialysis: no, H. Breast milk: unknown.

Administration and dosage
Adult

PO   1. Dosage should be initiated at a low level and increased gradually, particularly in elderly or debilitated patients. Increases in dosage should be made in the evening, since increased sedation is often present.

2. Initially, 150 mg/day in 3 divided doses. Increase in increments of 50 mg/day every 3 to 4 days while monitoring clinical response. Do not exceed 400 mg/day in outpatients or 600 mg/day in hospitalized patients.
3. Administer shortly after a meal or with a light snack to reduce adverse effects.
4. Sedation may be less of a problem if the majority of the daily dose is administered in the evening. This may also help induce sleep.

Pediatric

Safe use and effectiveness in patients under 18 years of age have not been determined.

Nurse and patient considerations

* Manifestations of depression may improve within a few days (that is, increase in appetite, sleep, and psychomotor activity). However, the depression still exists, and it usually takes several weeks of therapeutic doses of antidepressants and psychotherapy before improvement is noted. Suicide precautions should be maintained during this time.
* After an optimal response has been obtained, dosage should be reduced to the minimum necessary to maintain relief of depression.
* Drowsiness and decreased energy are the most commonly reported adverse effects. Other CNS effects reported are fatigue, lightheadedness, dizziness, ataxia, mild confusion, and inability to think clearly.
* Cardiovascular side effects reported are orthostatic hypotension, tachycardia, and palpitations. Syncope, arrhythmias, angina, and bradycardia have rarely occurred.
* Fetotoxicity and teratogenic effects have been reported in laboratory animals. Trazodone should not be administered to pregnant patients unless therapeutic benefits significantly outweigh possible adverse effects to the fetus.

Drug interactions

The sedative properties of trazodone will be enhanced by concomitant use of ethanol, barbiturates, narcotics, tranquilizers, antihistamines, sedative-hypnotics, and anesthetics. Use combined therapy with caution.

Trazodone may inhibit the antihypertensive activity of clonidine and guanethidine.

Tranylcypromine sulfate
(Parnate)

Action and use

Tranylcypromine sulfate is a nonhydrazine monoamine oxidase (MAO) inhibitor. It is used to treat severe depression when tricyclic antidepressants and electroconvulsive treatment have been unsuccessful or refused. It may also be used in certain neurotic illnesses that have a depressive component and in the treatment of certain phobias and anxiety states. The MAO inhibitors are somewhat like the tricyclic antidepressants in that they increase the level of norepinephrine and serotonin in the neuronal presynaptic cleft. The MAO inhibitors act, however, by inhibiting monoamine oxidase, the enzyme necessary to metabolize these biogenic amines, thus allowing accumulation in the presynaptic clefts.

Characteristics

Clinical improvement is observed 2 days to 3 weeks after initiation of therapy. When tranylcypromine is discontinued, monoamine oxidase activity returns in 3 to 5 days.

Administration and dosage

NOTE: Tranylcypromine is contraindicated in certain types of patients and in conjunction with certain foods and medications. See the Contraindications section (p. 402).

Tranylcypromine therapy should be initiated only in hospitalized or very closely observed outpatients.

PO 1. Initially, 10 mg in the morning and afternoon for at least 2 weeks.
2. If necessary, increase to 20 mg in the morning, and 10 mg in the afternoon. If inadequate response is noted in another week, consider other treatments. Higher dosages may be used, but the incidence of side effects increases significantly.
3. In conjunction with electroconvulsive therapy: 10 mg 2 times daily during treatment, followed by 10 mg daily for maintenance therapy.

Contraindications

Do not administer to any patient with confirmed or suspected cardiovascular disease or hypertension or a history of severe headaches.

Do not administer to patients over 60 years of age, because of the possibility of cerebral sclerosis with damaged vessels.

Do not administer to patients with a known or suspected pheochromocytoma. These tumors secrete catecholamines that produce severe hypertension.

Dietary restrictions: MAO inhibitors act throughout the body inhibiting monoamine oxidase. Foods and other drugs are not metabolized as rapidly and may accumulate to toxic levels. Foods with a high tyramine content must be avoided to prevent these serious interactions. Patients must be instructed not to ingest cheese (particularly strong or aged varieties), sour cream, Chianti wine, sherry, beer, pickled herring, liver, canned figs, raisins, bananas, or avocados (particularly if overripe), chocolate, soy sauce, the pods of broad beans (fava beans), yeast extracts, or meat prepared with tenderizers.

Concurrent administration of certain drugs is contraindicated, and other drugs must be used with extreme caution. See Drug interactions (p. 404).

Overdosage

Hypertensive crisis is the most important adverse reaction reported with MAO inhibitors. It is manifested by an occipital headache radiating frontally, palpitations, neck stiffness or soreness, sweating, occasionally hyperpyrexia, photophobia, dilated pupils, tachycardia or bradycardia, and chest pain, along with significantly elevated blood pressure. Intracranial hemorrhage may also develop. A few cases of severe hypertension with seizure activity, coma, and death have been reported. Tranylcypromine therapy should be discontinued immediately if patients experience palpitations or recurrent headaches.

Hypertensive episodes may be treated with phentolamine, 5 mg IV (Regitine, see p. 212). Monitor not only the blood pressure but the entire patient as well. The headache tends to subside as the blood pressure is reduced. Hyperpyrexia may be controlled by external cooling (sponge bath, fan, ice bath).

The characteristic symptoms of insidious overdosage by drug accumulation are usually increased anxiety, agitation, and manic activity. These symptoms may progress to insomnia, mental confusion, and incoherence. Some patients have developed hypotension, dizziness, weakness, drowsiness, seizure activity, and shock. Hypotension may be controlled with dopamine (Intropin) (p. 137) or levarterenol (Levophed) (p. 146). The starting dose in such patients should be reduced to at least one tenth the usual dose and then titrated upward, based on the patient's response. Keep in mind that the MAO inhibitors block the metabolism of dopamine and levarterenol. Monitor heart rate, rhythm, blood pressure, fluid input and output, and temperature on a regular basis. Seizure activity may be controlled with phenobarbital, but remember that the duration of activity is prolonged due to inhibition of barbiturate metabolism by MAO inhibitors.

Nurse and patient considerations

* Manifestations of depression may improve within a few days (that is, increase in appetite, sleep, and psychomotor activity). However, the depression still exists and usually takes several weeks of therapeutic doses of antidepressants and psychotherapy before improvement is noted. Suicide precautions should be maintained during this time.

* Postural hypotension and dizziness are observed more frequently as dosages exceed 30 mg/day. They may be relieved by having the patient lie down until blood pressure returns to normal. Patients should be taught to rise slowly from a horizontal position to a sitting position and then flex the arms and legs several times before standing. The patient should be forewarned to sit or lie down with the onset of weakness and dizziness.

* Other side effects reported with tranylcypromine include dizziness, tachycardia, drowsiness, dryness of mouth, nausea, anorexia, diarrhea, abdominal pain, and constipation.

* Administer tranylcypromine with caution to patients with hyperthyroidism. Patients with this disease are quite sensitive to increased levels of norepinephrine and serotonin.

* Administer with caution in patients with diabetes mellitus. Tranylcypromine has been reported to contribute to hypoglycemic episodes in diabetic patients being treated with insulin or oral hypoglycemic agents.

* Use with caution in patients at risk for angina pec-

toris. Tranylcypromine may suppress anginal pain that would otherwise serve as a warning of myocardial ischemia.

* It is recommended that tranylcypromine be discontinued 7 days before elective surgery to allow time for recovery of monoamine oxidase levels before anesthetic agents are administered.

* Use tranylcypromine with extreme caution in pregnancy and only when the benefits of therapy significantly outweigh the risk of exposure to MAO inhibitors to the fetus. Laboratory tests indicate that tranylcypromine crosses the placental barrier and is secreted into breast milk.

Drug interactions

Tranylcypromine must not be administered together or in rapid succession with other MAO inhibitors such as isocarboxazid (Marplan), pargyline (Eutonyl), and phenelzine (Nardil). Patients may suffer hypertensive crises or severe seizure activity as a result. A 1-week "washout" period is recommended before starting the new MAO inhibitor at one half the normal starting dose.

Concurrent administration with tricyclic antidepressants (amitriptyline [Elavil], desipramine [Pertofrane, Norpramin], imipramine [Imavate, Tofranil, Presamine], nortriptyline [Aventyl, Pamelor], protriptyline [Vivactil] doxepin, [Adapin, Sinequan], amoxepine [Asendin], maprotiline [Ludiomil], and trimipramine [Surmontil]) is not recommended.

Other agents with structural similarities to the tricyclic antidepressants are carbamazepine (Tegretol) and cyclobenzaprine (Flexeril). Patients are susceptible to severe hypertension and seizure activity when these agents and MAO inhibitors are used concurrently. A 2-week "washout" period is recommended.

Tranylcypromine must not be administered in conjunction with any type of sympathomimetic-like agents. These agents include amphetamines, methyldopa (Aldomet), dopamine (Intropin), dobutamine (Dobutrex), levarterenol (Levophed), ephedrine, methylphenidate (Ritalin), phenylephrine (Neo-Synephrine), phenylpropanolamine, epinephrine, metaraminol (Aramine), and levodopa (Dopar, Sinemet). Patients should be warned that this restriction includes over-the-counter weight reduction products, allergy, and cough and cold medications that may include pseudoephedrine (Sudafed), dextromethorphan (Romilar), phenylpropanolamine (Propadrine), ephedrine, or phenylephrine (Neo-Synephrine). All the agents listed above may produce severe hypertension and/or seizure activity when administered to patients concurrently receiving MAO inhibitors.

Concurrent administration of MAO inhibitors and meperidine (Demerol) may cause a stimulatory state manifested by excitation, sweating, rigidity, and hypertension or a depressed state characterized by hypotension and coma. Concurrent therapy is not recommended. Consider cautious administration of morphine.

CNS depressants such as barbiturates (phenobarbital, pentobarbital, secobarbital), alcohol, narcotics (morphine, codeine), and anticholinergic agents (trihexyphenidyl [Artane], procyclidine [Kemadrin], benztropine [Cogentin]) may all have prolonged activity when administered with MAO inhibitors. These agents must be used with caution and in reduced dosages.

Patients receiving hypoglycemic agents (insulin, tolbutamide [Orinase], tolazamide [Tolinase], chlorpropamide [Diabinese], others) should be closely observed for hypoglycemic effects when concurrently administered with MAO inhibitors. The inhibitors have been shown to enhance and/or prolong the hypoglycemic activity.

The MAO inhibitors may antagonize the antihypertensive effects of guanethidine (Ismelin).

Monitor blood pressures closely in patients receiving concomitant phenothiazine and tranylcypromine therapy. Both these agents may aggravate the other agent's orthostatic hypotensive effects.

Lithium carbonate
(Eskalith, Lithane, Lithonate)

AHFS 28:16.12
CATEGORY Psychotherapeutic agent

Action and use

Lithium carbonate is used for the prophylactic treatment of recurrent manic and depressive episodes in bipolar major affective disorders and for the recurrence of depressive episodes in unipolar illness. The exact mechanism of action is not known; however, lithium does replace intracellular and intraneuronal sodium, stabilizing the neuronal membrane. It also prevents the release of norepinephrine and increases the uptake of L-tryptophane, the precursor to serotonin. It has no sedative, depressant, or euphoric properties, differentiating it from all other psychotropic agents.

Characteristics

Peak serum levels: 2 to 4 hr. Protein binding: 0%. Half-life: 24 hr in younger adults; 36 hr in the elderly. Metabolism: none. Excretion: 95% in urine, 1% in feces, 4 to 5% in sweat. Therapeutic levels: 0.7 to 1.5 mEq/l. Toxic levels: >2 mEq/l. Dialysis: yes, H. Breast milk: yes.

Administration and dosage

NOTE: Before initiation of lithium therapy, the following laboratory tests should be completed for baseline information: fasting blood glucose, BUN, serum creatinine, creatinine clearance, urinalysis, and thyroid function tests (T_3 and T_4).

Lithium may enhance sodium depletion, and sodium depletion enhances lithium toxicity. It is very important that patients maintain a normal dietary intake of sodium with adequate maintenance fluids, especially during the initiation of therapy, to prevent toxicity.

It is quite important that lithium serum levels be monitored, especially during initiation of therapy. Do not allow levels to exceed 2 mEq/L. Maintenance levels are 0.7 to 1.5 mEq/L. There is great interpatient variation between particular serum levels and dosages; however, there is reasonable correlation between dosages and serum levels in individual patients. It is important that the serum levels are drawn at similar time intervals. Drawing blood samples before the morning dose provides greatest consistency and correlation. Serum levels should be obtained twice weekly during acute manic episodes, biweekly as the patient is stabilized, then monthly to quarterly as the patient is well stabilized on maintenance therapy.

Early signs of toxicity include nausea, vomiting, abdominal pain, diarrhea, mild ataxia, and tremor. Patients and their families should be informed to observe for these effects and to report these effects immediately. See below for treatment of overdosage.

For acute mania:

PO—Initially, 600 mg 3 times daily with food. Monitor patients clinically and with serum levels twice weekly. Do not exceed 2 mEq/L. Normalization of symptoms should be observed within 1 to 3 weeks. A phenothiazine or haloperidol is frequently prescribed concurrently for acute therapy.

For depressive states and maintenance therapy:

PO 1. 300 mg 3 to 4 times daily. Maintain serum levels in the range of 0.7 to 1.2 mEq/L. Interpatient variation requires individual dosage adjustment.

2. Elderly patients tend to accumulate lithium and are more sensitive to toxicities.
3. Administration with food or milk minimizes gastric distress.

Overdose

Manifestations of lithium toxicity include nausea, vomiting, drowsiness, lethargy, speech difficulty, tremor, ataxia, myoclonic activity, hypotension, hyperreflexia, and unconsciousness. Electrocardiographic changes may show flattening, isoelectricity, or inversion of T waves and arrhythmias. The serum levels may or may not be greater than 2 mEq/L. Treatment consists of gastric lavage, correction of fluid and electrolyte balance, and urinary alkalinization with sodium bicarbonate or acetazolamide to enhance lithium excretion. Urea, mannitol, or aminophylline infusions will also significantly increase urinary excretion. Hemodialysis is also quite useful.

Nurse and patient considerations

* Side effects frequently reported early in the course of therapy are nausea, anorexia, stomach irritation, and diarrhea. These effects are frequently minimized by administration with meals. Polyuria and excessive thirst are common in the first week of therapy because of sodium diuresis. Fine hand tremor and mild, transient ataxia are also occasionally observed.

* Persistent vomiting, profuse diarrhea, hyperreflexia, lethargy, and weakness are all signs of impending serious toxicity. Dosages should be reduced or discontinued.

* Rarely, long-term lithium therapy (greater than 6 months) produces hypothyroidism. The mechanism of action is unknown. The hypothyroid state should be treated with thyroid replacement.

* Chronic lithium therapy rarely initiates a diabetes insipidus–like syndrome characterized by polyuria and polydipsia. Temporarily discontinuing therapy for a few days corrects the problem. Reinitiation of therapy at lower doses rarely reactivates the syndrome. Monitor patients closely for fluid and electrolyte balance.

* Other adverse effects that have been reported with lithium therapy include albuminuria, oliguria, renal

tubular damage, transient hyperglycemia, leukocytosis, worsening of organic brain syndrome, generalized pruritus with and without rash, edematous swelling of the ankles and wrists, and metallic taste.

* Lithium should be avoided in pregnancy, especially in the first trimester, if at all possible. The use of lithium early in pregnancy may be associated with an increased incidence of cardiovascular abnormalities in the neonate. Breast-feeding during lithium therapy is also not recommended. Significant amounts of lithium are excreted in breast milk, and toxicities have been reported.

Drug interactions

Therapeutic activity and toxicity of lithium is highly dependent on sodium concentrations. Decreased sodium levels significantly enhance the toxicity of lithium. Patients who are to initiate diuretic therapy, a low sodium diet, or activities that will produce excessive, prolonged sweating should be observed particularly closely.

There is an increased incidence of lithium toxicity when methyldopa (Aldomet) therapy is initiated in patients on long-term lithium therapy. The mechanism is unknown. The serum lithium levels remain within the therapeutic range.

There is an increased incidence of lithium toxicity when indomethacin (Indocin) therapy is initiated in patients on long-term lithium therapy. Indomethacin reduces the renal clearance of lithium, allowing it to accumulate, possibly to toxic levels. When indomethacin therapy is discontinued after long-term concomitant use with lithium, lithium levels may fall below the therapeutic range because of increased urinary excretion.

Although frequently used concomitantly, several drug interactions are reported between lithium and phenothiazines. Interactions include increased cellular uptake of lithium, increased excretion of lithium, neurotoxicity (delirium, seizures), and extrapyramidal symptoms. Predictability of these sometimes conflicting interactions is difficult. Patients should be monitored closely for altered response to either drug with combined use.

CHAPTER ELEVEN

Anticonvulsant agents

Carbamazepine
Clonazepam
Diazepam

Phenytoin
Primidone
Valproic acid

Carbamazepine
(Tegretol)

AHFS 28:12
CATEGORY Anticonvulsant

Action and use

Carbamazepine is an anticonvulsant structurally related to the tricyclic antidepressants. Its mechanism for antiepileptic activity appears to be similar to that of the hydantoin derivatives (Dilantin); it elevates the convulsive threshold and limits the spread of the seizure discharge from its focus. Carbamazepine has been found to be effective in the prophylactic treatment of generalized tonic-clonic, simple partial, and complex partial seizures. It is not effective in the control of absence seizures. Carbamazepine has also been used to successfully treat the pain associated with trigeminal neuralgia (tic douloureaux).

Characteristics

Peak plasma levels: 2 to 4 hr. Protein binding: 75% to 90%; Half-life: 14 to 36 hr. Metabolism: liver to several metabolites, activity unknown. Excretion: less than 1% unchanged in urine. Therapeutic plasma level: 0.3 mg/100 ml. Toxic plasma level: 0.8 mg/100 ml to 1 mg/100 ml. Dialysis: unknown.

Administration and dosage
Adult

PO
1. Initial: 200 mg 2 times daily. Add up to 200 mg daily as tolerated until the best response is attained. Daily dosages above 1200 mg are not recommended; however, 1600 mg daily may be required in certain instances.
2. Maintenance: adjust dosage to the minimum effective level, usually 800 to 1200 mg daily.

Pediatric
Ages 12 to 15

PO—As for adults; dosage should generally not exceed 1000 mg daily.

Ages 15 and older

PO—As for adults; dosage should generally not exceed 1200 mg daily.

NOTE: Serious and sometimes fatal blood dyscrasias have been reported following treatment with carbamazepine. Use of this drug is not recommended unless other antiepileptic agents have been found to be ineffective or produce unacceptable side effects.

Patients sensitive to the tricyclic antidepressants must not receive carbamazepine. If serious side effects should require abrupt cessation of carbamazepine therapy, patients must be observed closely for increased seizure activity.

Nurse and patient considerations

* Side effects often observed on initiation of therapy include dizziness, drowsiness, nausea, and vomiting. Reduction in dosage or gradual increases in dosage will help minimize these adverse effects.
* As a result of serious adverse reactions the manufacturer recommends that the following baseline studies be repeated at regular intervals:

   Complete blood count with differential, platelet, and reticulocyte counts; serum iron determinations

   Liver function tests

   Urinalysis, BUN, and serum creatinine

   Ophthalmologic examination
* Congestive heart failure, hypertension, hypotension, edema, and aggravation of coronary artery disease have been reported. Although not reported specifically with carbamazepine, arrhythmias and myocardial infarction have been reported with other tricyclic compounds.
* Neurologic side effects include incoordination, nystagmus, visual hallucinations, and oculomotor and speech disturbances.
* Dermatologic manifestations of alopecia, pruritus, rashes, skin pigmentation, urticaria, and aggrava-

tion of systemic lupus erythematosus have been reported.

* Carbamazepine anticonvulsant therapy should only be used in pregnant women on a risk versus benefit basis. Carbamazepine crosses the placental barrier, and teratogenic abnormalities have been reported in laboratory animals. It is recommended that lactating women *not* nurse their infants. Carbamazepine does appear in breast milk.

Drug interactions

Carbamazepine causes hepatic microsomal enzyme induction. It may enhance the metabolism of other anticonvulsants (phenytoin [Dilantin], phenobarbital, valproic acid [Depakene], and primidone [Mysoline]) used concurrently with carbamazepine. Monitoring changes in serum levels should help warn of possible increased seizure activity.

Warfarin (Coumadin) metabolism may be increased by enzyme induction from carbamazepine. Monitor the prothrombin time more closely while carbamazepine therapy is being started or stopped.

The clinical effectiveness of doxycycline (Vibramycin) may be reduced by enhanced metabolism caused by carbamazepine.

MAO therapy should be discontinued at least 1 week before initiating carbamazepine therapy.

The contraceptive efficacy of oral contraceptives when taken with carbamazepine may be impaired. Breakthrough bleeding may be an indication of this interaction. Adjustment in dosage of oral contraceptives and use of alternative methods of contraception should be considered.

The combined use of propoxyphene (Darvon) and carbamazepine is not recommended. Propoxyphene may significantly increase serum levels of carbamazepine, resulting in toxicity manifested by dizziness, nausea, drowsiness, and headache.

Isoniazid inhibits the metabolism of carbamazepine, resulting in signs of carbamazepine toxicity (disorientation, ataxia, lethargy, headache, drowsiness, nausea, vomiting). The reaction may develop within 1 to 2 days of combined therapy and is more likely to occur in patients taking greater than 200 mg of isoniazid daily.

Clonazepam
(Clonopin)

AHFS 28:12; C-IV
CATEGORY Anticonvulsant

Action and use

Clonazepam is a benzodiazepine derivative used in the prophylactic treatment of akinetic and complex absence seizures. It is the first PO benzodiazepine derivative available for anticonvulsant use in the United States. Its mechanism of action is unknown. Investigationally, clonazepam has shown variable degrees of success in generalized tonic-clonic and complex partial seizures when other first-line therapy has failed. IV Clonazepam has been effective in various types of status epilepticus.

Characteristics

Onset: 20 to 60 min. Peak levels: 1 to 2 hr. Duration: 6 to 8 hr in infants and children, 12 hr in adults. Half-life: 19 to 50 hr. Metabolism: liver to 5 inactive metabolites. Excretion: 50% to 70% in urine, 13% to 30% in feces, as metabolites.

Administration and dosage
Adult

PO 1. Initial—up to 1.5 mg/day divided into 3 doses. Increase the dosage in increments of 0.5 to 1 mg every 3 days until seizures are controlled or side effects prevail.
    2. Maintenance: individualized for each patient. The maximum recommended daily dosage is 20 mg.

Pediatric (to 10 years of age or 30 kg)

PO 1. Initial: 0.01 to 0.03 mg/kg/day, not to exceed 0.05 mg/kg/day. Administer in 2 or 3 divided doses.
    2. Maintenance: increase dosage by no more than 0.25 to 0.5 mg every third day until the daily maintenance dose of 0.1 to 0.2 mg/kg is achieved, seizures are controlled, or side effects are unacceptable. Divide the dosage into 3 equal doses if possible. If not, administer the largest dose at bedtime.

NOTE: Dosage should be reduced slowly, especially after long-term, high-dose therapy, to avoid precipitating seizures or status epilepticus.

Nurse and patient considerations

* Addition of clonazepam to a therapeutic regimen of other anticonvulsants may allow reduction in dosage of the other anticonvulsants; however, paradoxic increases in seizure activity have also been reported.

* Patients may become refractory to clonazepam after months or years of therapy. In some cases, increased doses may be effective, if tolerated. Addition of other antiepileptic agents may also be required.

* The most commonly occurring side effects are related to CNS depression. Drowsiness and ataxia are frequently seen, especially on initiation of therapy. They do dissipate to some extent with time. They may be enhanced by the concurrent use of other anticonvulsants with CNS depressant effects.

* Behavioral disturbances such as aggressiveness, agitation, and hyperkinesis have been reported, especially in patients with preexisting brain damage, mental retardation, or psychiatric disturbances.

* Respiratory hypersecretion, chest congestion, shortness of breath, increased salivation, and rhinorrhea may occur.

* Numerous other neurologic side effects have been reported, including nystagmus, double vision, slurred speech, headache, tremor, and vertigo.

* Various dermatologic and hematologic effects have also been reported. Periodic blood counts and liver function tests should be performed on patients receiving long-term clonazepam therapy.

* Clonazepam therapy is not recommended for pregnant or nursing women. It crosses the placental barrier, and its relationship to birth defects is not fully known.

* See General information on benzodiazepines (p. 358).

Drug interactions

Ethanol, narcotics, barbiturates, anticonvulsants, sedative-hypnotics, tranquilizers, phenothiazines, and tricyclic antidepressants may potentiate the CNS depressant effects of clonazepam.

The concurrent use of clonazepam and valproic acid has been associated with the development of absence seizures. The incidence and mechanism of this interaction are unknown.

Diazepam
(Valium)

AHFS 28:16.08; C-IV
CATEGORY Tranquilizer, anticonvulsant

Action and use

Diazepam is a benzodiazepine derivative used in mild to moderate states of anxiety and tension. It may also be used as a tranquilizer for acute alcohol withdrawal syndrome.

Diazepam has beneficial tranquilizing and amnesic effects when administered parenterally for the relief of anxiety and tension before endoscopy, minor surgical procedures, and cardioversion of atrial fibrillation.

Diazepam is often effective in controlling various types of partial and generalized seizures and in controlling tonic-clonic status epilepticus.

Characteristics

Onset: immediate (IV), 15 to 30 min (IM), 30 to 60 min (PO). Peak plasma levels: 1 to 3 hr (PO). Protein binding: highly bound. Half-life: 1 to 2 days (parent compound and active metabolites). Metabolism: liver, active; Excretion: metabolites in urine and feces. Therapeutic level: 0.1 mg/100 ml to 0.25 mg/100 ml. Toxic level: 0.5 mg/100 ml to 2 mg/100 ml. Fatal level: 2 mg/100 ml. Dialysis: no, H.

Administration and dosage
Adult

PO—2 to 10 mg 2 to 4 times daily.

IM—Should be discouraged: it is painful, with erratic absorption.

IV—2 to 40 mg depending on use; added in small increments. Inject slowly, monitoring the patient's response. Take at least 1 min for each 5 mg (1 ml) given. A fine, white precipitate will develop when diazepam is added to other solutions, including dextrose 5% and saline solution. Administer as close to the venipuncture site as possible.

Pediatric

PO—0.12 to 0.8 mg/kg/24 hr divided into 3 or 4 doses.

IM—0.1 to 0.3 mg/kg repeated in 2 to 4 hr as needed.

NOTE: Diazepam is not recommended in infants less than 30 days of age. However, if seizure activity cannot be arrested with maximum dosages of phenobarbital, 0.1 to 0.8 mg/kg/24 hr may be used. Sodium benzoate, a preservative used in parenteral solutions of diazepam, has been associated with clinically significant displacement of bilirubin from protein-binding sites.

Nurse and patient considerations

* See General information on benzodiazepines (p. 358).
* Overdosage may be manifested by somnolence, confusion, coma, and respiratory depression. Treatment consists of general physiologic supportive measures including maintenance of an airway and administration of oxygen. Methylphenidate (Ritalin) or caffeine may be effective against severe CNS or respiratory depression. Do not use barbiturates in patients who develop excitation after ingestion of diazepam.
* Hypotension may occur, particularly on parenteral administration. Severe hypotensive effects may be reversed with levarterenol (Levophed) or metaraminol (Aramine).
* Use with caution in pregnant women. Fetal blood levels are similar to those in maternal circulation. Small amounts are found in breast milk.

Drug interactions

When diazepam is used with a narcotic analgesic, the dosage of the narcotic should be reduced by at least one third and administered in small increments.

Rare cases have been reported where diazepam has inhibited the metabolism of phenytoin (Dilantin), resulting in increased serum levels of phenytoin and potential toxicity.

Rifampin may significantly decrease serum levels of diazepam. Dosage adjustment for anticonvulsant therapy may be necessary.

Cimetidine inhibits the metabolism of diazepam, enhancing its sedative effects. A decrease in dosage of diazepam may be necessary.

Isoniazid may inhibit the metabolism of diazepam, causing moderately prolonged activity. Observe patients for altered response to diazepam when isoniazid therapy is started or stopped.

See General information on benzodiazepines (p. 358).

Phenytoin
(Dilantin)

AHFS 28:12
CATEGORY Anticonvulsant

Action and use

Phenytoin may be effective in the treatment of epilepsy. It appears to stabilize the normal seizure threshold and prevent the spread of seizure activity. It does not abolish the primary focus of seizure discharges. It is indicated for the control of generalized tonic-clonic, simple partial, and complex partial seizure activity. It is generally of little value in absence seizures.

Characteristics

Onset: 1 to 2 hr following an IV loading dose of 1 to 1.5 g, 2 to 24 hr following a PO loading dose of 1 g. Protein binding: 95%. Half-life: 18 to 24 hr. Metabolism: liver to inactive metabolites. Excretion: 1% unchanged in urine, 75% in urine as metabolites. Therapeutic levels: 7.5 to 20 μg/ml. Toxic level: 10 to 50 μg/ml. Dialysis: yes, H.

Administration and dosage
Adult

PO—Initial: 100 mg 3 times daily. For most adults the daily maintenance dosage is 100 to 400 mg.

IM—Avoid if at all possible: the dosage is painful and quite erratically absorbed.

IV—Status epilepticus: 750 to 1000 mg at *a rate no faster than 50 mg/min*, with monitoring of the ECG and pulse rate.

Pediatric

PO—Initial: 5 to 7 mg/kg/24 hr in 1 or 2 doses.

IM—Avoid if at all possible; the dosage is painful and quite erratically absorbed.

IV—Status epilepticus: 15 to 20 mg/kg at *a rate no faster than 50 mg/min*, with monitoring of the ECG and pulse rate. Maintain response with 5 to 8 mg/kg/day in 1 or 2 divided doses.

NOTE: If given too rapidly by the IV route, bradycardia and severe hypotension may result. The diluent, propylene glycol, will also potentiate the hypotensive effect of phenytoin and cause ECG changes. Cardiac and respiratory arrest may occur with excessive dosage and rate of administration. Blood pressure and the ECG should be monitored carefully, especially during administration.

Phenytoin should not be mixed with any drugs or added to any IV infusion solutions. The solubility is very pH dependent, and use with other medications or solutions will result in a white precipitate.

Each IV injection should be followed by an injection of sterile saline solution through the same needle or IV catheter to avoid local venous irritation.

Nurse and patient considerations

* Frequent side effects include nystagmus, ataxia, slurred speech, and mental confusion. Dizziness, insomnia, and transient nervousness may also occur. These side effects are usually dose related and disappear at reduced dosage levels.
* Phenytoin may elevate blood glucose levels, especially if larger doses are used. Patients with diabetes mellitus or renal insufficiency may be more susceptible to hyperglycemia.
* Fatal dermatologic manifestations sometimes accompanied by fever, blood dyscrasias, toxic hepatitis, and liver damage have been attributed to phenytoin.
* Gingival hyperplasia occurs frequently, but the incidence may be reduced by good oral hygiene including gum massage, frequent brushing, and proper dental care.
* There have been reports suggesting a correlation between birth defects and the aministration of anticonvulsant drugs. Use of phenytoin must be on a risk versus benefit basis.

Drug interactions

Barbiturates may enhance the rate of metabolism of phenytoin.

Warfarin (Coumadin), disulfiram (Antabuse), phenylbutazone (butazolidin), chloramphenicol (Chloromycetin), and isoniazid (INH) inhibit the metabolism of phenytoin, resulting in signs of phenytoin toxicity (nystagmus, ataxia, lethargy, and confusion).

Complex relationships exist between folic acid, phenytoin, and anticonvulsant activity. Phenytoin may induce folic acid deficiency, while folic acid replacement may result in partial loss of seizure control.

Phenytoin stimulates microsomal enzyme activity that enhances the metabolism of corticosteroids and theophylline. Serum theophylline levels should be monitored closely when phenytoin is either added or removed from the drug therapy of a patient who is also taking theophylline.

The contraceptive efficacy of oral contraceptives when taken with phenytoin may be impaired. Breakthrough bleeding may be an indication of this interaction. Adjustment in dosage of oral contraceptives and use of alternative methods of contraception should be considered.

Valproic acid (Depakene) may increase or decrease phenytoin serum levels. Serum phenytoin levels should be determined periodically and dosages should be adjusted if necessary.

Phenytoin may significantly decrease serum levels of disopyramide. Patients should be observed for redevelopment of arrhythmias that may require an increase in dosage of disopyramide.

Primidone
(Mysoline)

AHFS 28:12
CATEGORY Anticonvulsant

Action and use

Primidone is an anticonvulsant structurally related to phenobarbital. It has anticonvulsant properties of its own, but is also metabolized to phenobarbital and phenyethylmalonamide (PEMA), both of which are also active anticonvulsants. Primidone is a useful adjunct to the treatment of several types of seizures. It is effective in the prophylactic control of generalized tonic-clonic, temporal lobe, and cortical focal epileptic seizures and is often used in combination with phenytoin (Dilantin) therapy.

Characteristics

Peak serum levels: 3 to 4 hr (PO). Protein binding: insignificant. Metabolism: to phenobarbital, PEMA (active). Half-life: primidone, 3 to 24 hr; PEMA, 24 to 48 hr; phenobarbital, 48 to 120 hr. With chronic administration, patients may accumulate high serum levels of phenobarbital. Excretion of primidone: 15% to 25% unchanged in urine, 15% to 25% metabolized to phenobarbital, 50% to 70% excreted in urine as PEMA. Therapeutic serum level: of primidone, 1 mg/100 ml to 2 mg/100 ml; of phenobarbital, 1 mg/100 ml to 2.5 mg/100 ml. Toxic level of primidone: 5 mg/100 ml to 8 mg/100 ml. Dialysis of primidone: yes, H, P.

Administration and dosage
Adult

PO—Initial: 250 mg daily, with incremental increases of 250 mg at weekly intervals to tolerance or therapeutic effectiveness. The average adult dose is 0.75 to 1.5 g/day. Maximum daily doses should not exceed 2 g.

Pediatric
Under 8 years of age

PO—Initial: 125 mg daily, with incremental increases of 125 mg at weekly intervals to tolerance or therapeutic effectiveness. The average pediatric dosage is 500 to 750 mg/day.

Over 8 years of age

PO—As for adult dosages.

Nurse and patient considerations

* Common adverse effects include sedation, drowsiness, dizziness, ataxia, diplopia, and nystagmus. These symptoms tend to disappear with continued therapy and possible readjustment of dosage.
* Primidone has been reported to produce paradoxic hyperexcitability in children (as does phenobarbital).
* Severe adverse effects such as maculopapular and morbilliform rash, leukopenia, thrombocytopenia, megaloblastic anemia, and systemic lupus erythematosus are rare occurrences, but have been reported. A complete blood count is recommended every 6 months during prolonged therapy.
* Neonatal hemorrhage has been reported in newborns whose mothers were taking primidone. It is recommended that pregnant women under anticonvulsant therapy should receive prophylactic phytonadione (Mephyton) therapy for 1 month before and during delivery. Primidone also appears in breast milk in substantial quantities and may result in somnolence and drowsiness in nursing newborns.

Drug interactions

Phenytoin (Dilantin) appears to increase the phenobarbital serum levels when taken concurrently with primidone. This may be beneficial in the control of epilepsy, but patients must also be observed for increased signs of sedation and lethargy caused by high phenobarbital levels.

Primidone may interfere with oral contraceptive therapy. See General information on oral contraceptives (p. 499).

Valproic acid
(Depakene)

AHFS 28:12
CATEGORY Anticonvulsant

Action and use

Valproic acid is an anticonvulsant chemically unrelated to other agents used to treat seizure disorders. Its mechanism of action is unknown. Valproic acid is most effective, either alone or in combination with other anticonvulsants, in the management of simple and complex absence (petit mal) seizures.

Characteristics

Peak serum levels: 1 to 4 hr (PO). Protein binding: 90%. Half-life: 8 to 12 hr. Metabolism: liver to inactive metabolites. Excretion: primarily in urine, small amounts in feces and via lungs; Therapeutic levels: 50 to 100 µg/ml (estimated). Dialysis: unknown.

Administration and dosage
Adult and pediatric

PO—Initial: 5 mg/kg every 8 hr. The dosage may be increased by 5 to 10 mg/kg/day at weekly intervals, depending on patient response. The maximum recommended daily dosage is 30 mg/kg/day. Between 2 and 4 weeks are required to fully assess the effectiveness of therapy.

NOTE: Valproic acid may be given with food or milk to minimize gastric irritation.

Nurse and patient considerations

* Gastric irritation resulting in nausea, vomiting, and indigestion is a common side effect on initiation of valproic acid therapy. Gradual increases in therapy or dosage reduction usually controls gastrointestinal discomfort.

* Sedative effects have been reported, particularly when valproic acid is used in conjunction with other anticonvulsant therapy. Ataxia, dizziness, diplopia, nystagmus, "spots before eyes," and headache have occasionally been reported. These side effects are usually dose related and disappear when the dosage of valproic acid or other anticonvulsant therapy is reduced. Patients should also be warned against engaging in activities requiring mental alertness.

* As a result of rare reports of impaired platelet aggregation, thrombocytopenia, and elevated liver enzymes, the manufacturer recommends that the following baseline studies be completed before therapy is initiated and at regular intervals thereafter:
    Liver function tests
    Bleeding time determination
    Platelet count

* One of the metabolites of valproic acid is a ketone-containing derivative. It is excreted in the urine and may produce a false-positive test (Ketostix, Acetest) for urine ketones.

* Valproic acid anticonvulsant therapy should only be used in pregnant women on a risk versus benefit basis. Valproic acid crosses the placental barrier, and teratogenic abnormalities have been reported in laboratory animals. It is recommended that lactating women *not* nurse their infants. Valproic acid does appear in breast milk.

Drug interactions

Ethanol, narcotics, barbiturates, anticonvulsants, sedative-hypnotics, tranquilizers, phenothiazines, and tricyclic antidepressants may enhance the CNS depressant effects of valproic acid.

Valproic acid may increase serum phenobarbital levels and may increase or decrease phenytoin (Dilantin) serum levels. Serum phenobarbital and phenytoin levels should be determined periodically, and dosages should be adjusted if necessary.

Absence status (continuous absence seizure activity) has been induced when the benzodiazepine-derivative anticonvulsant clonazepam was used concomitantly with valproic acid. The incidence and mechanism of this interaction is unknown.,

Coagulation studies should be monitored closely when valproic acid is prescribed for concurrent use with medications such as warfarin (Coumadin), sulfinpyrazone (Anturane), and aspirin.

The concurrent use of carbamazepine (Tegretol) and valproic acid may result in subtherapeutic serum levels of valproic acid. Serum valproic acid levels should be determined periodically, and dosages should be adjusted if necessary.

CHAPTER TWELVE

Antiemetic agents

Benzquinamide
Cyclizine
Trimethobenzamide

Benzquinamide
(Emete-Con)

AHFS 56:20
CATEGORY Antiemetic

Action and use

Benzquinamide is structurally unrelated to other phe-nothiazine or antihistaminic antiemetics. Its mechanism of action in humans is unknown, but is believed to involve sup-pression of the chemoreceptor trigger zone in the medulla oblongata.

Characteristics

Onset: antiemetic 15 min (IM or IV). Peak blood levels: 30 min (IM). Duration of action: 3 to 4 hr. Protein binding: 55% to 60%. Half-life: 30 to 40 min. Metabolism: liver. Excretion: 3% to 10% unchanged in urine, metabolites in feces and urine. Dialysis: no, H, P.

Administration and dosage

Reconstitute benzquinamide 50 mg/vial with 2.2 ml of sterile water or bacteriostatic water for injection to yield a solution containing 25 mg benzquinamide/ml. Do not recon-stitute with 0.9% sodium chloride injection because precip-itation may result. Potency is maintained for 14 days at room temperature. *Do not refrigerate.*

IM—50 mg or 0.5 to 1 mg/kg by deep IM injection in a large muscle mass. May repeat in 1 hr, with subsequent doses every 3 to 4 hr.

IV—25 mg or 0.2 to 0.4 mg/kg. Subsequent doses should be given IM.

NOTE: Sudden increase in blood pressure and transient car-diac arrhythmias (premature atrial and ventricular contrac-tions) have been reported following IV use. Use with extreme caution in patients with heart disease or those patients receiving preanesthetic or cardiovascular agents.

NOTE: Safe use in children has not been established.

Nurse and patient considerations

* Drowsiness and sedation appear to be the most commonly observed side effects of benzquinamide. Others include dry mouth, blurred vision, hypertension, hypotension, dizziness, and arrhythmias. Hypersensitivity reactions, nausea, vomiting, tremor, weakness, and abdominal cramps have also been reported.

* Antiemetics may obscure signs of overdosage of other drugs or of symptoms of such conditions as appendicitis, intestinal obstruction, or brain tumor.

* Other measures to enhance the antiemetic effect include frequent small amounts of dry carbohydrate feedings when allowed by the patient's diet, avoidance of high-fat foods, and antacids. Decrease noxious stimuli in the environment such as odors, smoke, unpleasant sounds, drainage, and waste products. Good oral hygiene is frequently overlooked after emesis.

* Be aware of excessive vomiting, and observe for deficiencies in fluids, electrolytes, and nutrients. See Table 4-1, Indications of electrolyte imbalance (p. 237).

* No teratogenic effects have yet been reported, but use in pregnancy is not recommended. It is not known whether benzquinamide crosses the placental barrier or appears in breast milk.

Drug interactions

None have been specifically reported; however, additive anticholinergic, antihistaminic, and sedative effects may be expected with other drugs with similar properties.

Cyclizine
(Marezine)

AHFS 56:20
CATEGORY Antihistamine, antiemetic

Action and use

Cyclizine is a short-acting antihistaminic agent with CNS depressant, anticholinergic, and antiemetic properties. It is used in the prophylaxis and treatment of the nausea, vomiting, and dizziness of motion sickness and vestibular disease.

Characteristics

Duration of action: 4 to 6 hr. Dialysis: unknown.

Administration and dosage
Adult

PO

1. Motion sickness: 50 mg 30 min before departure; may be repeated every 4 to 6 hr as needed. Do not exceed 4 tablets daily.
2. Vertigo: 50 mg 3 to 4 times daily.

IM—As for PO administration.

RECTAL—100 mg suppository every 4 to 6 hr.

NOTE: Cyclizine is not recommended for the nausea and vomiting of pregnancy. Teratogenic effects have been observed in laboratory animals.

Pediatric
Under 6 years of age

PO AND RECTAL—One fourth the adult dosages.

Between 6 and 12 years of age

PO AND RECTAL—Half the adult dosages.

Nurse and patient considerations

* A common side effect of cyclizine is drowsiness. Patients must be warned about performing tasks requiring mental alertness and coordination.
* Other side effects may include blurred vision, dry mouth, constipation, and fatigue.

Drug interactions

Cyclizine may display additive anticholinergic side effects (dry mouth, constipation, and blurred vision) when administered with other antihistamines, phenothiazines, trihexyphenidyl (Artane), benztropine (Cogentin), and other agents with anticholinergic activity.

Trimethobenzamide
(Tigan)

AHFS 56:20
CATEGORY Antiemetic

Action and use

Trimethobenzamide is a nonphenothiazine antiemetic structurally related to diphenhydramine-like antihistamines.

It is believed to control nausea and vomiting by suppression of the chemoreceptor trigger zone in the medulla oblongata through which impulses pass to the vomiting center.

Characteristics

Onset: 10 to 40 min (PO), 15 to 30 min (IM). Duration: 2 to 3 hr (IM), 4 to 6 hr (PO), Metabolism: liver. Excretion: 30% to 50% unchanged in urine within 48 to 72 hr, metabolites in urine and feces. Therapeutic level: 0.1 to 0.2 mg/ 100 ml.

Administration and dosage
Adult

PO—250 mg 2 to 4 times daily.
IM—200 mg 3 to 4 times daily.
IV—Not recommended.
RECTAL—200 mg 3 to 4 times daily.
NOTE: The suppository form contains benzocaine. It should not be administered to patients known to be sensitive to local anesthetics.

Pediatric

NOTE: Trimethobenzamide should be used with caution when administered to children. There has been some suspicion that centrally acting antiemetics, in combination with viral illnesses, may contribute to the development of Reye's syndrome, a potentially fatal acute childhood disease. Administration of antiemetics is not recommended until the cause of vomiting can be determined.

Under 13.5 kg

RECTAL—½ suppository (100 mg) 3 or 4 times daily.

Between 13.5 and 40.5 kg

PO—100 to 200 mg 3 or 4 times daily.
RECTAL—½ to 1 suppository (100 to 200 mg) 3 or 4 times daily.
NOTE: Do not administer suppositories to premature or newborn infants.
NOTE: IM administration is not recommended for use in children.

Nurse and patient considerations

* CNS reactions (opisthotonos, convulsions, coma, and extrapyramidal symptoms) may occur with and without the use of antiemetics during the course of acute febrile illness, encephalopathies, gastroenteritis, dehydration, and electrolyte imbalance. Trimethobenzamide should be used with caution especially in patients who have recently received other CNS-acting agents such as phenothiazines, barbiturates, and belladonna derivatives.

* Drowsiness, dizziness, and hypotension may occur. Patients should be warned about performing hazardous tasks requiring mental alertness or physical coordination.

* Antiemetics may obscure signs of overdosage of other drugs or of symptoms of such conditions as appendicitis, intestinal obstruction, or brain tumor.

* Blood dyscrasias, blurring of vision, coma, convulsions, depression of mood, diarrhea, disorientation, jaundice, muscle cramps, and exacerbation of pre-existing nausea have also been reported.

* Safety in pregnancy and in nursing mothers has not been established. Teratogenic effects have been noted in animal studies.

Drug interactions

None have been specifically reported; however, additive anticholinergic, antihistaminic, and sedative effects may be expected with other drugs with similar properties.

CHAPTER THIRTEEN

Antidiabetic agents

GENERAL INFORMATION ON DIABETES MELLITUS

Diabetes mellitus has been defined classically as a chronic, progressive disease manifested by abnormalities in carbohydrate, protein, and fat metabolism resulting from a relative or absolute lack of insulin. Diabetes mellitus has now been redefined as a syndrome. It is thought not to be a single disease, but a genetically and clinically heterogeneous group of disorders that have glucose intolerance in common. Multiple genetic and etiologic mechanisms are probably involved, and clinically similar types of diabetes may have different pathologic mechanisms.

Diabetes mellitus is a common syndrome, appearing with increasing frequency as the population ages. In the United States, approximately 4.5 million persons are being treated for diabetes. Another 2 million have undiagnosed diabetes, and 5 million more will develop diabetes sometime during their lives. Undiagnosed diabetic adults with few or no symptoms present a major challenge to the health profession. Because early diabetic symptoms are minimal, the patient does not seek medical advice and indications of the disease are discovered only at the time of routine physical examination. Those persons with a predisposition to developing diabetes include (1) persons who have relatives with diabetes (2½ times greater incidence of developing the disease), (2) obese persons (85% of diabetic patients are overweight), and (3) older persons (4 out of 5 diabetics are over 45 years of age).

In 1979, the National Diabetes Data Group of the National Institutes of Health published a new classification system for diabetes that more accurately reflects the various pathogenetic mechanisms in the disease. The classification includes three clinical classes characterized by either fasting hyperglycemia or abnormalities of glucose tolerance and two statistical risk classes with normal glucose tolerance that are thought possibly to be stages in the natural course of diabetes (See Table 13-1).

Type I, insulin-dependent diabetes (IDDM) is present in 5% to 10% of the diabetic population. It frequently occurs in juveniles, but it is now recognized that patients can become symptomatic for the first time at any age. The onset of this form of diabetes usually has a rapid progression (a few days to a few weeks) of symptomatology characterized by polydipsia (increased thirst), polyphagia (increased appetite), and polyuria (increased urination), increased frequency of infections, loss of weight and strength, irritability, and often ketoacidosis. There is no insulin secretion from the pancreas, and patients require administration of exogenous insulin. Insulin dosage adjustment is easily influenced by inconsistent patterns of physical activity and dietary irregularities.

Type II, non-insulin-dependent diabetes (NIDDM) is present in about 90% of the diabetic population. It usually has a much more insidious onset. The pancreas still maintains some capability to produce and secrete insulin. Consequently, symptoms are minimal or absent for quite some time. The patient may seek medical attention several years later only after symptoms of the complications of the disease have become apparent. Patients may complain of weight gain or loss. Blurred vision may be an indication of diabetic retinopathy. Neuropathies may be first observed as numbness or tingling of the extremities (paresthesia), loss of sensation, orthostatic hypotension, impotence, and difficulty in controlling urination (neurogenic bladder). An indication of chronic vascular disease may be nonhealing ulcers of the lower extremities. Fasting hyperglycemia can be controlled by diet in some patients, but other patients will require the use of supplemental insulin or oral hypoglycemic agents such as tolbutamide or acetohexamide. Although the onset is usually after the fourth decade of life, NIDDM can occur in younger patients who are not ketotic and who do not require insulin for control.

The third subclass of diabetes mellitus is for other types of diabetes that are a part of other diseases that have features not generally associated with the diabetic state. Diseases that may have a diabetic component include pheochromocytoma, acromegaly, and Cushing's syndrome. Other disorders included in this category are malnutrition, drugs and chemicals that induce hyperglycemia, defects in insulin receptors, and certain genetic syndromes.

Table 13-1. National Diabetes Data Group classification of glucose intolerance

Class	Former terminology
CLINICAL CLASSES	
Diabetes mellitus (DM)	
Type I: Insulin dependent (IDDM)	Juvenile diabetes, juvenile-onset diabetes, JOD, ketosis-prone diabetes, brittle diabetes
Type II: Non-insulin-dependent (NIDDM)	Adult-onset diabetes, maturity-onset diabetes, ketosis-resistant diabetes, stable diabetes, MOD
1. Nonobese NIDDM	
2. Obese NIDDM	
Other types associated with certain conditions and syndromes:	Secondary diabetes
1. Pancreatic disease	
2. Hormonal	
3. Drug or chemical induced	
4. Insulin receptor abnormalities	
5. Certain genetic syndromes	
6. Other types	

Modified from: National Diabetes Data Group, Diabetes **28**:1039-1057, Dec. 1979.

The second clinical class (gestational diabetes [GDM]) is reserved for women who show abnormal glucose tolerance during pregnancy. It is not for diabetic women who become pregnant. The majority of gestational diabetics will have a normal glucose tolerance post partum. Gestational diabetics must be reclassified after delivery into the category of diabetes mellitus, impaired glucose tolerance, or previous abnormality of glucose tolerance. Gestational diabetics have been put into a separate category because of the special clinical features of diabetes that develop during pregnancy and the complications associated with fetal involvement. These women are also at a higher risk of developing diabetes 5 to 10 years after pregnancy.

Table 13-1. National Diabetes Data Group classification of glucose intolerance—cont'd

Class	Former terminology
Gestational diabetes (GDM)	Gestational diabetes
Impaired glucose tolerance (IGT) Nonobese IGT Obese IGT IGT associated with certain conditions and syndromes: 1. Pancreatic disease 2. Hormonal 3. Drug or chemical induced 4. Insulin receptor abnormalities 5. Certain genetic syndromes	Asymptomatic diabetes, chemical diabetes, subclinical diabetes, borderline diabetes, latent diabetes

STATISTICAL RISK CLASSES

Previous abnormality of glucose tolerance (PrevAGT)	Latent diabetes
Potential abnormality of glucose tolerance (PotAGT)	Prediabetes, potential diabetes

The third and last clinical class is for those patients found to have an impaired glucose tolerance (IGT). It is now thought that patients with IGT are at a higher risk for developing NIDDM or IDDM in the future. Many of these patients, however, have their glucose tolerance return to normal or persist in the intermediate range for years. Studies indicate that these patients have an increased susceptibility to atherosclerotic disease.

There are two groups of patients at risk for diabetes or impaired glucose tolerance—those with a previous abnormality and those with a potential abnormality of glucose tolerance. Therefore, the National Diabetes Data Group included two statistical risk classes in the new classification. The first risk class is for patients with a previous abnormality of glucose tolerance (PrevAGT). This class is for patients who now have a normal glucose tolerance but who have a history of previous diabetes mellitus or impaired glucose tolerance. Representatives of this class might be the gestational diabetic who has a normal glucose tolerance after delivery or an obese patient whose glucose tolerance has returned to normal because of diet control and weight loss. It is important to realize that PrevAGT patients are not diabetics and should not be labeled as such, but should be tested periodically for the development of diabetes.

The second statistical risk class is potential abnormality of glucose tolerance (PotAGT). This class is for patients who have never exhibited abnormal glucose tolerance but who are at an increased risk for developing abnormalities. Risk factors for the development of non-insulin-dependent diabetes include being the monozygotic twin of a diabetic of this type, having a close relative (sibling, parent or child) that is a non-insulin-dependent diabetic, and being obese. A person with islet cell antibodies, or who is a monozygotic twin of an insulin-dependent diabetic, or who is a sibling of an insulin-dependent diabetic has an increased probability of becoming an insulin-dependent diabetic.

Although the classification system of the National Diabetes Data Group was developed to facilitate clinical and epidemiologic investigation, the categorization of patients can also be helpful in determining general principles for therapy. Since a cure for diabetes mellitus is unknown at present, the minimal purpose of treatment is to prevent ketoacidosis and symptoms resulting from hyperglycemia. The lifelong objectives of control must involve mechanisms to stem the progression of the complications of the disease. Major determinants involve a balanced diet, insulin or oral hypoglycemic therapy, routine exercise, and good hygiene. Patient education and reinforcement are tantamount to successful therapy. The intelligence and motivation of the diabetic patient and an awareness of the potential complications contribute significantly to the ultimate outcome of the disease and the quality of life the patient may lead.

Control

Patients with diabetes can lead a full and satisfying life. However, free diets and unrestricted activities are not possible. Dietary treatment of diabetes constitutes the basis for management of most patients, especially those with the adult onset form of disease. With adequate weight reduction and dietary control, patients may not require the use of exogenous insulin or oral hypoglycemic drug therapy. Type I diabetics will always require exogenous insulin as well as dietary control because the pancreas has lost the capacity to produce and secrete insulin. The aims of dietary control are (1) the prevention of excessive postprandial hyperglycemia, (2) the prevention of hypoglycemia in those patients being treated with hypoglycemic agents or insulin, and (3) the achievement and maintenance of an ideal body weight. A return to normal weight is often accompanied by a reduction in hyperglycemia. The diet should also be adjusted to reduce elevated cholesterol and triglyceride levels in an attempt to retard the progression of atherosclerosis.

To help maintain adherence to dietary restrictions, the diet should be planned in relation to the patient's food preferences, economic status, occupation, and physical activity. Emphasis should be placed on what food the patient may have and what exchanges are acceptable. Food should be measured for balanced portions, and the patient should be cautioned not to omit meals or between-meal and bedtime snacks.

All diabetic patients must receive adequate instruction on personal hygiene, especially regarding care of the feet, skin, and teeth. Development of infection is a common precipitating cause of ketosis and acidosis and must be treated promptly.

Insulin is required in the control of type I diabetes and in those patients whose diabetes cannot be controlled by diet, weight reduction, or oral hypoglycemic agents. Patients normally controlled with oral hypoglycemic agents will require insulin during situations of increased physiologic and psychologic stress such as pregnancy, surgery, and infections. The dosage of insulin is usually adjusted according to the blood glucose levels and the degree of glucosuria. The patient should test the urine before each meal and at bedtime while the insulin is being regulated. See General information on insulins (p. 434) for types and dosages of insulin, monitoring guidelines, and other medications that may cause hyperglycemia or hypoglycemia.

Another adjunct in the therapy of type II diabetes is the use of oral hypoglycemic agents. They are recommended only in those patients who cannot be controlled by diet alone and who are not prone to develop ketosis, acidosis, and/or infections. Patients most likely to benefit from treatment are those who have developed diabetes after 40 years of age and who require less than 40 units of insulin/day. See General information on sulfonylureas (p. 447).

GENERAL INFORMATION ON INSULINS

Insulin is a hormone produced in the beta cells of the pancreas and is a key regulator of metabolism. The protein molecule is composed of 51 amino acids divided into two chains. Insulins of various animal species have similar biologic activity and differ only in the sequence of one to three amino acids on one of the chains. Factors that promote the secretion of insulin are increased blood levels of glucose, various amino acids, ketone bodies, glucagon, sulfonylureas, gastrin, secretin, beta-receptor stimulants such as isoproterenol (Isuprel) and alpha-receptor blockers such as phentolamine (Regitine). Alpha-receptor stimulants—norepinephrine (Levophed), epinephrine (Adrenalin), and diazoxide (Hyperstat)—may inhibit the release of insulin.

Insulin promotes the entry of glucose into skeletal and heart muscle and fat and plays a significant role in protein and lipid metabolism. It is not required for glucose transport into brain or liver tissue.

A deficiency of insulin results in a marked reduction in the rate of transport of glucose across certain cell membranes, a reduction in the activity of the enzyme system that catalyzes the conversion of glucose to glycogen, an abnormally high rate of conversion of protein to glucose, and hyperlipidemia, ketosis and acidosis.

Several preparations of insulin isolated from beef and pork pancreas are commercially available. In 1972, the American Diabetes Association recommended the elimination of production of U-40 and U-80 insulins. The U-80 insulins have been phased out and replaced by U-100 insulin. The U-40 concentration is still available for those patients who require very small doses of insulin and for those older type I diabetics whose dosages are adjusted to it. The replacement with the U-100 dosage form for all types of insulin will help reduce the chance of patient error in using multiple dosage forms and dually calibrated syringes. U-500 regular insulin (pork) is also available for those patients developing resistence to insulin.

Over the past decade, significant progress has been made in improving the purity of insulin in an attempt to reduce allergenicity. Conventional insulins have always contained varying concentrations (greater than 10,000 parts per million [ppm]) of proinsulin, glucagon, somatostatin, and pancreatic polypeptides. The FDA has named the more highly refined products with less than 10 ppm of proinsulin as "purified". All conventional insulins are now "cleaner," with less than 25 ppm of proinsulin content (See Table 13-

2). Because the "purified" insulins are more expensive and limited in supply, their use should be restricted to those patients with specific indications, such as those using insulin for a short period of time (for example, gestational diabetics, type II diabetics undergoing surgery, nondiabetics receiving insulin as part of hyperalimentation solutions), patients with insulin resistance (using more than 100 to 200 units/day), patients with local cutaneous allergic reactions, patients with significant lipodystrophy, patients with renal transplants, and patients desensitized to pork insulin. Patients must be monitored very closely when being switched from conventional insulin to purified insulin and from beef to pork insulin. The response is highly variable, but patients usually require less insulin.

Biosynthetic human insulin is now available to selected patients. It may have a slightly more rapid onset of action than pork insulin and is expected to be less immunogenic than beef and pork insulin. A major unanswered question at this time is whether it will induce its own immunogenicity due to small amounts of impurities that are present from the manufacturing processes. The primary long-range advantage of human insulin is that a new source of insulin is now available to help meet a predicted worldwide shortage in the next decade.

Insulin dosage forms

All preparations of insulin (except biosynthetic insulin) are first extracted from animal pancreas. The predominant sources are of beef and pork origin, but sheep and fish sources may also be used. It is bioassayed, and the potencies are adjusted to provide concentrations of 40 units/ml (U-40), 100 units/ml (U-100) or 500 units/ml (U-500). Insulin can be modified by adding a protein or protamine or by precipitating it in varying concentrations of zinc chloride. Depending on the amount of protamine used and the physical state present (amorphous form, crystalline form, and the size of the crystals), insulin can be adjusted to have a short, intermediate, or long duration of action. See Table 13-2 for a comparison of the commercially available forms of insulin.

Regular insulin

Regular insulin is produced by precipitating insulin from solution in the amorphous (noncrystalline) form (Insulin Injection, U.S.P.) or by precipitating with zinc chloride to derive the crystalline form (Insulin Injection U.S.P. "Insulin made from zinc-insulin crystals"). There is essentially no

Text continued on p. 440.

Table 13-2. Commercially available forms of insulin

Type of insulin	Manufacturer	Strength (units/ml)	Source	Impurities (PPM)	Onset* (hr)	Peak* (hr)	Duration* (hr)	Glycosuria†	Hypoglycemia†
FAST-ACTING									
Insulin injection Actrapid	Novo	100	Pork	<10	0.5	2.5-5	8	Early AM[1]	Before lunch[3]
Insulin ("new")	Squibb	100	Pork	<25	0.5-1	3-6	6-8	Early AM[1]	Before lunch[3]
Insulin ("purified")	Squibb	40,100	Pork	<10	0.5-1	3-6	6-8	Early AM[1]	Before lunch[3]
Regular Iletin I	Lilly	40,100	Beef and pork	<25	0.5-1	3-6	6-8	Early AM[1]	Before lunch[3]
Regular Iletin II (Beef)	Lilly	100	Beef	<10	0.5-1	3-6	6-8	Early AM[1]	Before lunch[3]
Regular Iletin II (Pork)	Lilly	100, 500	Pork	<10	0.5-1	3-6	6-8	Early AM[1]	Before lunch[3]
Velosulin	Nordisk-USA	100	Pork	<10	0.5	1-3	8	Early AM[1]	Before lunch[3]
Prompt insulin zinc suspension Semilente Iletin I ("new")	Lilly	40,100	Beef and pork	<25	0.5-1	4-6	12-16	Early AM[1]	Before lunch[3]

Semilente insulin	Squibb	100	Beef	<25	0.5-1	4-6	12-16	Early AM[1]	Before lunch[3]
Semitard	Novo	100	Pork	<10	1.5	5-10	16	Early AM[1]	Before lunch[3]

INTERMEDIATE-ACTING

Isophane insulin suspension (NPH)

Insulatard	Nordisk-USA	100	Pork	<10	1.5	4-12	24	Before lunch[2]	3 PM to supper[3]
Isophane insulin NPH ("purified")	Squibb	100	Beef	<10	1-1.5	8-12	24	Before lunch[2]	3 PM to supper[3]
NPH Iletin I	Lilly	40,100	Beef and Pork	<25	1-1.5	8-12	24	Before lunch[2]	3 PM to supper[3]
NPH Iletin II	Lilly	100	Beef or pork	<10	1-1.5	8-12	24	Before lunch[2]	3 PM to supper[3]
Protophane NPH	Novo	100	Pork	<10	1.5	4-12	24	Before lunch[2]	3 PM to supper[3]

*The times listed are averages based on a newly diagnosed diabetic patient. Factors modifying these times include patient variation, site and route of administration, and dosage.

†Most frequently occurs when insulin is administered at (1) bedtime the previous night, (2) before breakfast the previous day, (3) before breakfast the same day.

Continued.

Table 13-2. Commercially available forms of insulin—cont'd

Type of insulin	Manu- facturer	Strength (units/ml)	Source	Impurities (PPM)	Onset* (hr)	Peak* (hr)	Duration* (hr)	Glycosuria†	Hypo- glycemia†
Isophane insulin suspension and insulin injection									
Mixtard	Nordisk-USA	100	Pork	<10	0.5	4-8	24	Before lunch[2]	3 PM to supper[3]
Insulin zinc suspension									
Lentard	Nordisk-USA	100	Pork and beef	<10	2.5	7-15	24	Before lunch[2]	3 PM to supper[3]
Lente Iletin	Lilly	40,100	Pork and beef	<25	1-1.5	8-12	24	Before lunch[2]	3 PM to supper[3]
Lente Iletin I	Lilly	100	Beef or pork	<25	1-1.5	8-12	24	Before lunch[2]	3 PM to supper[3]
Lente Iletin II	Lilly	100	Beef or pork	<10	1-1.5	8-12	24	Before lunch[2]	3 PM to supper[3]
Lente insulin	Squibb	40,100	Beef	<10	1-1.5	8-12	24	Before lunch[2]	3 PM to supper[3]
Monotard	Novo	100	Pork	<10	2.5	7-15	22	Before lunch[2]	3 PM to supper[3]

LONG-ACTING

Protamine zinc insulin suspension

Protamine zinc Iletin I	Lilly	40,100	Beef and pork	<25	1-8	16-24	36+	Supper to bedtime[2]	2 AM to breakfast[3]
Protamine zinc Iletin II	Lilly	100	Beef or pork	<10	1-8	16-24	36+	Supper to bedtime[2]	2 AM to breakfast[3]
Protamine zinc insulin	Squibb	100	Beef and pork	<25	4-8	16-24	36+	Supper to bedtime[2]	2 AM to breakfast[3]

Extended insulin zinc suspension

Ultralente Iletin I	Lilly	40,100	Beef and pork	<25	4-8	16-18	36+	Supper to bedtime[2]	2 AM to breakfast[3]
Ultralente insulin	Squibb	100	Beef	<25	4-8	16-18	36+	Supper to bedtime[2]	2 AM to breakfast[3]
Ultratard	Novo	100	Beef	<10	4	10-30	36	Supper to bedtime[2]	2 AM to breakfast[3]

Table 13-3. Compatibility of insulin combinations

Combination	Ratio	Mix before administration
Regular + NPH	Any combination	2 to 3 months*
Regular + Lente	Any combination	2 to 3 months*
Regular + PZI†	1:1 = action like PZI alone	Immediately
	2:1 = action like NPH	Immediately
	3:1 = action like NPH + regular	Immediately
Lentes	Any combination	Stable indefinitely

*Must be used immediately to retain properties of regular insulin.
†PZI contains excess protamine that binds with regular insulin, prolonging the activity of regular insulin. Regular and PZI should not be mixed, but administered at separate sites at approximately the same time.

clinical difference in therapeutic activity of equipotent solutions. Regular insulin is used for its immediate onset of activity and short duration of action. It is the only form of insulin that is a clear solution, not a cloudy suspension, and is the only dosage form of insulin that may be injected by intravenous as well as subcutaneous routes of administration. See Table 13-2 for the activity of the regular insulins, and Table 13-3 for mixing compatibility with other insulins.

Lente insulins

Another manufacturing process using much higher concentrations of zinc and an acetate buffer (phosphate buffers are used with insulins containing protamine) produces two physical forms, one crystalline and the other amorphous, at a neutral pH. The long-acting crystalline form is marketed as Ultralente, and the amorphous fast-acting compound is available as Semilente. The intermediate-acting Lente insulin is a mixture containing approximately 30% Semilente and 70% crystalline Ultralente insulin.

See Table 13-2 for a comparison of the properties of available forms of insulin and Table 13-3 for the compatibility of insulin mixtures.

Neutral-protamine-hagedorn (NPH) insulin

NPH insulin is an intermediate-acting insulin containing specific amounts of insulin and protamine so that the crystals formed leave behind no protamine or insulin. The activity of NPH is similar to that of a mixture of regular insulin and protamine zinc insulin (Tables 13-2 and 13-3).

Protamine zinc insulin (PZI)

Insulin precipitated with zinc in the presence of a protein, protamine, produces protamine zinc insulin. PZI is poorly soluble and absorbed slowly when injected in subcutaneous tissue. See Table 13-2 for the activity of protamine zinc insulin.

Characteristics

Onset, peak activity, duration: see Table 13-2. Plasma half-life: less than 9 min. Metabolism: 40% liver, 40% kidney. Excretion: less than 10% unchanged in urine. Dialysis: unknown.

Administration and dosage
Adult

For ketoacidosis:

SC AND IV—Initially, 50 to 100 units of regular insulin SC and 50 to 100 units IV. Follow with doses of 50 to 100 units every 2 to 4 hr until the blood glucose level falls to 250 mg/100 mg. The total dose of insulin required generally ranges between 200 and 400 units. Maintain the patient on regular insulin every 4 to 6 hr as needed, then start intermediate-acting insulin the next morning if the patient is doing well.*

IM—Initially, 10 to 20 units of regular insulin, followed by 5 to 10 units hourly until the blood glucose is 150 to 300 mg/100 ml.†

IV—IV bolus: 0.1 units/kg. Infusion: 0.1 units/kg/hr. (Addition of 50 units regular insulin to 500 ml one-half saline solution administered at a rate of 1 ml/min provides an insulin dose of 6 units/hr.) Various studies indicate a 20% to 33% loss of insulin potency caused by adsorption of insulin to the bottle and tubing. The addition of 3.5 mg of human serum albumin/ml of solution (7 ml of 25% albumin/500 ml of solution) has been found to prevent clinically significant absorption.‡

---

*N. Eng. J. Med. **290**:1360, 1974.

†Lancet **2**:515, 1973.

‡Br. Med. J. **2**:687, 691, 694, 1974.

NOTE: Only regular insulin may be injected IV. All other forms are suspensions and are contraindicated for IV use. All the above methods may be successful in treating ketoacidosis. Hourly observations of the patient's fluids, electrolytes (especially potassium), blood sugar, ketone levels, and arterial blood gases are essential to the proper treatment of ketoacidosis.

For maintenance therapy:
1. Newly diagnosed diabetic patients: after ketoacidosis and hyperglycemia have been controlled and the patient can tolerate oral feedings, determine the total amount of regular insulin needed in 24 hr. The usual initial dose in the nonketotic patients is 10 to 20 units of regular insulin SC. Subsequent doses administered ½ hr before meals and at bedtime are based on the blood glucose and urine glucose levels. After control is established, the patient is converted to intermediate-acting insulin administered in a dose 65% to 75% of the total dose of regular insulin required in 24 hr. Regular insulin is used as a supplement based on urine glucose levels. Adjustments in the intermediate-acting insulin will be necessary. Divided doses (two-thirds in the morning, one-third in the evening) or combination therapy using a mixture of insulin (see Table 13-3) may be required to maintain control, especially after the patient leaves the hospital and has changes in exercise and diet.
2. Known diabetic patients: once ketoacidosis and hyperglycemia have been controlled and the patient can tolerate oral feedings, initiate maintenance therapy at one half to two thirds their previous dose of intermediate-acting or combination insulin. Supplemental regular insulin is given when indicated by blood sugar and urine glucose determinations. Adjust maintenance insulin until optimal control for the patient is achieved.

NOTE: "Control" of the hyperglycemia of diabetes in the hospital is usually easier than on an outpatient basis. Adjustments are almost always necessary after dismissal as a result of changes in exercise and diet. Some physicians will allow their patients to spill a ¾% to 1% urine glucose while in the hospital so that after discharge a patient will spill a trace to ¼% as a result of change in routine. Other physicians will stabilize a patient to a trace to ¼% urine glucose while in the hospital and drop the insulin dosage 5 units on discharge. There is less chance of a hypoglycemic reaction when using the second method, but regardless of which treatment program is used the discharged patient will have to be monitored frequently for medical and emotional adjustment to the new disease.

Nurse and patient considerations

Insulin overdosage or decreased carbohydrate intake may result in hypoglycemia. Early symptoms may include nausea, hunger, headache, irritability, lethargy, ataxia, and mental confusion. The patient may also experience tremor, sweating and tachycardia. Severe hypoglycemia may result in convulsions and coma. If untreated, irreversible brain damage may occur. Hypoglycemia occurs most frequently when the administered insulin reaches its peak action. Hypoglycemia must be treated immediately. Mild symptomatology may be controlled by the oral administration of lump sugar, orange juice, carbonated cola beverages, or candy. Severe symptoms may be relieved by the administration of 5 to 25 g of dextrose (10 to 50 ml of dextrose 50%). The following conditions may predispose a diabetic patient to a hypoglycemic (insulin) reaction: improper measurement of insulin dosage, excessive exercise, insufficient food intake, concurrent ingestion of hypoglycemic drugs and discontinuance of drugs (see Drug interactions, p. 447), or conditions (infection, stress) causing hyperglycemia.

Allergic reactions manifested by itching, redness, and swelling at the site of injection are common occurrences in patients beginning insulin therapy. These reactions may be caused by modifying proteins in NPH or PZI insulin, the insulin itself (pure pork insulin, which differs from human insulin by one amino acid, is less antigenic than insulin derived from beef, which differs from human insulin by three amino acids; human insulin is expected to be less antigenic than pork insulin; the use of "purified" insulins may also be beneficial), the alcohol used to cleanse the injection site or sterilize the syringe, the patient's injection technique, or the intermittent use of insulin. Spontaneous desensitization frequently occurs within a few weeks, but changing to insulin without protein modifiers (the Lente series) or to insulins derived from another animal source, using unscented alcohol swabs or disposable syringes and needles, and checking the patient's injection technique (inject at an angle, not perpendicularly) may reduce local irritation. Acute, whole-body rashes and anaphylactic symptoms must be treated with antihistamines, epinephrine, and steroids. The animal source of the insulin should then be changed.

Rotation of injection sites is important. Atrophy or

hypertrophy of subcutaneous fat tissue may occur at the site of frequent insulin injections. The hypertrophic areas tend to be used more frequently by diabetic patients because the fat pad becomes anesthetic. In addition to the adverse cosmetic effects, the absorption of insulin from these sites becomes significantly prolonged and erratic. Loss of diabetic control may result, particularly in unstable type I diabetes.

Insulin resistance is an infrequent complication in the control of diabetic symptoms. Acute resistance may develop if the patient acquires an infection or experiences serious trauma, surgery, or emotional disturbances. This type of resistance subsides with regression of the acute episode. Chronic insulin resistance may occur with the reinstitution of insulin therapy after a period of discontinuance. Resistance may be reduced by changing the animal source of the insulin, using "purified" insulins, changing the use of glucocorticoids, or using specially prepared dealanated or sulfated insulins.

Teaching the newly diagnosed diabetic patient to test for sugar content in the urine is essential for symptom-free control of the disease. A detailed discussion of the various products available for testing for glucosuria is beyond the scope of this chapter; however, there are a few points that should be mentioned:

1. Each method uses a different colorimetric system that shows color changes for different concentrations of glucose. Before 1980, the manufacturers converted the scales to an approximation of the percent of glucose present, allowing greater standardization among the tests and more meaningful data for closer control. Unfortunately, many older diabetics still refer to the "+" system. Table 13-4 illustrates how the "+" values for urine sugar concentration vary between products. Note that a ½% urine glucose measures a 1+ using Clinitest, a 2+ using Diastix and Keto-Diastix, and a 3+ using Tes-Tape. All patients should be encouraged to use the "percent" system.

2. The Clinitest 2-drop method is now recommended by the American Diabetic Association. It has the advantages of being able to measure up to 5% glucose concentrations versus 2% concentrations with the other urine testing systems, and the "pass through" phenomenon does not occur as frequently as with the Clinitest 5-drop method (See no. 4 on next page).

Table 13-4. Comparison of the values of urine glucose tests

	Negative	\(^1/_{10}\)	\(^1/_4\)	\(^1/_2\)	\(^3/_4\)	1	2
				Percent			
Clinitest (5-drop method)	0			Trace	1+	2+ 3+	4+
Diastix or Keto-Diastix	0	Trace	1+	2+		3+	4+
Tes-Tape	0	1+	2+	3+			4+

3. The patient should use a double-voided urine specimen, especially for the early morning determination. The second void provides a more accurate estimation of the urine glucose content at that time. It prevents the testing of glucose that may have accumulated over the last several hours.

4. When using Clinitest, the patient should watch the reaction to see if the bright orange "pass through" phenomenon occurs. This is caused by a urine glucose concentration of greater than 2%. If the patient is not observant, the final color will be misrecorded as a ¾% or 1%. It is important to read the results 15 sec after the boiling ceases. The color may begin to fade leading to a misinterpretation of the results.

5. Urine testing products should be stored properly. They are sensitive to temperature, light, and humidity. If subpotency is suspected, the products can be tested by using Coca-Cola. A 5% reading should result with the Clinitest 2-drop method, and a 2% with the other methods.

6. Clinitest tablets are poisonous and must not be taken internally. Treat ingestion with vinegar or lemon, grapefruit, or orange juice in large quantities. Follow with olive or mineral oil. The tablets should be handled by using the lid of the container. Do not use fingertips, because of the possibility of burns.

7. Several drugs interfere with glucose urine testing products. See Table 13-5 for the false values that may occur. A "false positive" does not mean the results will automatically be a 2% or 5%. The drug may induce small changes such as a ½% registering as a ¾%. The opposite may occur with those drugs inducing false-negative values; a 1% may be read as a ¾% or a ½%. It may not record as a negative. These

Table 13-5. Drugs that may alter urine glucose determinations as a result of interference with the test procedure

Drug	Clinitest	Tes-Tape, Diastix
Ascorbic acid (large doses)	False +	False −
Azo Gantrisin (see Phenazopyridine)		
Cephalosporins (first generation)	False +	
Chloral hydrate (large doses)	False +	
Chloramphenicol (Chloromycetin)	False +	
Isoniazid (INH)	False +	
Ketones		False −
Levodopa, L-dopa (Dopar)	False +	False −
Penicillin (large doses)	False +	
Phenazopyridine (Pyridium)		False + or −
Probenecid (Benemid)	False +	
Salicylates (40 to 90 grains/day)*	False +	False −

Modified from Hansten, P.D.: Drug interactions, ed. 3; Philadelphia, 1975, Lea & Febiger.
*8 to 18 325 mg tablets/day.

slight changes become significant to those patients who adjust their insulin dosages according to the glucose content in the urine (those using the "sliding" or "rainbow" scale).

A diabetic person whose urine glucose concentration is 2% or more should also test the urine for ketones. If a patient has symptoms indicating ketoacidosis, but the results of Acetest tablets of Ketostix indicates no urine ketones, the patient should be observed carefully anyway, because these in vitro tests measure only acetone and acetoacetic acid. Beta-hydroxybutyric acid is not measured, although it is the major ketone responsible for ketoacidosis. Levodopa (Dopar) and phenazopyridine (Pyridium) may cause false-positive Labstix and Ketostix results. Paraldehyde may cause false-positive Acetest results. Ether anesthesia and overdoses of isopropyl alcohol, isoniazid, and insulin (or decreased carbohydrate intake) lead to true elevations of urine ketone levels.

Pregnant diabetic women must be observed closely for changing insulin requirements. Insulin dosages increase especially in the last trimester of pregnancy. Following delivery, insulin requirements rapidly fall to prepregnancy levels.

Drug interactions

The following drugs may cause hyperglycemia, especially in prediabetic and diabetic patients. Insulin dosages may require adjustment.

Ethanol	Dextrothyroxine (Choloxin)
Corticosteroids	Diazoxide (Hyperstat)
Epinephrine	Phenytoin (Dilantin)
Oral contraceptives	Diuretics (thiazides,
Glucagon	chlorthalidone)
Acetazolamide (Diamox)	Lithium carbonate
Salicylates	Dobutamine (Dobutrex)
Phenothiazines	

The following drugs may cause hypoglycemia, decreasing insulin requirements in diabetic patients.

Ethanol	Mono-amine oxidase
Anabolic steroids	inhibitors
(Dianabol, Durabolin)	Salicylates
Guanethidine sulfate	Acetaminophen (Tylenol)
(Ismelin)	Propranolol (Inderal)

Although the mechanism is unknown, Beta-blocking agents (propranolol, nadolol, others) may produce hypoglycemia, especially in diabetic patients. The reaction may be particularly serious because propranolol may prevent signs of hypoglycemia (tremor, tachycardia).

GENERAL INFORMATION ON SULFONYLUREAS

AHFS 68:20

The sulfonylureas are a class of compounds capable of producing hypoglycemia by stimulating the release of insulin from the beta cells in the pancreas. The exact mechanism is unknown. They are of no benefit in pancreatectomized patients and in type I diabetic patients; however, they are effective in type II diabetic patients in whom the pancreas retains the capacity to secrete insulin.

Commercially available forms of sulfonylureas (Table 13-6) may be effective in the treatment of type II diabetes mellitus that cannot be controlled by diet alone and if the patient is not prone to develop ketosis, acidosis, and/or infections. Patients most likely to benefit from treatment are those who have developed signs of diabetes after 40 years of age and who require less than 40 units of insulin/day.

Nurse and patient considerations

The University Group Diabetes Program (UGDP) study concluded that there may be a higher incidence of cardio-

Table 13-6. Comparison of the sulfonylureas

Characteristics	Acetohexamide (Dymelor)	Chlorpropamide (Diabinese)	Tolazamide (Tolinase)	Tolbutamide (Orinase)
Dosage range (g)	0.25-1.5 (single or divided dose)	0.1-0.5 (single dose)	0.1-0.25 (single or divided dose)	0.5-3 (divided dose)
Onset (hr)	1	1	4-6	0.5-1
Peak (hr)	3	—	—	3.5
Duration (hr)	12-18	24-72	12-16	6-12
Half-life (hr)	6	36	7	5
Metabolism	Liver (active)	80% liver	Liver (active)	Liver (inactive)
Excretion	>80% urine	20% unchanged in urine	Urine	>75% metabolites in urine
Dialysis	?	P-NO*	?	H-NO†

*Peritoneal dialysis.
†Hemodialysis.

vascular death in diabetic patients treated with oral hypoglycemic agents than in those treated by diet or insulin alone.
The results of this study have been quite controversial, and
further studies have as yet not refuted or confirmed the
UGDP data. Until further studies are completed, it would be
wise to initiate oral hypoglycemic therapy only in those
patients whose diabetes truly can not be controlled by diet
and weight reduction alone and where risks of insulin therapy outweigh its benefits.

Patients on oral hypoglycemic therapy are as susceptible to hypoglycemia as those diabetic patients on insulin
therapy. Consequently blood sugar levels and urine sugar
levels must be monitored closely, especially in the early
stages of therapy.

Patient education and dosage compliance as well as
dietary restriction, exercise, and infection control are mandatory to ensure maintenance of therapy.

Individual dosage adjustment is essential for the successful use of oral hypoglycemic agents. A patient should be
given a 1-month trial on maximum doses of the sulfonylurea
being used before the patient can be considered a primary
failure. If a patient represents a secondary failure (a patient
initially controlled on oral agents), changing to an alternative sulfonylurea is occasionally successful.

If a patient develops severe hyperglycemia, acidosis,
ketosis, severe infection, or undergoes a surgical procedure,
the oral hypoglycemic should be discontinued temporarily
while diabetic control is maintained with insulin.

Side effects of the sulfonylureas are infrequent and generally mild. The more common adverse reactions include
allergic skin reactions (maculopapular, erythematous, and,
occasionally, pruritus) and gastrointestinal symptoms
(heartburn, fullness, nausea). Alcohol intolerance, manifested by facial flushing, pounding headache, feeling of breath-
lessness, and nausea, is occasionally noted, especially in
patients being treated with chlorpropamide. This disulfiram-
like reaction can be initiated by small amounts of alcohol in
mouthwashes and other over-the-counter products with a
hydroalcoholic base.

Sulfonylureas are not recommended for use in pregnant
women or nursing mothers.

Drug interactions

The following drugs may produce hypoglycemia and
may potentiate sulfonylureas. Propranolol may also mask
some of the symptoms of hypoglycemia such as tachycardia

and tremor. Dosage adjustment of the oral hypoglycemic may be necessary.

Ethanol	Sulfisoxazole (Gantrisin)
Methandrostenolone (Dianabol)	Guanethidine sulfate (Ismelin)
Chloramphenicol	Oxytetracycline (Terramycin)
(Chloromycetin)	MAO inhibitors (Marplan,
Warfarin (Coumadin)	Parnate, Eutonyl)
Propranolol (Inderal)	Phenylbutazone (Butazolidin)
Salicylates (aspirin)	

The following drugs may antagonize the hypoglycemic effects of sulfonylureas, possibly requiring increased dosages of the oral hypoglycemic agent to maintain control of the diabetes.

Corticosteroids (prednisone)	Phenytoin (Dilantin)
Phenothiazines (chlorpromazine)	Salicylates (aspirin)
Diuretics (thiazides, chlorthalidone)	Diazoxide (Hyperstat)
Oral contraceptives	Lithium carbonate
Thyroid replacement therapy	

CHAPTER FOURTEEN

Corticosteroids

General information on corticosteroids

GENERAL INFORMATION ON CORTICOSTEROIDS

AHFS 68:04

The corticosteroids are hormones secreted by the adrenal cortex. They are divided into two classes according to their structure and biologic activity. The activity of the mineralocorticoids (desoxycorticosterone, aldosterone) is limited primarily to regulating water and electrolyte balance. The glucocorticoids (hydrocortisone, prednisone) regulate carbohydrate metabolism, but also affect most other physiologic processes.

The major glucocorticoid of the adrenal cortex is cortisol. The hypothalamic-pituitary axis regulates the secretion of cortisol by increasing or decreasing the output of corticotropin-releasing factor (CRF) from the hypothalamus. CRF stimulates the release of adrenocorticotropic hormone (ACTH) from the pituitary gland. ACTH then stimulates the adrenal cortex to secrete cortisol. As serum levels of cortisol increase, the amount of CRF secreted by the hypothalamus is decreased, resulting in diminished secretion of cortisol from the adrenal cortex.

Corticosteroids are used most frequently for their antiinflammatory and antiallergic properties. While the underlying cause remains, the symptoms are suppressed. Corticosteroids nonspecifically inhibit inflammatory effects of many microorganisms, chemical or thermal irritants, allergens, and trauma. Although the precise mechanisms of action are unknown, steroids have been observed to inhibit the early inflammatory process (edema, capillary dilatation, migration of leukocytes into the inflamed area, and phagocytic activity), as well as the later processes (capillary proliferation, fibroblastic activity, deposition of collagen, and scar formation).

Corticosteroids are frequently used in rheumatic disorders (arthritis), collagen diseases (systemic lupus erythematosus), dermatologic disorders (pemphigus, exfoliative dermatitis), allergic states (bronchial asthma, drug hypersensitivity reactions), gastrointestinal diseases (ulcerative colitis, regional enteritis), diagnostic testing, and cerebral edema.

Glucocorticoids are thought to be effective in the treatment of septic shock when (1) doses are massive, (2) therapy is initiated early, and (3) supportive therapy includes fluids, electrolytes, antibiotics, plasma expanders, and pressor agents. The proposed mechanisms by which glucocorticoids may be effective in the treatment of shock (in addition to those above) include a positive inotropic effect on the myocardium, a decrease in peripheral vascular resistance, and chemical inactivation of endotoxins.

Administrative considerations

Clinicians should have firm therapeutic goals prior to initiation of therapy. Once control has been established, dosage should be tapered to the lowest effective amount possible.

Continuous daily therapy is usually reserved for acute conditions (for example, trauma, burns, septic shock, systemic lupus erythematosus). For chronic disorders such as rheumatoid disease or bronchial asthma, enough steroid should be administered to allow function, but usually not enough to provide complete symptomatic relief, since much higher dosages are often required.

The use of alternate-day therapy should be considered in chronic diseases treated with maintenance therapy. Patients receive a 2-day dosage in a single administration every other morning. This mode of administration may reduce side effects, particularly those of adrenal suppression. The theory of this method is that on the "off" days (when the patient receives no exogenous steroids), the patient has lower steroid blood levels, allowing a day of reactivation of the adrenal glands by the normal mechanism of CRF-ACTH and recovery of other tissues from the metabolic effects of exogenous steroids. Steroids that are inactivated in less than 30 to 36 hr (that is, prednisone, prednisolone, methylprednisolone) must be used to allow the body's own secretory mechanisms to prevail on the nontreatment days. The timing of dosage administration on the treatment days appears to be critical. The dose should be given in early morning to simulate the normal pattern of diurnal rhythm. In the normal individual ACTH accumulates in the circulation during sleep and produces peak serum levels of cortisol between 7 and 8 AM. By administering the shortacting steroid at about this time on the treatment day, the patient receives the benefit of high steroid serum levels that provide symptomatic relief. The high levels dissipate through normal metabolic mechanisms, allowing ACTH levels to accumulate through the night, which in turn stimulate the release of cortisol from the adrenal glands early in the morning of the nontreatment day.

When therapeutic dosages of steroids are administered for a week or longer, one must assume that endogenous cortisol production has been suppressed. Abrupt withdrawal of the glucocorticoids may result in adrenal insufficiency. Therapy should be withdrawn with gradual reductions in dosage. The length of time required to taper off glucocorticoids depends on the duration of treatment, the amount of the dosage, the mode of administration, and the corticosteroid being used. Symptoms of rapid taper include fever, malaise, fatigue, weakness, anorexia, nausea, orthostatic dizziness, hypotension, fainting, dyspnea, hypoglycemia, muscle and joint pain, and possible exacerbation of the disease process being treated.

Nurse and patient considerations

The glucocorticoids are very potent agents that produce many undesirable side effects as well as therapeutic benefits. Unless immediate life-threatening conditions exist, other methods of therapy should be given a good therapeutic trial before corticosteroid therapy is initiated. Many of the side effects of the steroids are related to dosage and duration of therapy.

Corticosteroids are quite valuable agents in the suppression of inflammation, but this action also eliminates the symptoms often necessary in monitoring the disease process and in evaluating the effectiveness of treatment. Corticoids may increase the susceptibility to infection, suppress skin sensitivity tests, and elevate serum amylase and blood glucose levels, while decreasing serum potassium and 24 hr ^{131}I thyroid uptake tests. Patients should be advised to avoid exposure to infections and to observe for evidence of recurring infections or delayed healing of wounds.

When glucocorticoids are administered over a prolonged period, the patient may display sodium and water retention, potassium depletion, and symptoms similar to Cushing's syndrome (hypersecretion of the adrenal cortex). These manifestations include hirsutism, cervicothoracic ("buffalo") hump, rounding of the face, hypertension, edema, amenorrhea, striae and thinning of the skin, hyperglycemia, hypokalemic, hypochloremic, metabolic alkalosis, and mental disturbances. Patients may also complain of increased appetite and weight gain, peptic ulcer, purpura, headache, and dizziness. Osteoporosis and vertebral com-

Table 14-1. Comparison chart of corticosteroid preparations

USP name	Structure of synthetic analog	Trade names	Approximate equivalent dose (mg)	Anti-inflammatory potency	Mineralo-corticoid potency	Usual starting dose (mg/day) Life-threatening illness	Usual starting dose (mg/day) Moderately severe illness
Hydrocortisone (cortisol)	—		20.0	1.0	1.0	—	80-120
Cortisone	—	Meticorten	25.0	0.8	0.8	—	100-150
Prednisone	delta-1-cortisone	Deltasone	5.0	3.0-5.0	0.8	50-100	20-30
Prednisolone	delta-1-cortisol	Meticortelone Hydeltra-T.B.A. Delta-Cortef	5.0	3.0-5.0	0.8	50-100	20-30
Triamcinolone	9-alpha fluoro-16-alpha-hydroxyprednisolone	Aristocort Kenacort	4.0	3.0-5.0	0	40-80	16-24
Dexamethasone	9-alpha fluoro-16-alpha-methyl-	Decadron Deronil Gammacorten Hexadrol	0.75	20.0-30.0	0	7.5-15.0	3.0-4.5

	prednisolone						
Methylprednisolone	6-alpha-methyl-prednisolone	Medrol	4.0	3.0-5.0	0	40-80	16-24
Fluprednisolone	6-alpha fluoro-prednisolone	Alphadrol	1.5	10.0-20.0	0	15-30	6-9
Betamethasone	9-alpha fluoro-16-beta-methyl-prednisolone	Celestone	0.6	20.0-30.0	0	6-12	2.4-3.6
Paramethasone	6-alpha-fluro-16-alpha-methyl-prednisolone 21-acetate	Haldrone Stemex	2.0	8.0-12.0	0	20-40	8-12
Meprednisone	16-beta-methyl-prednisone	Betapar	4	3.0-5.0	0	40-80	16-24

From Boedeker, E.C., and Dauber, J.H., editors: Manual of medical therapeutics, ed. 21, Boston, 1974, Little, Brown and Co.

pression are frequent serious complications in patients taking glucocorticoids for longer than a few months. Radiographic studies of the spine should be completed on a routine basis.

Glucocorticoids should be used with caution in the presence of diabetes mellitus (insulin therapy may require adjustment), hypertension, congestive heart failure, thrombophlebitis, infectious diseases, peptic ulcer disease, and tuberculosis.

Behavioral disturbances ranging from nervousness and insomnia to manic-depressive or schizophrenic psychoses and suicidal tendencies may develop, particularly with prolonged therapy. These psychotic manifestations are more likely to occur in patients with a previous history of mental instability.

Teratogenic effects have been reported in infants of women ingesting glucocorticoids during pregnancy. Glucocorticoids must be used only on a risk versus benefit basis during pregnancy as well as any other time.

Drug interactions

Although the mechanisms are only speculative, glucocorticoids may alter the coagulation status of patients ingesting oral anticoagulants such as warfarin (Coumadin). Anticoagulant therapy may have to be increased or decreased, depending on the response of the patient. The ulcerogenic potential of steroids requires even closer observation of anticoagulated patients to reduce the possibility of hemorrhage.

Patients may require an increase in dosage of insulin or oral hypoglycemic agents as a result of the intrinsic hyperglycemic effects of glucocorticoids.

Although the mechanisms are unknown, estrogen administration retards the metabolism of hydrocortisone. This may allow reduction of the glucocorticoid dosage.

Corticosteroids may enhance potassium loss when administered with ethacrynic acid (Edecrin), furosemide (Lasix), and thiazide diuretics. Observe for evidence of hypokalemia (see Table 14-1).

CHAPTER FIFTEEN

Antineoplastic agents

*General information on
    cancer chemotherapy*

GENERAL INFORMATION ON CANCER CHEMOTHERAPY

Cancer is a disorder of cellular growth. It is a collection of abnormal cells that generally proliferate more rapidly than do normal cells, lose the ability to perform specialized functions, invade surrounding tissues, and develop growths in other tissues (metastases).

Cancer is a leading cause of death in the United States. Unfortunately, the number of persons dying from malignant disease increases each year. Early diagnosis and treatment is still one of the most important factors in providing a more optimistic prognosis for those patients stricken with the many forms of neoplastic disease.

Treatment of cancer often requires a combination of surgery, radiation, and chemotherapy. Recent advancements in carcinogenesis, cellular and molecular biology, and tumor immunology have enhanced the role that antineoplastic agents may play in therapy. It is beyond the scope of this chapter to delve into the interrelationships of chemotherapy and neoplastic disease; however, a short discussion of the concepts of cancer chemotherapy will be presented. As a result of rapidly changing approaches to the treatment of specific malignancies and the changing nature of chemotherapeutic regimens, specific agents and dosages have not been discussed.

All cells, whether normal or malignant, pass through a similar series of phases during their lifetime, although the duration of time spent in each phase differs with the type of cell.

Mitosis (M) is that phase of cellular proliferation when the cell divides into two equal daughter cells. Phase G_1 follows mitosis and is considered a resting phase before the S phase, the stage of active DNA synthesis. G_2 is a postsynthetic phase wherein the cell contains a double complement of DNA. After a period of apparently minimal cellular activity in phase G_2, the M phase again divides the cell into two G_1 daughter cells. G_1 cells may advance again to the S phase or pass into a nonproliferative stage known as G_0. The time required to complete one cycle is called the "generation time."

Many antineoplastic agents are "cell-cycle specific"; that is, the drug is selectively toxic when the cell is in a specific phase of growth. Thus those malignancies most amenable to chemotherapy proliferate rapidly. "Cell-cycle nonspecific" drugs are active throughout the cell cycle and may be more effective against slowly proliferating neoplastic tissue. One implication of cell-cycle specificity is the importance of correlating the dosage schedule of anticancer therapy with the known cellular kinetics of that type of neoplasm. Drugs are usually administered when the cell is most susceptible to the cytotoxic effects of the agent. Table 15-1 lists the more common commercially available drugs, their dosage range, major toxicities, and major indications.

Pharmacology

Chemotherapeutic agents currently used are classified as (1) alkylating agents, (2) antimetabolites, (3) natural products, and (4) hormones. The mechanisms by which these agents cause cell death have not yet been fully determined.

Alkylating agents

The alkylating agents are highly reactive chemical compounds that unite with DNA molecules, causing cross-linking of DNA strands. The interstrand binding prevents the separation of the double-coiled DNA molecule that is necessary for cellular division. Alkylating agents are cell-cycle nonspecific, being capable of combining with cellular components at any phase of the cell cycle. Generally speaking, the development of resistance to one alkylating agent imparts cross-resistance to other alkylators.

Antimetabolites

The antimetabolites (subclassified as folic acid, purine, and pyrimidine antagonists) inhibit key enzymes in the biosynthetic pathways of DNA and RNA synthesis. Many of the antagonists are cell-cycle specific, killing cells during the S phase of cell maturation.

Natural products

1. Vinca alkaloids. Vincristine and Vinblastine are natural derivatives of the periwinkle plant. They are cell-cycle specific agents that block the formation of the mitotic spin-

Text continued on p. 469.

Table 15-1. Cancer chemotherapeutic agents

Drug	Usual dosage	Toxicity		Major indications
		Acute	Delayed	
ALKYLATING AGENTS				
Busulfan (Myleran)	2-8 mg/day for 2-3 weeks PO; stop for recovery; then maintenance	None	Bone marrow depression	Chronic granulocytic leukemia
Carmustine (BCNU)	As single agent: 100-200 mg/m^2 IV; over 1-2 hr infusion every 6-8 weeks In combination: 30-60 mg/m^2 IV Use gloves, since solution may cause skin discoloration	Nausea and vomiting; pain along vein of infusion	Granulocyte and platelet suppression Hepatic and renal toxicity	Brain, colon, breast, lung, Hodgkin's disease, lymphosarcoma, myeloma, malignant melanoma

Modified from Carter, S.K., and Kershner, L.M.: Pharmacy Times **41**(8):56, 1975.

Continued.

Table 15-1. Cancer chemotherapeutic agents—cont'd

Drug	Usual dosage	Toxicity		Major indications
		Acute	Delayed	
Chlorambucil (Leukeran)	Start 0.1-0.2 mg/kg/day PO; adjust for maintenace	None	Bone marrow depression (anemia, leukopenia, and thrombocytopenia) can be severe with excessive dosage	Chronic lymphocytic leukemia, Hodgkin's disease, non-Hodgkin's lymphoma, trophoblastic neoplasms
Cyclophosphamide (Cytoxan)	40 mg/kg IV in single or in 2-8 daily doses or 2-4 mg/kg/day PO for 10 days; adjust for maintenance	Nausea and vomiting	Bone marrow depression, alopecia, cystitis	Hodgkin's disease and other lymphomas, multiple myeloma, lymphocytic leukemia, many solid cancers
Lomustine (CCNU)	130 mg/m² PO once every 6 weeks	Severe nausea and vomiting; anorexia	Thrombocytopenia, leukopenia, alopecia, confusion, lethargy, ataxia	Brain, colon, Hodgkin's disease, lymphosarcoma, malignant melanoma

	Dosage	Acute toxicity	Chronic toxicity	Indications
Mechlorethamine (nitrogen mustard; HN₂, Mustargen)	0.4 mg/kg IV in single or divided doses	Nausea and vomiting	Moderate depression of peripheral blood count	Hodgkin's disease and other lymphomas, bronchogenic carcinoma
Melphalan (1-phenylalanine mustard; Alkeran)	0.25 mg/kg/day for 4 days PO; 2-4 mg/day as maintenance or 0.1-0.15 mg/kg/day for 2-3 weeks	None	Bone marrow depression	Multiple myeloma, malignant melanoma, ovarian carcinoma, testicular seminoma
Thiotepa (triethylenethiophosphoramide)	0.2 mg/kg IV for 5 days	None	Bone marrow depression	Hodgkin's disease, bronchogenic and breast carcinomas
ANTIMETABOLITES				
Cytarabine hydrochloride (arabinosyl cytosine; Cytosar)	2-3 mg/kg/day IV until response or toxicity or 1-3 mg/kg IV over 24 hr for up to 10 days	Nausea and vomiting	Bone marrow depression megaloblastosis	Acute leukemia

Continued.

Table 15-1. Cancer chemotherapeutic agents—cont'd

Drug	Usual dosage	Toxicity		Major indications
		Acute	Delayed	
Fluorouracil (5-FU, FU)	12.5 mg/kg/day IV for 3-5 days or 15 mg/kg/week for 6 weeks	Nausea	Oral and gastrointestinal ulceration, stomatitis and diarrhea, bone marrow depression	Breast, large bowel, and ovarian carcinoma
Mercaptopurine (6-MP, Purinethol)	2.5 mg/kg/day PO	Occasional nausea and vomiting, usually well tolerated	Bone marrow depression, occasional hepatic damage	Acute lymphocytic and granulocytic leukemia, chronic granulocytic leukemia
Methotrexate (amethopterin; MTX)	2.5-5.0 mg/day PO; 0.4 mg/kg rapid IV daily 4-5 days (not over 25 mg) or 0.4 mg/kg rapid IV twice/week	Occasional diarrhea, hepatic necrosis	Oral and gastrointestinal ulceration, bone marrow depression (anemia, leukopenia, thrombocytopenia), cirrhosis	Acute lymphocytic leukemia, choriocarcinoma, carcinoma of cervix and head and neck area, mycosis fungoides, solid cancers

Thioguanine (6-TG)	2 mg/kg/day PO	Occasional nausea and vomiting, usually well tolerated	Bone marrow depression	Acute leukemia
PLANT ALKALOIDS				
Vinblastine sulfate (Velban)	0.1-0.2 mg/kg/week IV or every 2 weeks	Nausea and vomiting, local irritant	Alopecia, stomatitis, bone marrow depression, loss of reflexes	Hodgkin's disease and other lymphomas, solid cancers
Vincristine sulfate (Oncovin)	0.01-0.03 mg/kg/week IV	Local irritant	Areflexia, peripheral neuritis, paralytic ileus, mild bone marrow depression	Acute lymphcytic leukemia, Hodgkin's disease and other lymphomas, solid cancers
ANTIBIOTICS				
Doxorubicin (Adriamycin)	60-90 mg/m^2 IV, single dose or over 3 days; repeat every 3 weeks up to total dose 500 mg/m^2	Nausea, red urine (not hematuria)	Bone marrow depression, cardiotoxicity, alopecia, stomatitis	Soft tissue, osteogenic and miscellaneous sarcomas, Hodgkin's disease, non-Hodgkin's lymphoma, bronchogenic and breast carcinoma, thyroid cancer

Continued.

Table 15-1. Cancer chemotherapeutic agents—cont'd

Drug	Usual dosage	Toxicity		Major indications
		Acute	*Delayed*	
Bleomycin (Blenoxane)	10-15 mg/m² once or twice a week, IV or IM to total dose 300-400 mg	Nausea and vomiting, fever, very toxic	Edema of hands, pulmonary fibrosis, stomatitis, alopecia	Hodgkin's disease, non-Hodgkin's lymphoma, squamous cell carcinoma of head and neck, testicular carcinoma
Dactinomycin (actinomycin D; Cosmegen)	0.015-0.05 mg/kg/week (1-2.5 mg) for 3-5 weeks IV; wait for marrow recovery (3-4 weeks), then repeat course	Nausea and vomiting, local irritant	Stomatitis, oral ulcers, diarrhea, alopecia, mental depression, bone marrow depression	Testicular carcinoma, Wilms' tumor, rhabdomyosarcoma, Ewing's and osteogenic sarcoma, and other solid tumors
Mithramycin (Mithracin)	0.025-0.050 mg/kg every 2 days for up to 8 doses, IV	Nausea and vomiting, hepatotoxicity	Bone marrow depression (thrombocytopenia), hypocalcemia	Testicular carcinoma, trophoblastic neoplasms

Mitomycin C (Mutamycin)	0.05 mg/kg/day IV for 5 days	Nausea and vomiting, "flulike syndrome"	Bone marrow depression, skin toxicity; pulmonary, renal, CNS effects	Squamous cell carcinoma of head and neck, lungs, and cervix; adenocarcinoma of the stomach, pancreas, colon, rectum; adenocarcinoma and duct cell carcinoma of the breast
Streptozocin (Zanosar)	As single agent: 1.0-1.5 mg/m²/week for 6 consecutive weeks with 4 weeks observation In combination: 400-500 mg/m² for 4-5 consecutive days with 6 weeks observation	Hypoglycemia, severe nausea and vomiting	Moderate but transient renal and hepatic toxicity, hypoglycemia, mild anemia, leukopenia	Pancreatic islet cell tumors

Continued.

Table 15-1. Cancer chemotherapeutic agents—cont'd

Drug	Usual dosage	Toxicity		Major indications
		Acute	Delayed	
OTHER SYNTHETIC AGENTS				
Dacarbazine (DTIC-Dome; DIC)	4.5 mg/kg/day IV for 10 days; repeated every 28 days	Nausea and vomiting, "flulike syndrome"	Bone marrow depression (rare)	Metastatic malignant melanoma
Hydroxyurea (Hydrea)	80 mg/kg PO single dose every 3 days or 20-30 mg/kg/day PO	Mild nausea and vomiting	Bone marrow depression	Chronic granulocytic leukemia
Mitotane (ortho para DDD o,p' DDD; Lysodren)	6-15 mg/kg/day PO	Nausea and vomiting	Dermatitis, diarrhea, mental depression	Adrenal cortical carcinoma
Procarbazine hydrochloride (Methyl hydrazine; ibenzmethylzin; Matulane)	Start 1-2 mg/kg/day PO; increase over 1 week to 3 mg/kg; maintain for 3 weeks, then reduce to 2 mg/kg/day until	Nausea and vomiting	Bone marrow depression, CNS depression	Hodgkin's disease, non-Hodgkin's lymphoma, bronchogenic carcinoma

Tamoxifen (Nolvadex)	20-40 mg daily in two divided doses	Nausea, vomiting, hot flashes	Increased bone and tumor pain; thrombocytopenia, leukopenia, edema, hypercalcemia	Breast cancer (estrogen sensitive)
HORMONES			
Diethylstilbestrol (DES)	15 mg/day PO (1 mg in prostate cancer)	None	Fluid retention, hypercalcemia, feminization, uterine bleeding; if during pregnancy, may cause vaginal carcinoma in offspring	Breast and prostate carcinomas
Dromostanolone propionate (Drolban)	100 mg 3 times a week IM	None	Fluid retention, masculinization, hypercalcemia	Breast carcinoma
Ethinyl estradiol	3 mg/day PO	None	Fluid retention, hypercalcemia, feminization, uterine bleeding	Breast and prostate carcinomas

Continued.

Table 15-1. Cancer chemotherapeutic agents—cont'd

| Drug | Usual dosage | Toxicity | | Major indications |
		Acute	Delayed	
Fluoxymesterone	10-20 mg/day PO	None	Fluid retention, masculinization, cholestatic jaundice	Breast carcinoma
Hydroxyprogesterone caproate	1 g IM twice a week	None	None	Endometrial carcinoma
Medroxyprogesterone acetate	100-200 mg/day PO; 200-600 mg twice a week	None	None	Endometrial carcinoma, renal cell, breast cancer
Prednisone	10-100 mg/day PO	None	Hyperadrenocorticism	Acute and chronic lymphocytic leukemia, Hodgkin's disease, non-Hodgkin's lymphomas
Testolactone (Teslac)	100 mg 3 times a week IM	None	Fluid retention, masculinization	Breast carcinoma
Testosterone enanthate	600-1200 mg/week IM	None	Fluid retention, masculinization	Breast carcinoma
Testosterone propionate	50-100 mg, IM 3 times a week	None	Fluid retention, masculinization	Breast carcinoma

dle during mitosis, thus inhibiting cell division. Even though there is close structural similarity, cross-resistance does not usually develop between the two agents.

2. Antibiotics. Through various mechanisms, the antibiotics bind with cellular DNA, preventing its replication as well as RNA synthesis, which is required for subsequent protein synthesis.

Hormones

Adrenocorticosteroids (usually prednisone) may be beneficial in treating lymphomas and acute leukemia because of their lympholytic effects and their ability to suppress mitosis in lymphocytes. Steroids are also used to help reduce edema secondary to radiation therapy and as palliative therapy in temporarily suppressing fever, sweats, and pain and in restoring, to some degree, appetite, lost weight, strength, and a sense of well-being in critically ill patients. With symptomatic relief, it is hoped that the patient's general physical condition may be improved sufficiently to permit further definitive therapy.

Estrogens and androgens are used in malignancies of sexual organs based on the assumption that these malignancies have hormonal requirements similar to those of nonmalignant sexual organs. Estrogens (usually diethylstilbestrol) are frequently used in prostatic carcinoma. There are regressions in the primary tumor and in soft tissue metastases, with significant symptomatic relief from the point of view of the patient. Androgens may be used in the treatment of metastatic breast cancer of any age group, and estrogens may be used in postmenopausal women with metastatic breast cancer.

Patients often may not complete a course of therapy because of the toxic effects of chemotherapeutic agents on normal as well as malignant cells. Malignant cells that were once susceptible may also develop a resistance to antineoplastic drugs. Several mechanisms may be involved, depending on the sites of action of the drug within the biochemical pathways of the cell. Theories about these mechanisms include a repair mechanism to damaged DNA molecules, altered permeability of the cell to the drug, and increased intracellular concentrations of protective chemicals.

Nurse and patient considerations

Before the treatment of neoplastic disease, several factors must be considered:

1. A tissue diagnosis to determine the type, extent, and grade of the malignancy, its natural history, and the most current results of chemotherapeutic studies is essential in selecting the most effective therapeutic regimen.

2. The physiologic and psychologic status of the patient must be considered. Patients in a good nutritional state with adequate renal, hepatic, and bone marrow function generally respond to therapy with fewer complications.

3. Location of the treatment center should also be considered. Some hospitals may be capable of providing special supportive measures such as isolation rooms to help protect the patient while taking immunosuppressive agents.

4. An "endpoint" or goal for therapy should be established. Is the malignancy in a stage that is "curable," or is remission or palliation of symptomatology the goal? The goal will help determine the approach to therapy and which adverse effects of therapy may be considered "acceptable" while the patient is receiving therapy.

Unlike antimicrobial therapy, in vitro sensitivity studies before the initiation of chemotherapy are unavailable. The physician must rely on previously collected data used in similar tumors to select a course of therapy, using one or more agents that appear to be most effective.

The scheduling of dosages may be of crucial importance in achieving therapeutic benefit and diminishing toxic response. Based on cell-cycle kinetics, only cells in a specific stage of nucleic acid production will be affected by some chemotherapeutic agents. Depending on the type of malignant tissue and the agents being used, dosages may be best given by continuous infusion or daily single administration. Frequency of repetition of therapy for maintenance of remission will also affect the course of the disease and the clinical condition of the patient.

Once therapy is initiated, the drug must be given an adequate therapeutic trial. A mechanism must be used to measure the success of therapy (such as reduction in tumor size). Generally speaking, if there is an objective response to therapy, the same regimen should be used until there is little or no objective change while the patient is taking the drug.

While a drug is being observed for therapeutic benefit, it must also be monitored for toxic effects. There are no predetermined dosage schedules that are universally therapeutic, and dosage may change according to the patient's response.

Most chemotherapeutic agents are nonselective in their activity and have clinical effects on normal as well as on malignant cells. Normal cells of the bone marrow, gastrointestinal tract, gonads, and hair follicles also have rapid rates of growth and are most susceptible to the action of antineoplastic agents.

Bone marrow depression characterized by leukopenia, thrombocytopenia, and anemia is a common adverse effect of most chemotherapeutic agents. Increased susceptibility to infection and thrombocytopenic purpura may result. Observe for easy bruisability, coffee-ground emesis, tarry stools, hematuria, and bleeding gums. White blood cell and platelet counts and serum uric acid levels must be monitored routinely.

Stomatitis, manifested by erythema, ulcerations, or white patchy membranes can be very uncomfortable and may interfere with the patient's nutrition. An anesthetic mouthwash, soft-bristled toothbrush, good oral hygiene, and bland, nonirritating foods may be beneficial.

Cellular damage to the intestinal mucosa may be characterized by diarrhea, abdominal cramps, or bleeding. Stools should be checked periodically for occult blood.

Nausea, vomiting, and anorexia are particularly troublesome to the patient's nutritional status as well as physical well-being. Small frequent meals planned at prime tolerance time may help. Administering oral medications with meals as well as using antiemetics before therapy may be beneficial.

Skin lesions, incisions, and wounds should be closely examined on a routine basis. Cellular growth necessary for normal healing processes as well as normal defense mechanisms may be suppressed by chemotherapy.

Infection is a serious problem in these patients and susceptibility is generally higher in those with hematologic malignancies. Infections may result from lowered resistance caused by either depressed host immunity resulting from the cancer, steroid therapy, or depressed granulocyte levels resulting from chemotherapy or bone marrow metastases. These patients are also more susceptible to "opportunistic pathogens" such as candidiasis and aspergillosis. Patients with a previous positive skin test for tuberculosis are often started on prophylactic isoniazid therapy.

Patients must be observed closely for signs of infection

(fever, sore throat, inflammation of cuts or abrasions), since many of the chemotherapeutic agents used alter clinical indications of infection. Analgesics (aspirin and acetaminophen) may also inadvertently suppress the fever response.

At the first sign of infection, urine, blood, and throat cultures should be obtained. Gram stains of the urine and throat cultures may give an indication of predominant microorganisms.

Antibiotic therapy based on the Gram stain and clinical judgment must often be initiated before the results of the cultures are known.

An area of patient care frequently neglected is the patient's emotional status. Information for the patient and family on matters of drug administration, expectations from therapy, and side effects should be discussed honestly. Hope of complete cure is usually unrealistic, while remission of symptoms and disease progression is more achievable. Patients and family should anticipate signs of fatigue and debilitation such as irritability, short attention span, and decreased pain threshold. Tell the patient what activity level to expect (shopping, occupational activities, driving) and how to plan and allow for frequent rest periods. Patients are usually interested in not what causes fatigue but rather what they can do in spite of it.

Long periods of therapy with frequent interruptions caused by adverse effects and short remissions may be expected to compound frustrations of both the patient and the family. Accept the patient's need to discuss feelings of anger, depression, and hopelessness. Verbal and nonverbal communications that convey feelings of interest and concern as well as positive progress in therapy help the patient retain a sense of dignity and self-respect.

CHAPTER SIXTEEN

Thyroactive agents

GENERAL INFORMATION ON THYROID THERAPY

The thyroid gland is an endocrine gland consisting of two oblong lobes connected by a narrow isthmus. In the mature adult it weighs between 25 and 35 g and is anatomically located in the anterior neck, overlying the larynx.

The gland is subdivided into pseudolobules made up of follicles or *acini*. The lumen of the acini contains a protein unique to the thyroid gland called "thyroglobulin." A primary function of thyroglobulin is the storage of triiodothyronine (T_3) and thyroxine (T_4, tetraiodothyronine), two hormones synthesized and secreted by the thyroid gland.

As with other endocrine glands, thyroid gland function is regulated by the hypothalamus and anterior pituitary gland. The hypothalamus secretes thyrotropin-releasing hormone (TRH), which stimulates the anterior pituitary gland to release thyroid-stimulating hormone (TSH thyrotropin). TSH mediates the synthesis and secretion of thyroid hormones from the thyroid gland. The release of TRH and TSH is controlled by complex feedback mechanisms that are based on demand for thyroid hormones and the circulating blood levels of T_3 and T_4.

Triiodothyronine and thyroxine regulate general body metabolism, more specifically, growth and maturation; CNS function; carbohydrate, protein, and lipid metabolism; fluid, and electrolyte balance; thermal regulation, cardiovascular function; gastrointestinal activity; and lactation and reproduction. Imbalance in hormone production may interfere with the regulation of any of these metabolic processes.

An in-depth discussion of the diagnosis and treatment of thyroid dysfunction is beyond the scope of this chapter; however, guidelines for the use of pharmacologic agents used to treat thyroid disorders will be presented.

Drugs used to treat thyroid disorders fall into two categories: (1) those used to replace thyroid hormones in such deficiency states as nontoxic goiter, hypothyroidism, myxedema, chronic thyroiditis, and cretinism and (2) those antithyroid agents used to suppress synthesis of thyroid hormones in hyperthyroid states. Thyroid hormone replacements discussed in this chapter include levothyroxine (T_4), liothyronine (T_3), liotrix, thyroglobulin, and thyroid, USP. Thyrolytic agents discussed are propylthiouracil and methimazole.

Action and use of thyroid replacement hormone medication

See individual monographs: levothyroxine (p. 478), liothyronine (p. 481), liotrix (p. 483), thyroglobulin (p. 484), and thyroid, USP (p. 485).

Nurse and patient considerations in the treatment of hypothyroidism

Recognize that the patient's cooperation may initially be difficult to achieve. Patients with decreased thyroid function are often apathetic and lack ambition secondary to their disease. Inform the patient that treatment must be a gradual process and that it may require several weeks or months to achieve a normal (euthyroid) state.

One of the first indications of therapeutic effect in the adult hypothyroid patient will be a diuresis with loss of puffiness and weight. This generally occurs within the first 2 to 4 days after therapy is initiated. Over the next 2 weeks the patient will notice an increased appetite, heart rate, and activity level and a sense of well-being. Skin and hair abnormalities will resolve within several weeks.

Changes initiated by thyroid hormone replacement in pediatric patients include increased activity levels, rapid growth, initial weight loss, and loss of hair. Height, weight, sleeping pulse, and morning temperature reading are all parameters that may be used to monitor pediatric therapy.

Patients with cardiovascular disease, hypertension, diabetes mellitus, adrenal insufficiency, hyperadrenalism, and pituitary dysfunction must be observed closely when thyroid hormone dosage adjustments are made. Adjustment in other medications may also be required. Patients should be counseled to report any cardiac palpitations or chest pain immediately.

Adverse effects of thyroid replacement preparations are dose related and may occur 1 to 3 weeks after changes in therapy have been initiated. Symptoms that may occur include cardiac palpitations, arrhythmias, angina pectoris, tachycardia, weight loss, abdominal cramping and diarrhea, headaches, insomnia, menstrual irregularities, fever, and intolerance to heat. Symptoms may require a discontinuation of therapy. Patients may require up to a month without use of medication for toxic effects to fully dissipate. Therapy must be reinstituted at lower dosages after symptoms have abated.

Inadequate patient counseling frequently leads to noncompliance and the renewal of symptoms of hypothyroidism. The need for lifelong replacement therapy, a review of the symptoms of overdosage, and the importance of periodic re-evaluation are facts that must be reinforced for successful therapy.

Action and use of antithyroid agents

Propylthiouracil (PTU) and methimazole are antithyroid agents that act by inhibiting the synthesis of T_3 and T_4. The drugs do not affect circulating hormone levels or hormones stored within the gland. Therefore there is usually a latent period of a few days to 2 weeks after antithyroid therapy has been initiated before symptoms improve. A euthyroid metabolic state is usually achieved within 6 to 8 weeks. Since PTU and methimazole do not alter the underlying thyroid disease, therapy is either continued for 1 to 2 years at reduced dosages or at the same dosage but with levothyroxine (T_4) supplementation added to prevent hypothyroidism. The combination of PTU or methimazole and thyroxine helps control the symptoms of the ophthalmopathy that is characteristic of Graves' disease. After long-term therapy, antithyroid medication is gradually withdrawn to determine whether there has been a spontaneous remission of the underlying disease.

Propylthiouracil and methimazole also serve a role in preparing the hyperthyroid patient for thyroidectomy. Rendering the patient euthyroid prior to surgery reduces the risk of thyrotoxic crisis during and after surgery.

Nurse and patient considerations in the treatment of hyperthyroidism

Propylthiouracil and methimazole may rarely cause bone marrow suppression, hepatotoxicity, or a lupuslike syndrome, usually within the first few months of therapy. Patients should notify their physician if symptoms such as sore throat, enlargement of cervical lymph nodes, fever, jaundice, nausea, vomiting, rash, sore joints, or headache occur.

Propylthiouracil may rarely cause hypoprothrombinemia. Patients should be warned to report signs of bleeding such as easy bruisability, petechiae, purpura, ecchymoses, and bleeding gums immediately. These patients should be monitored particularly closely if receiving anticoagulant therapy.

The most common reaction (5%) that occurs with PTU and methimazole is a purpuric, maculopapular skin eruption. It often occurs during the first 2 weeks of therapy and usually resolves spontaneously without treatment. If pruritus becomes severe, a change to the other agent (PTU or methimazole) may be necessary. Cross-sensitivity is uncommon.

Evidence of therapeutic activity is usually seen within 2 to 3 weeks, although 6 to 8 weeks are required to return the patient to a euthyroid state. Early subjective indications are weight gain and reduced heart rate. Objectively the PBI and serum T_4 level will be reduced. A patient may participate in monitoring therapy by recording weight and pulse rate on a chart 2 or 3 times a week. Once the euthyroid state is attained, patients must be encouraged to remain on therapy as prescribed. Follow-up examinations and hematologic studies should be repeated every 2 to 3 months.

Hyperthyroidism during pregnancy may be treated with small dosages (100 to 300 mg) of propylthiouracil. PTU does cross the placenta and can induce hypothyroid goiter in the neonate, particularly when larger dosages are used. Thyroid hormone replacement therapy should not be given to prevent fetal goiter, since thyroid hormones do not cross the placenta and will increase antithyroid medication for the mother.

Both PTU and methimazole are secreted in breast milk. Postpartum patients receiving antithyroid therapy should not breast-feed their infants.

Drugs that may alter thyroid function tests

Lithium carbonate may cause a decrease in PBI, free thyroxine, and T_4 by column and an increase in ^{131}I uptake; however, the incidence of clinical hypothyroidism is very rare.

Phenytoin (Dilantin) displaces levothyroxine from protein-binding sites, causing decreases in PBI, T_4 by column, and T_4 by Murphy-Pattee. The T_3 resin uptake is occasionally elevated, while the ^{131}I uptake and free thyroxine index are normal.

Salicylates (6 to 8 g/day) may displace thyroxine from protein-binding sites, resulting in a decreased PBI, T_4 by Murphy-Pattee, and ^{131}I uptake and a slight increase in T_3 red cell uptake.

Although the mechanism of action is unknown, heparin administration results in an increase in free thyroxine levels and an increased T_3 uptake.

Para-aminosalicylic acid (PAS) reduces PBI and ^{131}I uptake by decreasing thyroxine production. The decrease in 24 hr ^{131}I uptake may last 2 weeks after PAS is discontinued.

Estrogens, including oral contraceptives, increase circulating proteins (thyroxine-binding globulin [TBG]), thus increasing circulating thyroxin levels. PBI, T_4 by column, and T_4 by Murphy-Pattee are increased and T_3 uptake is decreased, but ^{131}I thyroidal uptake is not affected. The alterations in laboratory tests may last for 2 to 4 weeks after discontinuation of therapy.

Phenylbutazone (Butazolidin, Azolid) competes with thyroxine for protein-binding sites. T_3 uptake is increased, and PBI and 24 hr ^{131}I thyroidal uptake are decreased.

Androgens and anabolic steroids may decrease TBG levels, resulting in a decrease in serum thyroxine and an increase in T_3 uptake. The 24 hr ^{131}I uptake is not affected.

Propylthiouracil (PTU) and methimazole (Tapazole) induce clinical hypothyroidism with reduced circulating thyroxine and T_3 uptake levels. The 24 hr ^{131}I thyroidal uptake may also be decreased.

Desiccated thyroid, levothyroxine, triiodothyronine, and liotrix, all products containing thyroid hormones, will alter thyroid function tests.

The protein-bound iodine (PBI) test measures the iodine content of precipitated protein as an indicator of the amount of bound thyroxine (T_4). The PBI may be falsely elevated by compounds containing iodides. (The T_4 by Murphy-Pattee method of measuring thyroxine is not altered by products containing iodides.) The following products have been reported to interfere with the PBI test:

Barium sulfate	Lugol's solution
Barium bromide	Suntan lotions
Diiodohydroxyquin (Diodoquin)	Antidandruff agents
Iodochlorhydroxyquin (Vioform)	Salt substitutes
Iodophor antiseptics (Betadine)	Cod liver oil
Cough syrups	Contrast media
Gargles	

Drug interactions associated with thyroid hormone replacement therapy

The toxicity of digitalis glycosides (digoxin, digitoxin, others) may be enhanced when thyroid therapy is initiated. Dosage adjustments with digitalis preparations are frequently necessary as a patient returns to a euthyroid state. Hypothyroid patients often require small dosages of digitalis, whereas hyperthyroid patients require high dosages because of rapid metabolic turnover in the hyperthyroid state.

Patients with hypothyroidism are "resistant" to warfarin (Coumadin) anticoagulant therapy and will require larger dosages of anticoagulant. If thyroid replacement therapy is initiated while the patient is receiving warfarin therapy, the patient should have frequent prothrombin time determinations and should be counseled to observe closely for signs of overanticoagulation. The dosage of warfarin may have to be reduced by one third to half over the next 1 to 4 weeks.

Estrogens (Premarin, oral contraceptives) increase the amount of circulating TBG. Those patients already receiving thyroid hormone replacement may require an increase in thyroid hormone, since the increase in TBG induced by estrogens may reduce the amount of free (active) thyroxine in circulation.

Cholestyramine (Questran) binds triiodothyronine and thyroxine in the gastrointestinal tract, preventing absorption and enterohepatic recirculation of thyroid hormones. Studies indicate that at least 4 hr should separate the administration of cholestyramine and thyroid hormones.

Patients with diabetes mellitus being treated with insulin or oral hypoglycemic agents should test urine for glucosuria and ketonuria more frequently when thyroid hormone replacement therapy is initiated. The hyperglycemic effects of thyroid therapy may require an increase in dosage of the antidiabetic agent.

Drug interactions associated with antithyroid therapy

Hyperthyroid patients with congestive heart failure require higher than normal dosages of digitalis glycosides (digitoxin, digoxin) to be effective. As a euthyroid state is approached, the dosages of digitalis must be reduced to prevent toxicity.

Thyrotoxic patients appear to metabolize warfarin (Coumadin) and clotting factors more rapidly than euthyroid patients. The anticoagulant response to warfarin should be monitored carefully in patients with thyrotoxicosis and the dosage adjusted as the thyroid status changes.

THYROID HORMONES

Levothyroxine sodium
(Letter, Synthroid, others)

AHFS 68:36
CATEGORY Thyroid
hormone

Action and use

Levothyroxine (L-thyroxine, T_4) is one of two primary hormones produced and secreted by the thyroid gland. It is partially metabolized to triiodothyronine (T_3, liothyronine), the other primary thyroid hormone, so that therapy with levothyroxine provides physiologic replacement of both thyroid hormones. Chemical purity, uniform potency, long half-life, and catabolic pathways make levothyroxine the drug of choice for hormone replacement in patients with an inadequately functioning thyroid gland (hypothyroidism).

Characteristics

Absorption: 50% to 60% (PO). Onset: 3 to 5 days (PO), 6 to 8 hr (IV). Duration: 6 to 10 days after discontinuation of therapy. Protein binding: 99.98% bound—80% to thyroxine-binding globulin (TGB), 15% to thyroxine binding prealbumin (TBPA), 4% to 5% to albumin. Half-life: euthyroid, 6 to 7 days: hypothyroid, 9 to 10 days; hyperthyroid, 3 to 4 days. Metabolism and excretion: 30% to 40% metabolized to triiodothyronine, 20% to 40% conjugated in liver and excreted in stool as sulfates and glucuronides.

Administration and dosage

NOTE: The age of the patient, severity of hypothyroidism, and other concurrent medical conditions will determine the initial dosage and the interval of time necessary before increasing the dosage. Hypothyroid patients are quite sensitive to replacement of thyroid hormones. Monitor patients closely for adverse effects.

NOTE: When transferring patients already stabilized on thyroid, USP to levothyroxine, 1 grain (60 mg) of thyroid, USP is approximately equivalent to 100 μg (0.1 mg) of levothyroxine. When converting a patient to levothyroxine, administer 50 μg (0.05 mg) of levothyroxine less than calculated. Thyroid, USP has variable potency. Adjust the dosage as necessary in 2 to 3 weeks.

Adult

PO 1. Normal, otherwise healthy adults with recent onset of hypothyroidism: initially, 100 μg (0.1 mg) daily. Reevaluate therapy in 30 days and adjust dosage in increments of 50 μg (0.05 mg) every 3 to 4 weeks. The average maintenance dosage range is 100 to 200 μg (0.1 to 0.2 mg)/day.

2. Patients with cardiovascular disease and long-standing hypothyroidism: initially, 25 μg (0.025 mg) daily. Increase the dosage by 25 μg (0.025 mg) every 3 to 4 weeks.

IM—Generally not recommended due to erratic absorption.

IV—Myxedema stupor or coma without severe heart disease: 200 to 500 μg (0.2 to 0.5 mg) on the first day, followed by 100 to 300 μg (0.1 to 0.3 mg) on the second day.

NOTE: Parenteral levothyroxine can be substituted for the PO dosage form when ingestion is unacceptable. When administering levothyroxine parenterally, one should be aware that PO absorption is incomplete. Therefore only 50% to 60% of the PO dosage should be administered IV. When reconstituting the levothyroxine powder, add 5 ml of 0.9% sodium chloride injection, USP to the vial. Do not use bacteriostatic water for injection, because the bacteriostatic agent may interfere with complete dissolution. *Use immediately after dissolution and discard any unused portion.*

Pediatric

PO—Initially, 25 to 50 μg (0.025 to 0.05 mg) daily, with dosage increases of 25 to 50 μg (0.025 to 0.05 mg) every 2 weeks. The maintenance dosage may range from 0.3 to 0.4 mg daily.

IV—As for PO dosage: observe precautions for adult IV administration.

Nurse and patient considerations

* Laboratory tests commonly used to monitor levothyroxine therapy are the protein-bound iodine (PBI), the Murphy-Pattee T_4, and the T_3 resin uptake (T_3RU). A patient's clinical status must be assessed when thyroid function tests are interpreted. Variations in laboratory tests may indicate slight hyper-

thyroidism even though the patient is clinically euthyroid. Dosage should not be altered unless the patient displays symptoms of hyperthyroidism.

✳ See General information on thyroid therapy (p. 473).

Drug interactions

See General information on thyroid therapy (p. 473).

Liothyronine sodium
(Cytomel)

AHFS 68:36
CATEGORY Thyroid hormone

Action and use

Liothyronine is a synthetic reproduction of triiodothyronine (T_3), one of two primary hormones synthesized by the thyroid gland. Triiodothyronine is about four times more potent in thyroid activity than thyroxine (T_4), the other biologically active thyroid hormone; however, circulating serum levels of T_3 are lower. Liothyronine has an onset of action more rapid than levothyroxine and is occasionally used as a thyroid hormone replacement when prompt activity is necessary. Liothyronine is also used as a diagnostic agent for thyroid function in the T_3 suppression test.

Characteristics

Absorption: 85% (PO). Onset: a few hours; maximal response in 2 or 3 days. Duration: 3 to 5 days after discontinuation of therapy. Protein binding: 99.8% to thyroxine-binding globulin (TBG), thyroxine-binding prealbumin (TBPA), and albumin. Half-life: euthyroid, 1 day; hypothyroid, up to 2 days; hyperthyroid, 0.6 day. Metabolism and excretion: deiodinated, inactive metabolites in urine and feces.

Administration and dosage

NOTE: Liothyronine therapy should not be used in patients with cardiovascular disease unless a rapid onset of activity is deemed essential. Initiate therapy at low dosages (see p. 482) and observe patients particularly for tachycardia, palpitations, cardiac arrhythmias, and angina pectoris.

Adult

PO 1. Mild hypothyroidism: initially, 25 µg daily, with increases of 12.5 to 25 µg every 1 to 2 weeks. The usual maintenance dose is 25 to 75 µg daily. Occasionally 100 µg daily may be required.

2. Myxedema: initially, 5 µg daily, increased by 5 to 10 µg daily every 1 to 2 weeks. When 25 µg daily is attained, the dosage may be increased by 12.5 to 25 µg every 1 to 2 weeks. The usual maintenance dose is 50 to 100 µg daily.

Pediatric

PO 1. Initially, 5µg daily, with increases of 5 µg every 4 to 5 days until the desired response is attained.

2. Maintenance:
   a. Infants: approximately 20 µg daily.
   b. Ages 1 to 3: approximately 50 µg daily.
   c. Over 3 years of age: as for adult dosage.

When transferring a patient from thyroid, levothyroxine, or thyroglobulin therapy to liothyronine therapy, discontinue the initial thyroid therapy and start liothyronine therapy at a low dosage. Liothyronine has a rapid onset of action, and the residual effects of the initial thyroid therapy may be evident for several weeks. Liothyronine, 25 µg, is equivalent to approximately 1 grain (60 mg) of desiccated thyroid or thyroglobulin and 0.1 mg (100 µg) of levothyroxine.

Nurse and patient considerations

* The PBI usually remains at levels below normal during full replacement therapy with liothyronine. Observe the clinical status of patients on liothyronine closely. Do not make dosage adjustments based solely on laboratory function tests.

* See General information on thyroid therapy (p. 473).

Drug interactions

See General information on thyroid therapy (p. 473).

Liotrix
(Thyrolar, Euthroid)

AHFS 68:36
CATEGORY Thyroid hormone

Action and use

Liotrix is a combination of synthetically produced levo-thyroxine (T_4) and liothyronine (T_3) in a ratio of 4:1. Chemical purity, stability, and predictable potency are advantages of this combination product. These two thyroid hormones are marketed in this ratio because until a few years ago it was thought that the thyroid gland secreted these hormones in a ratio of 4:1. However, since it has been shown that a significant amount of active T_3 is produced from the peripheral catabolism of T_4, there is no longer a rationale for the use of this product.

Characteristics

See Levothyroxine (p. 479). and Liothyronine (p. 481) for the specific characteristics of T_4 and T_3.

Administration and dosage

NOTE: Do not use in patients with cardiovascular disease unless thyroid replacement is indicated. Initiate therapy at low dosages and observe patients for tachycardia, palpitations, cardiac arrhythmias, and angina pectoris.

Adult

PO—Newly diagnosed or untreated hypothyroidism: initially, ¼ to ½ grain daily. Increase dosage by ¼ to ½ grain every 2 to 4 weeks. The maintenance dosage range is 1 to 3 grains daily.

Nurse and patient considerations

* Some individuals who are euthyroid while receiving liotrix complain of recurrent headaches. The dosage should be reduced in these patients. If the headaches persist or symptoms of hypoglycemia develop, another thyroid preparation should be substituted.
* The PBI, T_3, and T_4 laboratory tests usually remain at levels in the normal range during full replacement therapy with liotrix. Observe the clinical status of patients closely. Do not make any dosage adjustments based solely on laboratory function tests.
* See General information on thyroid therapy (p. 473).

Table 16-1. Comparison of Thyrolar and Euthroid

Product (grains)	T_4/T_3 content	Approximate equivalence thyroid, USP (grains)
Thyrolar, ¼	12.5 µg/3.1 µg	¼
Thyrolar, ½	25 µg/6.25 µg	½
Euthroid, ½	30 µg/7.5 µg	½
Thyrolar, 1	50 µg/12.5 µg	1
Euthroid, 1	60 µg/15 µg	1
Thyrolar, 2	100 µg/25 µg	2
Euthroid, 2	120 µg/30 µg	2
Thyrolar, 3	150 µg/37.5 µg	3
Euthroid, 3	180 µg/45 µg	3
Thyrolar, 5	250 µg/62.5 µg	5

NOTE: Euthroid contains 20% more active T_3 and T_4 per approximate equivalent to thyroid, USP than Thyrolar.

Drug interactions

See General information on thyroid therapy (p. 473).

Thyroglobulin
(Proloid)

AHFS 68:36
CATEGORY Thyroid hormone

Action and use

Thyroglobulin is a purified protein extract from hog thyroid glands. It contains the active thyroid hormones thyroxine (T_4) and triiodothyronine (T_3) in a ratio of 2.5:1. Its potency is adjusted to be equivalent to thyroid, USP, but it is considerably more expensive. Thyroglobulin is used clinically for thyroid hormone replacement therapy in patients with hypothyroidism.

Characteristics

See Levothyroxine (p. 479) and Liothyronine (p. 481) for the specific characteristics of T_4 and T_3.

Administration and dosage

NOTE: Thyroglobulin should not be used in patients with cardiovascular disease unless thyroid replacement is indicated. Initiate therapy at low dosages (see below) and observe patients particularly for tachycardia, palpitations, cardiac arrhythmias, and angina pectoris.

Adult

PO 1. Mild hypothyroidism with no other apparent disorders: initially, 65 mg (1 grain) daily, with increases of 30 mg (0.5 grain) every 1 to 2 weeks. The maintenance dosage range is 30 to 200 mg (0.5 to 3 grains) daily.
2. Cardiovascular disease: 15 to 30 mg (0.25 to 0.5 grain) daily, with increases of 15 to 30 mg (0.25 to 0.5 grain) every 2 weeks.

Nurse and patient considerations

* The PBI usually remains at levels in the normal range during full replacement therapy with thyroglobulin. Observe the clinical status of patients closely. Do not make dosage adjustments based solely on laboratory function tests.

* See General information on thyroid therapy (p. 473).

Drug interactions

See General information on thyroid therapy (p. 473).

Thyroid, USP
(Various)

AHFS 68:36
CATEGORY Thyroid hormone

Action and use

Thyroid, USP (desiccated thyroid) is derived from pig, beef, and sheep thyroid glands. It contains the active thyroid hormones thyroxine (T_4) and triiodothyronine (T_3) in a ratio of about 2:1. There is some variation in potency, since the content of iodine and T_4 and T_3 vary slightly. Thyroid, USP is the oldest thyroid hormone replacement available and the least expensive. Due to its lack of purity, uniformity, and stability, it is generally not the drug of choice for the initiation of thyroid replacement therapy.

Administration and dosage

NOTE: Thyroid, USP should not be used in patients with cardiovascular disease unless thyroid replacement is indicated. Initiate therapy at low dosages (see p. 486) and observe patients particularly for tachycardia, palpitations, cardiac arrhythmias, and angina pectoris.

Adult

PO 1. Mild hypothyroidism with no other apparent disorders: initially, 60 mg (1 grain) daily, with increases of 60 mg every month until the desired result is obtained. The maintenance dosage range is 30 to 200 mg (0.5 to 3 grains) daily.
2. Myxedema or cardiovascular disease: initially, 15 mg (0.25 grain) daily, with increases of 15 mg every 2 weeks to a total dosage of 60 mg (1 grain) daily. The patient should continue to receive this dosage for 1 month and then be reassessed for further dosage adjustment. The usual maintenance dosage is 30 to 200 mg (0.5 to 3 grains) daily.

Pediatric

PO—As for adults with myxedema. Maintenance dosages may be greater than those for adults.

Nurse and patient considerations

∗ The PBI usually remains at levels in the normal range during full replacement therapy with thyroid, USP. Observe the clinical status of patients closely. Do not make any dosage adjustments based solely on laboratory function tests.
∗ See General information on thyroid therapy (p. 473).

Drug interactions

See General information on thyroid therapy (p. 473).

ANTITHYROID AGENTS

Methimazole
(Tapazole)

AHFS 68:36
CATEGORY Antithyroid agent

Action and use

Methimazole is an antithyroid agent used in the treatment of hyperthyroidism. For further information, see General information on thyroid therapy (p. 473).

Characteristics

Onset of clinical activity: dependent on thyroid hormone storage levels. Half-life: 6 to 8 hr. Metabolism: extensive. Excretion: in urine. Dialysis: unknown.

Administration and dosage
Adult

PO 1. Initial daily dosage:
   a. Mild hyperthyroidism: 5 mg every 8 hr.
   b. Moderate to severe hyperthyroidism: 10 to 15 mg every 8 hr.
   c. Severe hyperthyroidism: 20 mg every 8 hr.
  2. Maintenance daily dosage: 5 to 15 mg.

Pediatric

PO 1. Initial daily dosage: 0.4 mg/kg divided into 3 doses and administered every 9 hr.
  2. Maintenance daily dosage: approximately half the initial dosage.

Nurse and patient considerations

∗ See General information on thyroid therapy (p. 473).

Drug interactions

See General information on thyroid therapy (p. 473).

Propylthiouracil
(Propacil)

AHFS 68:36
CATEGORY Antithyroid agent

Action and use

Propylthiouracil (PTU) is a thyrolytic agent used in the treatment of hyperthyroidism. For further information, see General information on thyroid therapy (p. 473).

Characteristics

Onset: rapid absorption (PO); onset of clinical activity dependent on thyroid hormone storage levels. Half-life: less than 2 hr. Metabolism: extensive. Excretion: in urine. Dialysis: unknown.

Administration and dosage
Adult

PO—Initially, 100 to 150 mg every 6 to 8 hr. Dosage range: to 900 mg daily (150 mg every 4 hr). The maintenance dosage is 50 mg 2 or 3 times daily.

Pediatric
Ages 6 to 10

PO—Initially, 50 to 150 mg daily. The maintenance dosage is 50 to 100 mg daily, dependent on response.

Over 10 years of age

PO—Initially, 150 to 300 mg daily. The maintenance dosage is as for ages 6 to 10.

Nurse and patient considerations

* See General information on thyroid therapy (p. 473).

Drug interactions

See General information on thyroid therapy (p. 473).

CHAPTER SEVENTEEN

Agents used in the treatment of gout

Allopurinol
Colchicine
Probenecid
Sulfinpyrazone

Allopurinol
(Zyloprim)

AHFS 92:00
CATEGORY Xanthine oxidase inhibitor

Action and use

Allopurinol is used in the treatment of hyperuricemia. In contrast to the uricosuric agents (probenecid, sulfinpyrazone) that enhance the excretion of uric acid, allopurinol inhibits the enzyme xanthine oxidase, reducing the formation of uric acid from xanthine and hypoxanthine. Xanthine and hypoxanthine are then excreted unchanged in the urine. Allopurinol is indicated for use in the long-term management of the primary hyperuricemia of gout and the secondary hyperuricemia of antineoplastic therapy. It is not effective in treating acute attacks of gouty arthritis.

Characteristics

Onset: serum levels of uric acid start falling within 2 to 3 days after therapy is initiated. Duration: serum levels of uric acid return to pretreatment levels within 7 to 10 days after discontinuation of therapy. Protein binding: 0%. Half-life: allopurinol, 2 to 3 hr; oxipurinol, 18 to 30 hr. Metabolism: allopurinol is metabolized by xanthine oxidase to oxipurinol (active). Dialysis: unknown.

Administration and dosage

For primary hyperuricemia:

Adult

PO—Initially, 100 mg daily. Increase the daily dosage by 100 mg/week until the serum urate level falls to 60 mg/100 ml or a maximum dosage of 800 mg daily is achieved. The average maintenance dose is 300 mg daily. Allopurinol may be better tolerated if it is taken after meals. Dosage must be reduced in patients with renal failure (see chart below).

Creatine clearance (ml/min)	Recommended dosage
10-20	200 mg daily
<10	100 mg daily
<3	100 mg every 36-48 hr

For secondary hyperuricemia during antineoplastic therapy:

Adult

PO—600 to 800 mg daily for 2 or 3 days.

Pediatric
Under 6 years of age

PO—150 mg daily.

Ages 6 to 10

PO—300 mg daily.

Readjust therapy after 48 hr.

NOTE: Initiate allopurinol therapy 1 or 2 days before starting oncologic chemotherapy. Urine output should be maintained at 2 to 3 L/day. Alkalinization of the urine may also be beneficial.

Nurse and patient considerations

* The frequency of gouty attacks may increase during the first 6 to 12 months of therapy. During these attacks, continue allopurinol therapy without changing dosages. Treat the attack with full therapeutic courses of colchicine or other antiinflammatory agents. Alkalinization of the urine increases the solubility of urates, reducing the possibility of renal stone formation.

* Therapy should be discontinued immediately if any form of skin rash should develop. Skin rashes may be an early indication of hypersensitivity reactions and may occur months or years after therapy has begun (usually within 1 to 6 weeks).

* Hepatotoxicity manifested by hepatomegaly, hepatitis, and jaundice with abnormal liver function tests (SGOT, SGPT, alkaline phosphatase) have occurred. Symptoms are reversible on discontinuation of therapy. Liver function tests should be performed before initiating therapy and periodically thereafter, especially during the first few months of therapy.
* Blood dyscrasias manifested by anemia, thrombocytopenia, and granulocytopenia have been reported. Periodic blood cell counts should be performed before initiating therapy and periodically thereafter, especially during the first few months of therapy.
* Allopurinol is contraindicated in patients with idiopathic hemochromatosis. The manufacturer also states that iron salts should not be administered to patients who are receiving allopurinol therapy.
* Allopurinol should not be administered to pregnant or nursing women. The effects of xanthine oxidase inhibition on the fetus and infant are not known.

Drug interactions

Allopurinol inhibits the metabolism of azathioprine (Imuran) and mercaptopurine (Purinethol). When initiating therapy with azathioprine or mercaptopurine, start at one fourth to one third of the normal dosage and adjust subsequent dosages to the patient's response.

Allopurinol may increase the frequency of bone marrow depression in patients receiving cyclophosphamide. The mechanism of action is unknown. When concomitant therapy is used, monitor patients closely for bone marrow depression.

Allopurinol may prolong the half-life of the oral hypoglycemic agent chlorpropamide (Diabinese). The patient should be advised of signs of hypoglycemia (faintness, pallor, diaphoresis, increased irritability, seizures, or coma). Reduction of the dosage of chlorpropamide may be required.

Allopurinol may prolong the half-life of dicumarol. This interaction has not been shown to take place with warfarin (Coumadin); however, patients receiving both allopurinol and warfarin must be observed closely for signs of hemorrhage (bruises, bleeding gums, hematuria, or petechial hemorrhages).

There has been an increased incidence of rash reported in patients receiving concomitant therapy with ampicillin and allopurinol. If a rash occurs, evaluate patient carefully for penicillin and allopurinol hypersensitivity.

Allopurinol alters the metabolism of vidarabine, producing neurotoxicity manifested by pain, itching, tremors of the extremities and facial muscles, and impaired mentation. Patients should be observed closely when receiving both drugs for more than 4 days.

Allopurinol significantly reduces the metabolism of theophylline. See General information on theophylline derivatives (p. 271).

Colchicine

AHFS 92:00
CATEGORY Unclassified

Action and use

Colchicine is a unique agent known for two centuries to be effective in the treatment of acute attacks of gouty arthritis. It has mild antiinflammatory but no analgesic activity.

Colchicine evokes several pharmacologic responses such as hypothermia, respiratory depression, vasoconstriction, and gastrointestinal stimulation. It is an antimitotic agent, arresting cell division in metaphase by blocking spindle formation. It inhibits migration of granulocytes (white blood cells) to inflamed tissue and reduces urate crystal deposition in inflamed joints, but its mechanism of action in the treatment of gouty arthritis has not been completely determined. It does not enhance renal excretion of uric acid or reduce its concentration in the blood.

Because of its broad pharmacologic activity, colchicine has been used investigationally in the treatment of neoplastic and inflammatory diseases but is currently a drug of choice only for preventing and aborting acute attacks of gouty arthritis.

Characteristics

Absorption: well absorbed after administration (PO). Protein binding: 31%. Half-life: plasma, 20 min; leukocytes, several days. Metabolism: deacetylated in the liver. Excretion: 10% to 30% renal excretion, remainder by fecal elimination. Dialysis: unknown.

Administration and dosage
Adult

PO

1. Acute gout: initially, 0.5 to 1.2 mg, followed by 0.6 mg every 1 to 2 hr until pain subsides or nausea, vomiting and diarrhea develop. A total dosage of 4 to 10 mg may be required. Joint pain and swelling begin to subside within 12 hr and are usually gone within 48 to 72 hr following initiation of therapy. After the acute attack, 0.5 to 0.6 mg should be administered every 6 hr for a few days to prevent relapse. Do not repeat high-dosage therapy for at least 3 days.
2. Prophylaxis for recurrent gout: 0.5 to 0.6 mg every 1 to 3 days depending on the frequency of gouty attacks.

IV—Acute gout: initially, 2 mg diluted in 20 ml saline solution, administered slowly over 5 min, and followed by 0.5 mg every 6 to 12 hr to a maximum of 4 mg in 24 hr. If pain recurs, daily doses of 1 to 2 mg may be administered for several days. Do not repeat high-dosage therapy for at least 3 days. *Avoid extravasation.*

SC OR IM—*Do not administer SC or IM.* Severe local reactions may occur.

NOTE: Use with extreme caution in elderly or debilitated patients and in those patients with impaired renal, cardiac, or gastrointestinal function.

Nurse and patient considerations

* Nausea, vomiting, and diarrhea are common adverse effects of colchicine therapy. Discontinue therapy when gastrointestinal symptoms develop. Symptoms tend to be less severe when IV therapy is used. Antidiarrheal agents such as diphenoxylate (Lomotil), loperamide (Imodium), or paregoric may be required to control severe diarrhea. Black tarry stools or bright red blood in the stools may indicate gastrointestinal bleeding and should be reported immediately.

* Although it occurs infrequently, chronic administration of colchicine may result in bone marrow depression, leading to aganulocytosis, thrombocytopenia, and aplastic anemia.

Drug interactions

Although not specifically a drug-drug interaction, salicylates should be used with caution in patients suffering from gouty arthritis. Salicylates reduce the solubility and renal tubular secretion of urates.

Probenecid
(Benemid, Probalan)

AHFS 40:40
CATEGORY Uricosuric agent

Action and use

Probenecid is a sulfonamide derivative that increases uric acid excretion by inhibiting renal tubular reabsorption of uric acid. Probenecid is used in the long-term management of hyperuricemia associated with gout and gouty arthritis.

Probenecid also blocks the secretion of weak organic acids into the proximal and distal renal tubules. This activity can be used to advantage clinically by blocking the secretion of penicillins and cephalosporins into the urine. Antibiotic plasma concentrations are maintained at higher levels for a longer duration, allowing more effective antibiotic therapy with less frequent dosage administration. Combination therapy with probenecid and a penicillin antibiotic is routinely used in the treatment of *Neisseria gonorrhoeae*.

Characteristics

Peak plasma levels: 2 to 4 hr. Protein-binding: greater than 75%. Half-life: 4 to 17 hr. Metabolism: liver to several active metabolites. Excretion: 5% to 10% unchanged, 90% to 95% as metabolites, in urine. Dialysis: unknown.

Administration and dosage

For hyperuricemia:

PO—Initially, 250 mg twice daily for 1 week, then 500 mg twice daily. Dosage may be increased by 500 mg every few weeks to a maximum of 2 to 3 g daily. Probenecid may be administered with food or milk to diminish gastric irritation.

NOTE: Do not start probenecid therapy during an attack of acute gout; wait 2 to 3 weeks before initiating treatment.

Patient fluid intake should be maintained at 2 to 3L/day.

Do not administer to patients with a creatine clearance of less than 40 ml/min or a BUN greater than 40 mg/100 ml.

Do not administer to patients with a history of blood dyscrasias or uric acid kidney stones.

In combination with penicillins or cephalosporins:

Adult

PO—500 mg 4 times daily.

Pediatric (2 to 14 years of age)

PO—25 mg/kg initially, followed by 10 mg/kg 4 times daily. Children weighing more than 50 kg (110 lb) may receive the adult dosage.

For acute, uncomplicated gonorrhea:
1. Probenecid, 1 g PO, plus 4.8 million units of IM aqueous procaine penicillin G injected at 2 different sites.
2. Probenecid, 1 g PO, plus 3.5 g of ampicillin PO.

Nurse and patient considerations

* The frequency of gouty attacks may increase during the first 6 to 12 months of therapy. During these attacks, continue probenecid therapy without changing dosages. Treat the acute attack with full therapeutic regimens of colchicine or other antiinflammatory agents. Alkalinization of the urine increases the solubility of urates, reducing the possibility of renal stone formation.
* Gastrointestinal complaints are the most common adverse effects of probenecid therapy. About 8% of patients will suffer from anorexia, nausea, and vomiting. Use with caution in patients with a history of peptic ulcer disease.
* Hypersensitivity reactions manifesting as fever, pruritus, and rashes occur in about 5% of patients. Discontinue probenecid therapy.
* A false-positive reaction for glucose in the urine may occur with Clinitest tablets, but not with Tes-Tape.
* There are no reports of adverse effects to either mother or fetus when probenecid is used during pregnancy.

Drug interactions

Probenecid may reduce the renal excretion of nitrofurantoin, diminishing its effectiveness as a urinary antiinfective agent as well as increasing the potential for toxicity.

It may prolong the half-life of oral hypoglycemic agents (chloropromide, tolbutamide). Reduction of the dosage of the oral hypoglycemic may be required, and the patient should be advised of signs of hypoglycemia (faintness, pallor, diaphoresis, increased irritability, seizures, or coma).

Probenecid may block the renal excretion of indomethacin (Indocin) dapsone (Avlosulfon), sulfinpyrazone (Anturane), and para-aminosalicylic acid (PAS), increasing the possibility of adverse effects from these agents. Dosage reduction may be all that is necessary to reduce toxicity while maintaining therapeutic activity.

Salicylates inhibit the uricosuric activity of probenecid. Any more than an occasional small dose of salicylate should be avoided in patients receiving probenecid.

Antineoplastic therapy frequently elevates serum uric acid levels. Probenecid is *not* recommended in these patients because of the possibility of their developing uric acid stones in the kidneys.

Probenecid inhibits the metabolism of clofibrate (Atromid S). Patients complaining of the development of muscle weakness and pain while taking clofibrate and probenecid concommitantly should be evaluated with the possibility of reducing the clofibrate dosage.

Sulfinpyrazone
(Anturane)

AHFS 40:40
CATEGORY Uricosuric agent

Action and use

Sulfinpyrazone is a renal tubular blocking agent. It inhibits the reabsorption of urate from the proximal renal tubules, increasing the urinary excretion of uric acid and decreasing serum urate levels. Sulfinpyrazone is used in the long-term management of hyperuricemia associated with gout and gouty arthritis.

Sulfinpyrazone also inhibits platelet adhesiveness and prolongs platelet life. Studies are now under way to determine whether sulfinpyrazone is effective in the prevention of thromboembolic diseases such as angina pectoris, transient ischemic attacks, and myocardial infarction.

Characteristics

Peak plasma levels: 1 to 2 hr. Duration: 4 to 10 hr. Protein-binding: 98%. Half-life: 1 to 9 hr. Metabolism: liver, active and inactive metabolites. Excretion: 95% excreted in urine as unchanged drug, active and inactive metabolites. Dialysis: unknown.

Administration and dosage

PO—Initially, 100 to 200 mg 2 times daily during the first week of therapy. The maintenance dosage is usually 200 to 400 mg twice daily. Sulfinpyrazone may be administered with food or milk to diminish gastric irritation.

NOTE: Do not start sulfinpyrazone therapy during an attack of acute gout. Wait 2 to 3 weeks before initiating therapy.

Patient fluid intake should be maintained at 2 to 3 L/day.

Do not administer to patients with a creatinine clearance of less than 40 ml/min or a BUN greater than 40 mg/100 ml.

Do not administer to patients with a history of blood dyscrasias or uric acid kidney stones.

Nurse and patient considerations

* The frequency of gouty attacks may increase during the first 6 to 12 months of therapy. During these attacks, continue sulfinpyrazone therapy without changing dosages. Treat the acute attack with full therapeutic regimens of colchicine or other antiinflammatory agents. Alkalinization of the urine increases the solubility of urates, reducing the possibility of renal stone formation.

* Gastrointestinal complaints are the most common adverse effects of sulfinpyrazone therapy. Use with caution in patients with a history of peptic ulcer disease.

* Hypersensitivity reactions manifesting as fever, pruritis, and rashes occur in less than 3% of patients. Sulfinpyrazone therapy should be discontinued. Patients who have developed hypersensitivities to oxyphenbutazone (Oxalid, Tandearil) or phenylbutazone (Azolid, Butazolidin) should not be placed on sulfinpyrazone therapy. All are pyrazolone derivatives and carry cross-sensitivities.

* Serious and fatal blood dyscrasias including anemia, agranulocytosis, and thrombocytopenia have been associated with sulfinpyrazone therapy. Although the development of blood dyscrasias is quite rare, periodic differential blood counts are recommended.

Drug interactions

Sulfinpyrazone may reduce the renal excretion of nitro-furantoin, diminishing its effectiveness as a urinary antiinfective agent as well as increasing the potential for toxicity.

Salicylates inhibit the uricosuric activity of sulfinpyrazone. Patients receiving sulfinpyrazone therapy should refrain from using salicylates.

Antineoplastic therapy frequently elevates serum uric acid levels. Sulfinpyrazone is *not* recommended in these patients because of the possibility of their developing uric acid stones in the kidneys.

CHAPTER EIGHTEEN

Oral contraceptives

General information on oral contraceptives

GENERAL INFORMATION ON ORAL CONTRACEPTIVES

Oral (hormonal) contraception is one of the most common forms of artificial birth control now in use in the United States; it is used by approximately one third of all women between 18 and 44 years of age.

There are two types of oral hormonal contraceptives in general use: (1) the combination pill, which is taken for 21 days of the menstrual cycle and contains both an estrogen and a progestin and (2) the "mini-pill," which is taken every day and contains only a progestin. The approximately 24 "combination"-type oral contraceptives currently available contain one of five progestins (norethynodrel, norethindrone, norethindrone acetate, ethynodiol diacetate, or norgestrel) and either of two estrogens (ethinyl estradiol or mestranol). The progestin-only pills contain either norethindrone or norgestrel.

Estrogens and progestins, to some extent, induce contraception by inhibiting ovulation. The estrogens block pituitary release of follicle-stimulating hormone (FSH), preventing the ovary from developing a follicle from which the ovum is released. Progestins inhibit pituitary release of luteinizing hormone (LH), the hormone responsible for release of the ovum from the follicle.

Other mechanisms play an ancillary role in preventing conception. Estrogens and progestins alter (1) cervical mucus by making it thick and viscous, inhibiting sperm migration; (2) mobility of uterine and oviduct muscle, reducing transport of both sperm and ovum; and (3) the endometrium, impairing implantation of the fertilized ovum.

The mini-pills or progestin-only pills represent a relatively new direction in oral contraceptive therapy. Many of the adverse effects of combination-type contraceptives are due to the estrogen component of the tablet. For those patients particularly susceptible to adverse effects of estrogen therapy, the mini-pill provides an alternative. Women who might prefer the mini-pill are those with a history of migraine headaches, hypertension, mental depression, weight gain, and breast tenderness and those who want to breast-feed post-partum. The mini-pill is not without its disadvantages, however. Between 30% and 40% of patients on the mini-pill continue to intermittently ovulate. Birth control is maintained by progestin activity on cervical mucus, uterine and fallopian transport, and implantation. There is a slightly higher incidence of both uterine and ectopic (tubal) pregnancy. Dysmenorrhea, manifested by irregular periods, infrequent periods, and spotting between periods, is common among women taking the mini-pill.

Adverse effects associated with oral contraceptive therapy

Two decades of clinical experience have shown that birth control pills (BCP) are not as "safe" as indicated by earlier studies. Use of oral contraceptives must be considered in light of the potential risks and complications stemming from pregnancy. There are (1) minor side effects, (2) major adverse effects, and (3) contraindications to use associated with oral contraceptives.

About 40% of patients using BCP will suffer some side effects. Hormones such as estrogens and progestins have many other actions that affect nearly every organ system within the body. It is beyond the scope of this general introduction to list every adverse effect associated with oral contraceptives. Only the more frequent minor side effects and the major adverse effects are listed (Table 18-1).

The most common side effects are related to the dose of estrogen and progestin in each product (see Table 18-2). The patient should return for reevaluation and a possible change in product if many early effects have not resolved by the third month. Nausea, headaches, weight gain, spotting, decreased menstrual flow, missed periods, mood changes, depression, fatigue, chloasma, yeast infection, vaginal itching or discharge, and changes in libido are common side effects.

Disease states that may be aggravated by continued use of oral contraceptives are hypertension (it may require 3 to 6 months to reverse hypertension after BCP are discontinued), gallbladder disease, diabetes mellitus, severe varicose veins, seizure disorders, oligomenorrhea or amenorrhea, and rheumatic heart disease.

The list of absolute contraindications to the use of BCP is somewhat variable depending on the clinician and the particular case history of each patient. However, patients with any of the following conditions should strongly consider oth-

Text continued on p. 506.

Table 18-1. Pill side effects: a time framework

Worse in first 3 months	Over time: steady-constant	Worse over time	Worse after discontinuation
Nausea plus dizziness	Headaches during 3 weeks that pills are being taken	Headaches during week pills are not taken	Infertility, amenorrhea; hypothalmic and endometrial† suppression, and miscalculation of the expected date of confinement
Thrombophlebitis (venous)	Arterial thromboembolic events, blurred vision, stroke*	Weight gain	One form of acne
Leg veins	Anxiety, fatigue, depression	Monilial vaginitis	Hair loss—alopecia
Pulmonary emboli*		Periodic missed menses while on oral contraceptives	
Pelvic vein thrombosis*	Thyroid function studies	Chloasma*	
Retinal vein thrombosis*	Elevated PBI	Myocardial infarction*	
Cyclic weight gain, edema	Depressed T₃ resin uptake	Spider angiomata	
Breast fullness, tenderness	Susceptibility to amenorrhea after discontinuation of pill	Growth of myoma	
		Predisposition to gallbladder disease	
Breakthrough bleeding	Change in cervical secretions—mucorrhea	Hirsutism	
Elevated serum lipid levels even to the extent of pancreatitis	Decrease in libido	Decreased menstrual flow	
		Small uterus, pelvic relaxation, cystocele, rectocele, atropic vaginitis	

From Hatcher, R.A., et al.: Contraceptive technology, 1978-1979, ed. 9, New York, 1978, Halstead Press. *Continued.*
*May be irreversible or produce permanent damage.
†To avoid this complication in many patients, advise women desiring to become pregnant to discontinue pills 3-6 months before desired pregnancy.

Table 18-1. Pill side effects: a time framework

Worse in first 3 months	Over time: steady-constant	Worse over time	Worse after discontinuation
Abnormal glucose tolerance test*	Autophonia, chronic dilatation of eustachian tubes rather than cyclic opening and closing	Cystic breast changes	
Contact lenses fail to fit because of fluid retention	Acne	Photodermatitis—sunlight sensitivity with hypopigmentation	
Abdominal cramping		One form of hair loss—alopecia	
Suppression of lactation		Hypertension	
Failure to understand correct use of oral contraceptives; pregnancy		Focal hyperplasia of liver and hepatic adenomas	

Table 18-2. Pill side effects: hormone etiology

Estrogen excess	Progestin excess	Androgen excess	Estrogen deficiency	Progestin deficiency
Nausea, dizziness	Increased appetite and weight gain (non-cyclic)	Increased appetite and weight gain	Irritability, nervousness	Late breakthrough bleeding
Edema and abdominal or leg pain with cyclic weight gain	Tiredness and fatigue and feeling weak	Hirsutism	Hot flushes	Heavy menstrual flow and clots
Leukorrhea		Acne	Uterine prolapse	Delayed onset of
		Oily skin, rash	Early and midcycle spotting	

Increase in leiomyoma size	Depression and decrease in libido	Increased libido	Decreased amount of menstrual flow	menses following last pill
Chloasma	Oily scalp, acne	Cholestatic jaundice	No withdrawal bleeding	Dysmenorrhea
Uterine cramps	Loss of hair	Pruritus	Decreased libido	Weight loss
Irritability	Cholestatic jaundice		Diminished breast size	
Increase female fat disposition	Decreased length of menstrual flow		Dry vaginal mucosa and dyspareunia	
Cervical exotrophia	Hypertension(?)		Headaches	
Contact lenses fail to fit	Headaches between pill packages		Depression	
Telangiectasia	Monilial vaginitis, cervicitis			
Vascular type headache	Increase in breast size (areolar tissue)			
Hypertension(?)	Breast tenderness without fluid retention			
Lactation suppression	Decreased carbohydrate tolerance			
Headaches while taking pills				
Cystic breast changes				
Breast tenderness with fluid retention				
Thrombophlebitis				
Cerebrovascular accidents				
Hepatic adenoma				

From Hatcher, R.A., et al.: Contraceptive technology, 1978-1979, ed. 9, New York, 1978, Halstead Press.

Table 18-3. Oral contraceptives

Brand name	Progestin					Estrogen		Other
	Norethindrone (mg)	Norethindrone acetate (mg)	Norgestrel (mg)	Ethynodiol diacetate (mg)	Norethynodrel (mg)	Ethinyl estradiol (μg)	Mestranol (μg)	
COMBINATION-TYPE*								
Brevicon (21, 28)†	0.5					35		
Demulen (21, 28)				1		50		
Enovid, 5 mg (20)					5		75	
Enovid-E (20, 21)					2.5		100	
Loestrin 1/20 (21, 28)		1				20		
Loestrin 1.5/3.0 (28)		1.5				30		
Lo/Ovral (21)			0.3			30		
Modicon (21, 28)	0.5					35		
Norinyl 1 + 35 (21, 28)	1					35		
Norinyl 1 + 50 (21, 28)	1						50	
Norinyl 1 + 80 (21, 28)	1						80	
Norinyl, 2 mg (21)	2						100	
Norlestrin 1/50 (21, 28)		1				50		

	Progestin (mg)	Estrogen (mcg)		Other
				75 mg ferrous fumarate
Norlestrin Fe 1/50 (28)	1	50		75 mg ferrous fumarate
Norlestrin 2.5/50 (21)	2.5	50		
Norlestrin Fe 2.5/50 (28)	2.5	50		75 mg ferrous fumarate
Ortho-Novum 1/35 (21, 28)	1	35		
Ortho-Novum 1/50 (21, 28)	1		50	
Ortho-Novum 1/80 (21, 28)	1		80	
Ortho-Novum 2 (21)	2		100	
Ortho-Novum 10/11 (21, 28)	10 Tablets—0.5 11 Tablets—1	35 35		
Ovcon-35 (28)	0.4	35		
Ovcon-50 (28)	1	50		
Ovral (21, 28)	0.5	50		
Ovulen (20, 21, 28)	1		100	
PROGESTIN ONLY‡				
Micronor (35)	0.35			
Nor-QD (42)	0.35			
Ovrette (28)	0.075			

*Products contain 20 or 21 hormone tablets/package.
†21 hormone tablets/package plus 7 inert tablets.
‡Products contain all active hormone tablets.

Continued.

er forms of contraception: a history of thromboembolic disease, stroke, malignancy of breast or reproductive system, renal or liver disease, severe mental depression, suspected pregnancy, and repeated contraceptive failure.

Administration and dosage

See Table 18-3 for products and range of hormone concentrations available. The estrogenic component of the combination-type pills is responsible for most of the major and minor side effects associated with oral contraceptive therapy. The FDA has recommended that therapy be initiated with a product containing a lower dose of estrogen. Side effects must be reviewed in relation to individual case histories, but many physicians initiate therapy with Norinyl 1 + 50 or Ortho Novum 1/50. Therapy and therefore products may be adjusted based on incidence of side effects.

Combination oral contraceptives: patient instructions

When to start the pill: start the first pill on the first Sunday after your period begins. Take 1 pill daily, at the same time daily, until the pack is gone. If using a 21-day pack, wait 1 week and restart on the next Sunday. If using a 28-day pack, start a new pack the day after finishing the last pack. Use another form of birth control (condoms, foam) during this first month. You may not be fully protected by the pill during the first month.

Missed pills: if you miss *1* pill, take it as soon as you remember it; take the next pill at the regularly scheduled time. If you miss 2 pills, take two pills as soon as you remember, and 2 the next day. Spotting may occur when 2 pills are missed. Use another form of birth control (condoms, foam) until you finish this pack of pills. If you miss *3 or more* pills, start using another form of birth control immediately. Start a new pack of pills on the next Sunday even if you are menstruating. Discard your old pack of pills. Use other forms of birth control through the next month after missing 3 or more pills.

Missed pills and skipped periods: return to your physician for a pregnancy test.

Skipping one period but no missed pills: it is not uncommon for a woman to occasionally miss a period when on the pill. Start the next pack on the appropriate Sunday.

Spotting for two or more cycles: see your physician.

Periodic examinations: a yearly examination should include tests for blood pressure, pelvic examination, urinalysis, breast examination, and Papanicolaou smear.

Discontinuing the pill for conception: because of a possibility of birth defects, discontinue the pill 3 months before attempting pregnancy. Use other methods of contraception for these 3 months.

Duration of oral contraceptive therapy: many physicians prefer to have their patients discontinue the pill for 3 out of every 18 months. This allows the body to return to a normal cycle. Be sure to use other forms of contraception during this time. Long-term use (3 or more years) must be determined on an individual basis.

Side effects to be reported as soon as possible: severe headaches, dizziness, blurred vision, leg pain, shortness of breath, chest pain, and acute abdominal pain. Although these side effects are usually of minor consequence, absence of serious adverse effects must be confirmed.

NOTE: When being seen by a physician or dentist for other reasons, be sure to mention that you are currently taking BCP.

Mini-pill: patient instructions

Starting the mini-pill: start on the first day of menstruation. Take 1 tablet daily, every day, regardless of when your next period is. Tablets should be taken at about the same time every day.

Missing 1 pill: take it as soon as you remember, and take your next pill at the regularly scheduled time. Use another form of birth control until your next period.

Missing 2 pills: take one of the missed pills immediately and take your regularly scheduled pill that day on time. The next day, take the regularly scheduled pill as well as the other missed pill. Use another method of birth control until your next period.

Missed periods: some women note changes in the time as well as duration of their periods while using mini-pills. These changes are to be expected. If menses occurs every 28 to 30 days, ovulation may still be occurring. For maximal safety, use alternate forms of contraception on days 10 through 18. If irregular bleeding occurs every 25 to 45 days, ovulation is probably not occurring on a regular basis. You may feel more comfortable if you use other forms of contraception with the mini-pill or discuss switching to an estrogen-containing (combination) contraceptive.

If you have taken all tablets correctly, but do not have a period for over 60 days, speak to your physician concerning a pregnancy test.

NOTE: Report sudden, severe abdominal pain, with or without nausea and vomiting, to your physician immediately. There is a higher incidence of ectopic pregnancy with the mini-pill, since ovulation is not inhibited in all women.

Side effects to be reported as soon as possible: severe headaches, dizziness, blurred vision, leg pain, shortness of breath, chest pain, and acute abdominal pain. Although these side effects are usually of minor consequence, absence of serious adverse effects must be confirmed.

Duration of oral contraceptive therapy: many physicians prefer to have their patients discontinue the pill for 3 out of every 18 months. This allows the body to return to a normal cycle. Be sure to use other forms of contraception during this time. Long-term use (3 or more years) must be determined on an individual basis.

Discontinuing the pill for conception: because of a possibility of birth defects, discontinue the pill 3 months before attempting pregnancy. Use other methods of contraception for these 3 months.

NOTE: When being seen by a physician or dentist for other reasons, be sure to mention that you are currently taking oral contraceptives.

Nurse and patient considerations

Before initiating therapy the patient should have a complete physical examination that includes blood pressure, pelvic and breast examination, Papanicolaou smear, urinalysis, and hemoglobin or hematocrit.

Patients planning elective surgery should discontinue oral contraceptive therapy 2 weeks before surgery. Studies indicate that there is an increased incidence of postsurgical thrombosis in patients taking oral contraceptives.

There is some evidence suggesting that the hormones used as oral contraceptives may carry tetratogenic risks. Therefore if pregnancy is suspected, a pregnancy test should be completed and contraceptive therapy should be discontinued as soon as possible. It is also recommended that patients stop taking the pill 3 months before pregnancy is planned.

Combination-type BCP tend to reduce the volume of breast milk produced and shorten the duration of lactation. For mothers wishing to breast-feed, low-dose estrogen combination pills or progestin-only mini-pills should be used.

No adverse effects secondary to hormone therapy have been noted in infants of nursing mothers using BCP. However, many clinicians recommend that mothers use other forms of contraception so that infants are not exposed to potentially harmful side effects from ingestion of hormones.

Laboratory tests altered by oral contraceptive therapy

The acute onset of pancreatitis with elevated serum amylase levels has been reported in several patients following the initiation of oral contraceptive therapy.

Oral contraceptive therapy tends to lower serum cholesterol levels in those patients with baseline cholesterol levels greater than 200 mg/100 ml. Elevations in serum cholesterol levels have been reported in those patients with baseline levels of about 160 mg/100 ml.

Abnormal glucose tolerance tests have been reported many times. However, the significance must be determined on an individual patient basis. The mechanism is not known, and variables appear to depend on estrogen content, duration of therapy, and patients.

Estrogens, including oral contraceptives, increase circulating proteins (TBG), thus increasing circulating thyroxine levels, PBI, T_4 by column, and T_4 by Murphy-Pattee are increased and T_3 uptake is decreased, but ^{131}I thyroidal uptake is not affected. The alterations in laboratory tests may last for 2 to 4 weeks after discontinuation of therapy.

Oral contraceptives decrease the urinary excretion of 17-hydroxycorticosteroids, 17-ketosteroids, and 17-ketogenic steroids.

Values in the following laboratory tests may be *increased* by estrogens and progestins contained in oral contraceptives. The changes may vary in magnitude, depending on the preparation.

Laboratory test
Blood serum, blood plasma

Aldosterone	Platelets
Ceruloplasmin	Prolactin
Coagulation factors (II, VII, IX, X)	Renin activity
Cortisol	Transaminases
Fibrinogen	Transferrin
Gamma-glutamyl transpeptidase	Triglycerides
Iron-binding capacity	Vitamin A
Plasminogen	

Urine

Delta-aminolevulinic acid	Porphyrins

Values in the following laboratory tests may be *decreased* by estrogens and progestins contained in oral contraceptives. The changes may vary in magnitude, depending on the preparation.

Laboratory test
Blood serum, blood plasma

Albumin	Folate	Magnesium
Cholinesterase	Haptoglobin	Vitamin B_{12}
		Zinc

Urine

Ascorbic acid	Calcium

Drug interactions

Oral contraceptives may increase the activity of clotting factors in the blood. Those patients requiring oral anticoagulation may need increased dosages of warfarin (Coumadin) to maintain anticoagulation.

Although it rarely occurs, patients with seizure disorders may have increased seizure activity while receiving oral contraceptives.

Although the mechanism of action is unknown, estrogens may inhibit phenytoin (Dilantin) metabolism, resulting in phenytoin toxicity.

Phenobarbital appears to increase the rate of metabolism of estrogens. Patients receiving low estrogen-content birth control pills may not have adequate contraceptive coverage if they are also taking barbiturates on a regular basis.

Estrogens, by unknown mechanisms, appear to diminish the metabolism of hydrocortisone. Patients receiving both estrogens and hydrocortisone should be observed for evidence of excessive hydrocortisone effects.

Patients who have no thyroid function and who start on BCP may require an increase in their thyroid hormone replacement dosage. Estrogens tend to increase serum thyroxine-binding globulin (TBG), leaving less unbound, active thyroxine in circulation. Do not alter thyroid therapy unless the patient shows clinical signs of hypothyroidism.

The contraceptive efficacy of oral contraceptives when taken with ampicillin, isoniazid, or rifampin may be impaired. Alternative contraceptive methods should be considered.

Oral contraceptives appear to have a variable effect on the metabolism of the benzodiazepines. Those that have reduced metabolism with an increase in therapeutic response are alprazolam (Xanax), chlorazepate (Tranxene), chlordiazepoxide (Librium), diazepam (Valium), flurazepam (Dalmane), halazepam (Paxipam), and prazepam (Centrax). Benzodiazepines that have enhanced metabolism and reduced therapeutic activity when taken with oral contraceptives are lorazepam (Ativan), oxazepam (Serax), and temazepam (Restoril).

The contraceptive efficacy of oral contraceptives when taken with phenytoin (Dilantin), primidone (Mysoline), or carbamazepine (Tegretol) may be impaired. Breakthrough bleeding may be an indication of this interaction. Adjustment in dosage of oral contraceptives and use of alternate methods of contraception should be considered.

CHAPTER NINETEEN

Agents used in obstetrics

Chlorotrianisene
Clomiphene citrate
Deladumone OB (testosterone
    enanthate and estradiol
    valerate)
Dinoprostone
    (prostaglandin E_2)

Ergonovine maleate,
    methylergonovine
    maleate
Hydroxyprogesterone
    caproate
Oxytocin
Ritodrine hydrochloride

Chlorotrianisene
(Tace)

AHFS 68:16
CATEGORY Estrogen

Action and use

Chlorotrianisene is a long-acting, synthetic estrogen used in obstetrics to inhibit lactation and reduce the frequency of postpartum breast engorgement in patients who do not wish to breast-feed. It acts by inhibiting the action of prolactin, a pituitary hormone that is necessary for milk production.

Administration dosage

NOTE: Do not administer during pregnancy. Chlorotrianisene has not been shown to be effective for any purpose during pregnancy, and its use may have potential teratogenic risks to the fetus. There is also a higher incidence of carcinoma in females later in life when exposed to estrogens in utero.

PO—72 mg every 12 hr for 4 doses. The first dose should be given as soon as possible after delivery but within 8 hr.

Nurse and patient considerations

∗ Side effects associated with short-term estrogen therapy are usually quite minimal. The most common side effect is nausea. There is a slightly increased incidence of blood clot formation and thrombophlebitis. Patients should be encouraged to

> report any symptoms of pain in the calves or chest,
> sudden shortness of breath, coughing of blood,
> severe headache, dizziness, faintness, or changes in
> vision as soon as possible.

Drug interactions

The following drugs elevate serum prolactin levels and thereby may antagonize the prolactin-inhibiting effects of chlorotrianisene: carbidopa (Sinemet), ethanol, haloperidol (Haldol), methyldopa (Aldomet), metoclopramide (Reglan), phenothiazines (Thorazine, Mellaril, others), reserpine (Sandril, others), and thiothixene (Navane).

Clomiphene citrate
(Clomid)

AHFS 92:00
CATEGORY Antiestrogen

Action and use

Clomiphene is a nonsteroidal compound that has antiestrogenic properties with no discernable progestational or androgenic activity. Clomiphene is structurally similar to estrogens, and binds to estrogen-receptor sites, reducing the number of sites available for circulating estrogens. The receptors send back false signals to the hypothalamus and pituitary gland, indicating a lack of circulating estrogens. The hypothalamus and pituitary gland respond by increasing the secretion of luteinizing hormone, follicle-stimulating hormone, and gonadotropins. The increased levels of gonadotropins cause ovarian stimulation, ovulation, and sustained function of the corpora lutea. Thus clomiphene is used to induce ovulation in women that are anovulatory secondary to reduced circulatory gonadotropin levels.

Characteristics

Clomiphene is well absorbed orally and excreted primarily in the feces. Fifty-one percent is recovered in 5 days, but the remaining drug and its metabolites are excreted over the next several weeks.

Administration and dosage

NOTE: It is mandatory that patients have had a complete physical examination to rule out other pathologic causes for anovulation before the initiation of clomiphene therapy.

PO 1. Initial dosage regimen: 50 mg/day for 5 days. Start therapy at any time if there has been no recent bleeding. If spontaneous bleeding occurs before therapy, start on or about the fifth day for 5 days. If ovulation occurs at this dosage, there is no advantage to increasing the dose in subsequent cycles of treatment.

2. If ovulation did not occur after the first course, give a second course of 100 mg/day for 5 days. Start this course no earlier than 30 days after the previous course.

3. A third course may be administered at 100 mg/day for 5 days, but most patients who respond will have done so in the first 2 courses. Reevaluation of the patient is necessary.

NOTE: Patient counseling: Patients must be informed of the possibility of multiple pregnancy (8% to 10%) and the importance of timing intercourse at the time of ovulation, usually 6 to 10 days after the last day of treatment.

Clomiphene should not be administered if pregnancy is suspected. Basal temperatures should be followed for the month following therapy. If the body temperature follows a biphasic distribution and is not followed by menses, the next course of clomiphene therapy should not be scheduled until pregnancy has been ruled out.

Patients should also be informed to report significant abdominal or pelvic pain and bloating that develops during therapy.

Patients developing visual blurring, spots, or flashes should use caution in performing activities requiring alert vision and should report for an ophthalmologic examination. Visual disturbances usually resolve within a few days of discontinuation of therapy.

Nurse and patient considerations

* Side effects of clomiphene therapy tend to be quite mild and are generally dose related. Common side effects include flushing resembling menopausal hot flashes and abdominal symptoms resembling Mittelschmerz and premenstrual symptoms. Nausea, vomiting, diarrhea, and constipation have been reported less often.
* Clomiphene may increase levels of serum thyroxine and thyroxine-binding globulin (TBG).

✳ Birth defects have been reported in laboratory animals, although there is no causative evidence of such effects on human fetuses. To avoid administration in early pregnancy, daily basal temperatures should be determined. If a biphasic pattern is observed and the next menses does not start, withhold clomiphene therapy until the possibility of pregnancy or the formation of an ovarian cyst has been eliminated.

Drug interactions

No specific drug interactions have been reported.

Testosterone enanthate and estradiol valerate
(Deladumone OB)

AHFS 68:16
CATEGORY Estrogen-androgen combination

Action and use

Deladumone OB is a long-acting combination estrogen-androgen product used in obstetrics to inhibit lactation and postpartum breast engorgement in patients who do not wish to breast-feed. Both estrogens and androgens may inhibit the secretion of prolactin, a pituitary hormone that stimulates milk synthesis.

Administration and dosage

NOTE: Do not administer during pregnancy. Deladumone OB has not been shown to be effective for any purpose during pregnancy, and its use may have potential teratogenic effects on the fetus. There is also a higher incidence of carcinoma in females later in life when exposed to estrogens in utero.

IM—2 ml of Deladumone OB (360 mg of testosterone enanthate and 16 mg of estradiol valerate). Administer just before the second stage of labor (complete cervical dilatation and effacement) by deep injection into the upper, outer quadrant of the gluteal muscle.

Nurse and patient considerations

* There are essentially no side effects associated with a single injection of Deladumone OB other than pain at the site of injection. There is a slightly increased incidence of blood clot formation and thrombophlebitis. Patients should be encouraged to report any symptoms of pain in the calves or chest, sudden shortness of breath, coughing of blood, severe headache, dizziness, faintness, or changes in vision as soon as possible.

Drug interactions

The following drugs elevate serum prolactin levels and thereby may antagonize the prolactin-inhibiting effects of Deladumone OB: carbidopa (Sinemet), ethanol, haloperidol (Haldol), methyldopa (Aldomet), metoclopramide (Reglan), phenothiazines (Thorazine, Mellaril, others), reserpine (Sandril, others), and thiothixene (Navane).

Dinoprostone (prostaglandin E$_2$)
(Prostin E$_2$)

AHFS 76:00
CATEGORY Oxytocic

Action and use

Dinoprostone, or prostaglandin E$_2$ (PGE$_2$), is a uterine and gastrointestinal circular smooth muscle stimulant. The exact mechanism of action is not known. When used during pregnancy, it increases the amplitude and frequency of uterine contractions and produces cervical softening and dilatation.

Dinoprostone is used to evacuate uterine contents in cases of intrauterine fetal death, benign hydatidiform mole, missed spontaneous miscarriage, and second trimester abortion. An advantage to the use of dinoprostone before full term is its uterine activity. Although uterine response to dinoprostone and oxytocin increases with the duration of pregnancy, the uterus is considerably more sensitive to dinoprostone than to oxytocin. Occasionally, oxytocin and dinoprostone are used concurrently to shorten the duration of uterine evacuation.

Characteristics

Onset of mild uterine contractions: 10 to 15 min. Duration: 2 to 3 hr. Metabolism: extensive, by lungs, kidneys, spleen, and other tissues to at least 9 inactive metabolites. Excretion: active drug and metabolites primarily in urine; small amounts in feces.

Administration and dosage

NOTE: Dinoprostone vaginal suppositories are stored in the freezer. Before removing the foil wrap, allow to warm to room temperature. Suppositories warmed to room temperature but unopened may be refrozen once for later use.

INTRAVAGINAL

1. Insert 1 suppository high into the posterior vaginal fornix. Patients should remain supine for at least 10 min after each insertion. Suppositories should be inserted every 2 to 5 hr, depending on uterine activity and tolerance to side effects.
2. Concurrent IV infusion of oxytocin may begin after at least 1 hr of dinoprostone therapy and should be adjusted to the response of the patient.
3. If complete uterine evacuation has not occurred within 24 to 36 hr, additional oxytocin, intraamniotic dinoprost tromethamine, or dilatation and evacuation should be considered.

Nurse and patient considerations

* Gastrointestinal side effects manifested by nausea, vomiting, and diarrhea are most frequently observed. Premedication with an antiemetic (prochlorperazine [Compazine]) and antidiarrheal (loperamide [Immodium] or diphenoxylate with atropine [Lomotil]) will reduce but usually not completely eliminate these adverse effects.
* Temperature elevations above 38° C (100.6° F) occur within 15 to 45 min and continue for up to 6 hr in 50% to 70% of patients. Sponge bathing with water or alcohol and maintaining fluid intake may provide symptomatic relief. Aspirin does not inhibit dinoprostone-induced pyrexia. Patients should be observed for clinical indications of intrauterine infection.

* Headache, chills, and shivering occur in about 10% of the patients receiving dinoprostone. Transient hypotension with drops in diastolic pressure of 20 mm Hg, dizziness, flushing, syncope, cardiac arrhythmias, bronchospasm, wheezing, dyspnea, chest pain, and coughing have all been reported.
* Fragments of uterine contents are frequently left in the uterus after evacuation. Patients should be manually examined to prevent the development of fever, infection, and hemorrhage.

Drug interactions

No specific drug interactions have been reported.

Ergonovine maleate, methylergonovine maleate

AHFS 76:00
CATEGORY Oxytocic

(Ergotrate, Methergine)

Action and use

Ergonovine and methylergonovine are structurally similar ergot alkaloid derivatives that share similar mechanisms of action and activities. Both drugs directly stimulate contractions of uterine and vascular smooth muscle by interacting with tryptaminergic, dopaminergic, and alpha-adrenergic receptors. Small doses produce uterine contractions with increased force and frequency with normal resting muscle tone; intermediate doses cause more forceful and prolonged contractions with an elevated resting muscle tone; and large doses cause sustained contractions and tetany. This sudden, intense uterine activity precludes these agents from being used for induction or augmentation of delivery. However, since these agents produce more sustained contractions and higher uterine tonus than does oxytocin, small doses of ergonovine and methylergonovine are used post partum to control bleeding and maintain uterine firmness. Methylergonovine is generally preferred because it tends to cause less hypertension than ergonovine.

Characteristics (similar for both agents)

Onset: immediate (IV); 2 to 5 min (IM); 5 to 15 min (PO). Duration: 3 hr or longer (PO, IM); 45 min (IV). Metabolism: liver.

Administration and dosage (same for both agents)

NOTE: Use with extreme caution in patients with hypertension, toxemia, heart disease, venoatrial shunts, mitral valve stenosis, obliterative vascular disease, sepsis, or hepatic or renal impairment.

PO—0.2 mg every 6 to 8 hr after delivery for a maximum of 1 week. Monitor the character and amount of vaginal discharge.

IM—0.2 mg every 2 to 4 hr, to a maximum of 5 doses. Monitor the character and amount of vaginal discharge.

IV   1. Use only for excessive uterine bleeding and emergency situations. Sudden hypertensive and cerebrovascular accidents have occurred, especially after rapid administration. If used, dilute the 1 ml dosage to 5 ml and inject over at least 60 sec. Monitor blood pressure, pulse, and uterine activity closely.

   2. Dosage: 0.2 mg (1 ml).

Nurse and patient considerations

* The most common side effects are nausea and vomiting, and these are fairly infrequent. Other side effects reported include dizziness, dyspnea, tinnitus, headache, palpitations, and chest pain. Patients may also complain of abdominal cramping. This is normally an indication of therapeutic activity, but, if severe, reduction in dosage may be necessary.
* Certain patients, especially those who are eclamptic or previously hypertensive, may be particularly sensitive to the hypertensive effects of these agents. These patients have a higher incidence of developing generalized headaches, severe arrhythmias, and cerebrovascular accidents.
* Ergonovine, but not methylergonovine, may inhibit prolactin secretion. This may inhibit the mother's ability to breast-feed her infant.

Drug interactions

Hypertension and headache may develop in patients who had received caudal or spinal anesthesia, followed by a dose of either methylergonovine or ergonovine.

Hydroxyprogesterone caproate
(Delalutin)

AHFS 68:32
CATEGORY Progestin

Action and use

Hydroxyprogesterone is a hormone that inhibits the secretion of pituitary gonadotropins, luteinizing hormone (LH), and follicle-stimulating hormone (FSH); transforms the proliferative endometrium into a secretory endometrium; and induces mammary duct development. It also inhibits spontaneous uterine contractions in the pregnant uterus and is therefore used in obstetrics as a possible prophylactic tocolytic agent to prevent habitual miscarriage. It is not effective once premature labor has started, but it may possibly be effective if administered periodically after the twentieth week of pregnancy.

Administration and dosage

NOTE: Do not administer during the first 4 months of pregnancy. Teratogenicity may result.

Adult

IM—250 mg once weekly injected deeply into the upper outer quadrant of the gluteal muscle.

Nurse and patient considerations

* The frequency of adverse effects with hydroxyprogesterone therapy is quite small. The most frequent adverse effect is pain at the site of injection.
* Hydroxyprogesterone may induce fluid retention. Patients with medical conditions such as asthma, migraine, epilepsy, or cardiac or renal dysfunction should be monitored closely.
* There is a slightly increased incidence of blood clot formation and thrombophlebitis. Patients should be encouraged to report any symptoms of pain in the calves or chest, sudden shortness of breath, coughing of blood, severe headache, dizziness, faintness, or changes in vision as soon as possible.

Drug interactions

No specific drug interactions have been reported.

Oxytocin
(Pitocin, Syntocinon)

AHFS 76:00
CATEGORY Oxytocic

Action and use

Oxytocin is a hormone produced in the hypothalamus and stored in the posterior pituitary gland (neurohypophysis). It has selective stimulatory effects on the smooth muscle of the uterus, blood vessels, and mammary myoepithelium. Oxytocin apparently induces and augments muscular contractility by increasing the permeability of muscle cell membranes to sodium ions, increasing the number of contracting myofibrils. The dosage required to initiate muscular contractions is dependent on the excitability of the muscle tissue. A very low level of muscular activity is present in the human uterus during the first and second trimesters of pregnancy, and the uterus is fairly resistant to the effects of oxytocin. As the third trimester progresses, however, uterine excitability increases significantly, and active labor may be initiated with relatively small doses of exogenous oxytocin.

Oxytocin is the current drug of choice for inducing labor at term and for augmenting uterine contractions during the first and second stages of labor. Oxytocin is routinely administered immediately postpartum to control uterine atony and postpartum hemorrhage. Oxytocin may also be applied intranasally to promote milk ejection and treat breast engorgement during lactation.

Characteristics

Onset of uterine activity: 3 to 7 min (IM), immediate (IV). Duration of uterine activity: 2 to 3 hr (IM), 45 to 60 min (IV). Plasma half-life: 3 to 5 min. Metabolism: lactating mammary gland, liver, kidneys, placenta, uterus. Excretion: small amounts excreted unchanged in urine.

Administration and dosage

For induction of labor:

IV INFUSION—Initial rate: 1 to 2 mU/min. It is strongly recommended that an infusion pump be used to help control the rate of oxytocin infusion. Most pregnancies close to term will respond well to 2 to 10 mU/min. Rarely will a patient require more than 20 mU/min. Those patients at 32 to 36 weeks of gestation often require 20 to 30 mU/min or more to develop a laborlike contractility pattern. Rates of infusion should not be altered more frequently than every 20 to 30 min. It is frequently necessary to reduce or discontinue the infusion as spontaneous uterine activity develops and labor progresses.

For augmentation of labor:

IV INFUSION—Occasionally a labor that started spontaneously may not progress satisfactorily. Labor may be augmented by oxytocin infusions at rates of 0.5 to 2 mU/min.

For milk ejection:

INTRANASAL OXYTOCIN (40 units/ml)—1 spray or 3 drops may be instilled into 1 or both nostrils 2 to 3 min before nursing or pumping of the breasts. The patient should sit upright if using nasal spray and recline if using nasal drops.

Nurse and patient considerations

* Most clinicians now recommend that fetal monitors be used during infusions of oxytocin. Overdosage of oxytocin may cause hyperstimulation of the uterus, resulting in tetanic contractions with possible abruptio placentae, cervical lacerations, impaired uterine blood flow, and fetal trauma and hypoxia manifested by fetal bradycardia, tachycardia, and arrhythmias.
* Oxytocin has some minor antidiuretic activity. When administered in large dosages or over prolonged periods with electrolyte-free solutions, water intoxication manifested by drowsiness, listlessness, headache, confusion, anuria, edema, and seizure activity may develop.
* Side effects that may occur include nausea, vomiting, hypotension, tachycardia, and cardiac arrhythmias.

Drug interactions

Anesthetics used during labor and delivery may modify the cardiovascular effects (blood pressure, heart rate) of oxytocin.

Ritodrine hydrochloride
(Yutopar)

AHFS 12:12
CATEGORY Beta$_2$-adrenergic
stimulant

Action and use

Ritodrine is a beta-receptor stimulant, acting predominantly on the beta$_2$ receptors but, especially in higher dosages, the beta$_1$ receptors as well. Stimulation of the beta$_2$ receptors produces relaxation of the uterine, bronchial, and vascular smooth muscle. Beta$_1$-receptor stimulation causes an increased heart rate.

Because of its selective relaxant properties on the uterus, causing a reduction in the intensity and frequency of uterine contractions, ritodrine is approved for use as a tocolytic agent. It is used in cases of premature labor where it has been determined that there is no underlying pathology that would dictate that pregnancy be terminated.

Characteristics

(Nonpregnant females) Bioavailability: 30% (PO). Onset: 30 to 60 min (PO). Protein binding: 30% to 32%. Half-life: first phase—6 to 9 min; second phase—1.7 to 2.6 hr; third phase—10 to 12 hr. Metabolism: hepatic, to sulfates and glucuronides. Excretion: 70% to 90% as active drug and inactive metabolites in urine within 10 to 12 hr. Dialysis: yes, H. Breast milk: unknown.

Administration and dosage

NOTE: Ritodrine should be used with extreme caution, with very close clinical observation of both the mother and fetus, in cases of hypertension, mild to moderate preeclampsia, premature rupture of the membranes, and diabetes mellitus. Ritodrine should not be used in cases where continuation of pregnancy is hazardous to the mother or fetus, such as antepartum hemorrhage, severe preeclampsia or eclampsia, intrauterine fetal death, chorioamnionitis, abruptio placentae, placenta previa, and with fetal anomalies incompatible with life.

Adult

Guidelines for use in premature labor:
1. Initiate a control IV of dextrose 5%, Ringer's lactate, or saline solution and administer 400 to 500 ml in 15 to 20 min before the initiation of the medication. Then decrease to 100 to 125 ml/hr.

Table 19-1. Ritodrine administration*

5 ml amps/500 ml†		1	2	3	4	5
mg/500 ml		50	100	150	200	250
µg/ml		100	200	300	400	500
µgtts/min	ml/min	µg/min	µg/min	µg/min	µg/min	µg/min
5	0.08	8	16	24	32	40
10	0.16	16	32	48	64	80
15	0.25	25	50	75	100	125
20	0.33	33	66	99	132	165
25	0.41	41	82	123	164	205
30	0.5	50	100	150	200	250
35	0.58	58	116	174	232	290
40	0.66	66	132	198	264	330
45	0.75	75	150	225	300	375
50	0.83	83	166	249	332	415
55	0.91	91	182	273	364	455
60	1.00	100	200	300	400	500

*Using a microdrip administration set—60 gtts/ml.

†Dilute in 500 ml of 0.9% sodium chloride, dextrose 5%, 10% dextran 40 in 0.9% sodium chloride, 10% fructose, Ringer's solution, or Hartmann's solution.

Usual initial dose is 50 to 100 µg/min. Increase by 50 µg/min every 10 min until desired result is attained. The effective dose usually lies between 150 and 350 µg/min. Frequent monitoring of maternal uterine contractions, heart rate, and blood pressure and of fetal heart rate is mandatory, with dosage individually titrated according to response.

2. Make a ritodrine infusion solution using Table 19-1. The usual concentration is 3 ampules in 500 ml of parenteral solution, but weaker or stronger concentrations may be used depending on the patient's fluid requirements.
3. Have the patient recline in a left lateral position.
4. The usual initial dosage is 50 to 100 μg/minute. Increase by 50 μg/min every 10 min until labor is inhibited or side effects preclude further increases in dosage. The effective dose is usually 150 to 350 μg/min. Frequent monitoring of maternal uterine contractions, heart rate, and blood pressure and fetal heart rate is mandatory, with dosage individually titrated according to response.
5. Fluid input and output, breath sounds, and blood glucose and serum electrolyte levels must be monitored periodically to prevent fluid overload, hyperglycemia, or hypokalemia.
6. The IV infusion is maintained for 8 to 12 hr after cessation of uterine contractions.
7. Start oral ritodrine tablets 30 to 60 min before discontinuation of IV therapy. The initial doses are 10 mg every 2 hr for the first 24 hr, then 10 to 20 mg every 4 to 6 hr, depending on uterine activity and side effects.
8. Recurrence of premature labor may be treated by starting the guidelines over again. Labor may be arrested on lower IV dosages, depending on the compliance of the oral medication regimen by the patient.

Nurse and patient considerations

* Side effects are frequent with ritodrine, particularly with IV administration. Most adverse effects relate to sympathomimetic activity and are dose related. Maternal and fetal tachycardia is common, averaging 130 and 164 beats/min, respectively. Maternal systolic blood pressure increases an average of 12 mm Hg to 96 to 162 mm Hg (average 128 mm Hg), while diastolic pressures drop an average of 23 mm Hg to an average of 48 mm Hg (range 0 to 76 mm Hg).

* Ritodrine routinely increases serum glucose and insulin levels, though they tend to return to normal within 48 to 72 hr with continued infusion. Diabetic patients should be monitored closely. Insulin requirements may double in these patients during ritodrine infusion.

* Serum potassium levels may drop during ritodrine therapy. Urinary losses generally do not increase; much of the losses are actually due to intracellular redistribution, which will return to the vascular compartment after discontinuation of therapy. Usually, only maintenance potassium needs to be administered, but if potassium-depleting diuretics are used, the potassium serum levels are low, or the ritodrine infusion time is particularly long, supplemental potassium may be necessary.

* Palpitations are reported in about one third of patients receiving IV ritodrine. Ten to fifteen percent complain of tremor, nausea, vomiting, headache, or erythema. Nervousness, jitteriness, restlessness, and emotional instability are noted in 5% to 6% of patients. Adverse cardiac effects of arrhythmias and/or chest pain are observed in 1% to 2% of patients.

* Adverse effects reported with oral ritodrine therapy include palpitations, tremor, nausea, jitteriness, and infrequent arrhythmias.

* Neonatal adverse effects are infrequent, but hyperglycemia, hypoglycemia, hypocalcemia, hypotension, and paralytic ileus have been reported.

Drug interactions

Beta-adrenergic blocking agents (propranolol, metoprolol, timolol, nadolol, others) will inhibit the pharmacologic effects of ritodrine.

Administration of ritodrine in conjunction with other sympathomimetic agents may enhance cardiovascular side effects. Use ritodrine with caution.

Concurrent administration of corticosteroids (betamethasone, dexamethasone, others) with IV ritodrine may result in pulmonary edema. This adverse interaction is infrequently reported, but there is a higher incidence in patients with multiple pregnancy, occult cardiac disease, and fluid overload. Persistent tachycardia may be a sign of impending pulmonary edema. Observe patients closely, monitoring fluid input and output, breath sounds, and heart rate, as well as the patient's anxiety level and state of well-being.

Concomitant administration of ritodrine with general anesthetics may result in additive hypotensive effects.

CHAPTER TWENTY

Local anesthetics

*General information on local
anesthetics*

GENERAL INFORMATION ON LOCAL ANESTHETICS

Local anesthetics are synthetic compounds that when applied in appropriate concentrations, block nerve conduction in the area of application. Two major advantages of local anesthetics are that (1) all types of nervous tissue are affected, and (2) their action is reversible; their use is followed by complete recovery in nerve function with no residual damage to nerve fibers or cells.

Local anesthetics apparently prevent depolarization (and therefore prevent propagation of nerve impulses) by displacing calcium ions from binding sites on the nerve cell membrane. Loss of bound calcium inhibits permeability of the cell membrane to sodium ions. The influx of sodium ions is necessary for depolarization of the nerve membrane and propagation of the action potential or nerve impulse.

The primary uses of parenteral local anesthetics include:

Spinal anesthesia: injection into the spinal theca or subarachnoid space, blocking nerve impulses in the sensory roots (pain, temperature, touch), sympathetic and parasympathetic fibers, and motor nerves.

Epidural anesthesia: injection of anesthetic into the epidural space (between the dura mater and the vertebral canal). Although somewhat similar to spinal anesthesia, an epidural block differs from a subarachnoid block in time of onset, duration, dose and extent of anesthesia.

Regional nerve blocks: injection into the vicinity of a specific nerve such as the pudendal nerve for obstetric procedures or a nerve plexus such as the brachial plexus for anesthesia of the arm, hand, and fingers.

Infiltration anesthesia: intradermal or subcutaneous injection of anesthetic to anesthetize nerve endings in a localized area.

Characteristics of local anesthetics

Local anesthetics for parenteral administration are the water-soluble salts (usually hydrochloride) of lipid-soluble substances. Each drug has its own specific pharmacologic properties that determine the duration of action, potency, and toxicity of the agent. Duration of anesthesia depends on the time that the drug is in contact with nerve tissue, the pH of the solution, and the electrolyte status of the tissue. After injection it is that fraction of the drug that is present as the lipid-soluble free base at the pH of the extracellular fluid that is active. A lowering of the pH by inflammation greatly decreases the amount of active free base present. Conversely, alkalinization enhances drug penetration and onset of activity. Many local anesthetics inherently cause vasodilatation, which will shorten the contact time and duration of action of local anesthetics. Local anesthetics are frequently administered in combination with vasoconstrictors, such as epinephrine, to prolong the duration of action.

Other factors that influence anesthetic activity include the diameter of the nerve fiber and the extent of myelination of the nerve. Larger nerves require greater amounts of anesthetic because of a larger surface area with more pores to be blocked. Local anesthetics also work only on unmyelinated neurons; nodes are more distant and require a larger volume and concentration of anesthetic to block an adequate number of nodes to render the neurons inexcitable.

From a structural standpoint there are two classes of local anesthetics: the ester type and amide type (Table 20-1). The ester-type anesthetics are metabolize primarily in the plasma by pseudocholinesterases and esterases in the liver. Patients susceptible to prolonged duration of action are those with atypical pseudocholinesterases or hepatic dysfunction. Microsomal enzymes within the liver metabolize local anesthetics of the amide type. Both the ester and the amide types are excreted primarily as metabolites in the urine.

Administration and dosage

The dosage of local anesthetics varies with the anesthetic procedure, the degree of anesthesia required, and the individual patient response. The smallest dosage and lowest concentration required to produce the desired effect should be used. See Table 20-1 for the concentrations generally used and the maximum dosages that should be administered. Resuscitative equipment should be immediately available to treat adverse reactions should they occur.

Local anesthetic solutions containing preservatives should not be used for spinal or epidural anesthesia. Partially used bottles of anesthetic that do not contain preservatives should be discarded immediately after use.

Table 20-1. Comparison of local anesthetics

Drug	Anesthesia	Percent concentration	Onset (min)	Duration (hr)	Maximum dose (mg)	Comments
ESTER TYPE						
Chloroprocaine hydrochloride (Nesacaine)	Infiltration; peripheral or sympathetic nerve block; epidural	1-2 1-2 2-3	6-12	½-1	800	Do not autoclave; do not use as spinal anesthetic
Procaine hydrochloride (Novocain)	Infiltration; peripheral or sympathetic nerve block; epidural; spinal	0.5 1.2 2	2-5	1	1000	Produces vasodilatation Do not exceed 14 mg/kg/dose
Tetracaine hydrochloride (Pontocaine)	Topical; epidural; spinal	10 0.5-2 0.15 0.2-0.3	15	1½-3	75	Slowest rate of metabolism of ester-type anesthetics
AMIDE TYPE						
Bupivacaine hydrochloride (Marcaine)	Infiltration; peripheral or sympathetic nerve block; epidural	0.25 0.25 0.5 0.50-0.75	4-17 6-9	3-17	400	Do not repeat doses more often than every 3 hr; accumulation occurs with multiple doses Has lowest degree of placental tranfer of local anesthetic

Agent	Use	Concentration (%)	Onset (min)	Duration (hr)	Maximum dose (mg)	Comments
Dibucaine hydrochloride (Nupercaine)	Spinal	0.5	10-15	6	10	Produces vasodilation
Etidocaine hydrochloride (Duranest)	Infiltration; peripheral or sympathetic nerve block; epidural	0.5; 0.5-1	2-8	4-13	400	Very rapid onset of action. Maximum single dose: 400 mg. May repeat in 2-3 hr. Also used as an antiarrhythmic agent
Lidocaine hydrochloride (Xylocaine)	Topical; infiltration; peripheral or sympathetic nerve block; epidural; spinal	2-4; 1; 1-2; 5	1	$1\frac{1}{2}$; $1\frac{1}{2}$-2	300	
Mepivacaine hydrochloride (Carbocaine)	Infiltration; peripheral or sympathetic nerve block; epidural; caudal	1-2; 1-2; 1-2; 1-2	7-15	2-$2\frac{2}{10}$; $1\frac{3}{5}$-$2\frac{9}{10}$	400	Accumulation occurs with multiple doses. No vasodilatory effect on injection
Prilocaine hydrochloride (Citanest)	Infiltration; peripheral or sympathetic nerve block; epidural	1-2; 2-3	?	2-$2\frac{3}{5}$	600	May produce methemoglobinemia, resulting in hypoxia. Do not use in patients with anemia or methemoglobinemia. Maximum single dose: 600 mg. May repeat in 2 hr

Nurse and patient considerations

It is essential that when local anesthetics are to be injected, the plunger of the syringe is pulled back first to determine blood return. Do not inject local anesthetics if there is blood return.

Local anesthetics eventually pass into the vascular system and are distributed to all tissues within the body. Adverse effects to other organ systems include:

1. Central nervous system: early signs of toxicity are stimulant in nature. Anxiety, apprehension, nervousness, confusion, disorientation, and seizure activity may be followed by CNS depression manifested by drowsiness, sedation, unconsciousness, and respiratory arrest.

2. Cardiovascular system: cardiovascular effects are usually seen only after high systemic concentrations have been achieved. After absorption, local anesthetics may cause direct myocardial depression, arterial vasodilatation, and autonomic nerve blockade that may result in bradycardia, cardiac arrhythmias, hypotension, and cardiac arrest. When anesthetics are administered by epidural or subarachnoid routes, cardiovascular and respiratory effects may be secondary to the effects of these agents on the vasomotor center in the medulla.

3. Rare allergic or hypersensitivity reactions manifested by skin rashes, edema, and status asthmaticus may occur. Most allergic reactions are associated with the ester-type anesthetics (Table 20-1). Reactions to the amide type are very infrequent, and cross-sensitivity between the two types of anesthetics is quite rare.

Patients with hepatic disease, myasthenia gravis, cardiac or respiratory disease, hyperthyroidism, and other neuromuscular disorders are more susceptible to the toxic effects of local anesthetics. Particular attention to the selection of the agent and the route and dosage used is required.

Possible localized and systemic adverse effects of vasoconstrictors (such as epinephrine) must always be considered when they are used in conjunction with local anesthetics. Vasoconstrictors must not be used when local anesthesia of the penis, nose, fingers, ears, or toes is required. Mepivacaine and prilocaine produce little or no vasodilatation and usually do not require the use of vasoconstrictors.

Drug interactions

Local anesthetics that are derivatives of para-aminobenzoic acid (PABA) such as benzocaine, procaine, and tetracaine may antagonize the antibacterial activity of sulfonamides (Gantrisin, Gantanol, Bactrim, Septra). Anesthetics that may be substituted instead include lidocaine and dibucaine.

Patients with glaucoma who are treated with echothiopate iodide (Phospholine iodide) may develop lower levels of circulating pseudocholinesterase. These patients are susceptible to prolonged anesthesia from the ester-type anesthetics.

CHAPTER TWENTY-ONE

Skeletal muscle relaxants

GENERAL INFORMATION ON NEUROMUSCULAR BLOCKING AGENTS

Neuromuscular blocking agents, also known as skeletal muscle relaxants, have a long history. South American Indians have used crude extracts (known generically as curare) from plants for centuries as arrow poisons. Use of neuromuscular blocking agents as adjuvants to anesthesia during surgery, however, has evolved only over the last 30 years. Neuromuscular blocking agents are now used extensively as muscle relaxants during surgical procedures to allow milder levels of anesthesia to be employed.

Neuromuscular blocking agents act by interrupting the transmission of impulses from motor nerves to muscles at the skeletal neuromuscular junction. These agents have no CNS activity and do not alter the patient's level of consciousness, memory, or pain threshold.

All neuromuscular blocking agents are quaternary ammonium compounds; however, the apparent mechanisms by which sensitivity to acetylcholine (the neurotransmitter released from the nerve terminal membrane) is reduced subdivide this category of drugs into two classes: (1) the competitve or nondepolarizing agents such as tubocurarine chloride and pancuronium bromide and (2) the depolarizing agents, represented by succinylcholine chloride.

The competitive neuromuscular blocking agents bind to the acetylcholine receptor site on the postjunctional membrane, competitively inhibiting the released acetylcholine from contacting the receptors on the postjunctional membrane, thus preventing depolarization and muscle contraction. The acetylcholine released into the synaptic cleft is rapidly metabolized to acetate and choline by the enzyme acetylcholinesterase. Recent investigations indicate that the competitive blockers also reduce the amount of acetylcholine released from the nerve terminal membrane.

Depolarizing agents also induce paralysis by blocking the acetylcholine receptors of the postjunctional membrane. However, the initial effect is to depolarize the membrane, resulting in a brief period of fine muscular contractions or fasciculations, followed by paralysis.

Selection of a neuromuscular blocking agent is dependent on (1) the pharmacokinetic properties of a particular drug, (2) the mechanism of action of the drug at the neuromuscular junction and at other sites, (3) the length of the surgical procedure, (4) the anesthetic to be used, and (5) conditions of the patient that might alter response to the blocking agent. Anesthesiologists frequently use a combination of premedicants, neuromuscular blocking agents, and anesthesia to produce a "balanced" anesthesia appropriate for the patient and the required surgery.

Nurse and patient considerations

The human body contains at least three different types of neuromuscular junctions. They differ in the size and shape of nerve terminals and postjunctional membranes, the density of neuromuscular junctions per muscle, and the amount of metabolic enzymes present. Therefore a differential response to neuromuscular blocking agents by different muscle groups is to be expected. The muscles of the eyelids are the most easily paralyzed, while the last muscles to become affected are usually the intercostal muscles and the diaphragm. There is considerable overlapping of these effects, however, and even small doses may depress respiration. Patients receiving neuromuscular blocking agents often require assisted ventilation and must be observed closely for evidence of inadequate respiratory effort.

Neuromuscular blocking agents may have significant effects on the autonomic nervous system. See the individual monographs for specific cardiovascular effects of each agent.

All neuromuscular blocking agents cause some release of histamine. The relative potential for histamine release is (1) tubocurarine, (2) succinylcholine, and (3) decamethonium, with gallamine and pancuronium being the least potent. Histamine release may cause bronchospasm, bronchial and salivary secretions, flushing, edema, and urticaria.

Electrolyte imbalance may have a profound effect on the depth and duration of neuromuscular blockade. Competitive blockers may be potentiated by hypokalemia. Hypocalcemia, hyponatremia, and hypermagnesemia may potentiate both competitive and depolarizing agents.

A fall in body temperature enhances the duration and intensity of depolarizing agents, but diminishes the effect of the competitive agents. Higher dosages of tubocurarine or pancuronium may be necessary with hypothermia, but may be excessive when the patient's temperature rises.

Patients with hepatic, pulmonary, or renal impairment or neurologic disorders such as myasthenia gravis, spinal cord injury, or multiple sclerosis must be fully evaluated to assess their ability to tolerate neuromuscular blocking agents. Much smaller dosages are often necessary when these diseases are present. Neonates and elderly patients also require adjustments in dosage because of the insensitivity of their neuromuscular junctions. Their volumes of distribution also differ from those of children and young adults.

Reversal of neuromuscular blockade

The blockade induced by the competitive neuromuscular blocking agents may be antagonized by acetylcholinesterase inhibitors. When enzyme inhibitors are used, acetylcholine accumulates in the synaptic cleft, competing with the blocking agent for receptor sites on the postjunctional membrane. Agents that may be used are neostigmine methylsulfate (Prostigmin), pyridostigmine bromide (Mestinon, Regonal) and edrophonium chloride (Tensilon). Atropine must usually be administered with neostigmine or pyridostigmine to block bradycardia, hypotension, and salivation induced by these agents.

The early blockade induced by succinylcholine is not reversible. Cholinesterase inhibitors may actually prolong it. Fortunately the early succinylcholine blockade is of short duration and thus does not require reversal.

Drug interactions

General anesthetics (ether, fluroxene [Fluoromar], methoxyflurane [Penthrane], enflurane [Ethrane], halothane [Fluothane], and cyclopropane) produce muscle relaxation by both CNS depression and neuromuscular junctional blockade. General anesthetics (except nitrous oxide) may thus add to or potentiate neuromuscular blocking agents.

Competitive and depolarizing neuromuscular blocking agents may be used to either antagonize or potentiate blockade:

1. Subblocking dosages of tubocurarine or pancuronium are occasionally administered to prevent muscle fasciculations induced by succinylcholine.
2. Small dosages of succinylcholine may be adminis-

tered to facilitate neuromuscular transmission during the recovery phase from a competitive blocking agent.
3. A synergistic blocking effect results when a competitive blocker is administered after a depolarizing agent.

Aminoglycoside antibiotics (kanamycin, gentamicin, neomycin, and streptomycin [possibly amikacin and tobramycin, although as yet unreported]) act synergistically with neuromuscular blocking agents to enhance blockade. Cases have been reported to occur up to 48 hr after recovery. IV calcium administration reverses the blockade.

The central respiratory depressant effects of narcotic analgesics may add to the respiratory depressant effects of the neuromuscular blocking agents.

Propranolol (Inderal) has been reported to prolong the activity of neuromuscular blocking agents.

Quinidine and quinine potentiate both competitive and depolarizing muscle relaxants. Patients requiring quinidine after surgery must be observed closely for unresponsiveness and apnea.

Pancuronium bromide
(Pavulon)

AHFS 12:20
CATEGORY Skeletal muscle relaxant

Action and use

Pancuronium bromide is a synthetic, competitive (nondepolarizing) neuromuscular blocking agent. It differs from other competitive blocking agents in that it has little or no histamine-releasing effect, does not block sympathetic ganglia (and therefore does not cause hypotension or bronchospasm), and has vagolytic effects on the heart, resulting in a rise in pulse of about 20%, a 10% to 20% rise in systolic blood pressure, and an increase in cardiac output. Pancuronium bromide may be used to produce skeletal muscle relaxation in surgical procedures, to aid in mechanical ventilation in patients with status asthmaticus, and to control spasms in electroconvulsive therapy.

See also General information on neuromuscular blocking agents (p. 532).

Characteristics

Onset: 3 to 5 min (IV). Duration: dose related; supplemental dosages increase the magnitude and duration of blockade. Protein binding: insignificant. Metabolism: minimal. Excretion: single doses lost by redistribution to non-reactive tissues, multiple doses excreted unchanged primarily by glomerular filtration; when renal impairment is present, larger portions are excreted via the bile.

Administration and dosage

NOTE: There is wide patient variation in response to neuromuscular blocking agents. Dosages must be individualized based on the length of surgery, anesthetics used, and the clinical condition of the patient. The following dosages are to be used as guidelines only.

Adult

IV—Initially, 40 to 100 µg/kg. Additional doses of 10 µg/kg may be administered every 20 to 60 min to maintain skeletal muscle relaxation.

Pediatric
Neonates

IV—Initially, 40 to 100 µg/kg. Additional doses of 20 to 40 µg/kg may be administered as needed.

Children

IV—Initially, 40 to 100 µg/kg. Additional doses of 16 to 20 µg/kg may be administered as needed.

Nurse and patient considerations

* The cardiac effects and excess salivation may be blocked by atropine.
* See General information on neuromuscular blocking agents (p. 532).

Drug interactions

See General information on neuromuscular blocking agents (p. 532).

Succinylcholine chloride
(Anectine, Quelicin, SUX-CERT)

AHFS 12:20
CATEGORY Skeletal muscle relaxant

Action and use

Succinylcholine is a short-acting depolarizing neuromuscular blocking agent. Other pharmacologic actions attributed to the use of succinylcholine include histamine release and bronchospasm; vagal stimulation with resultant bradycardia, hypotension, and cardiac arrhythmias; and increased gastric and salivary secretions. Because of its short duration of action, succinylcholine is particularly useful in providing muscular relaxation for procedures such as endoscopies, endotracheal intubation, manipulations, and electroconvulsive therapy. See also General information on neuromuscular blocking agents (p. 532).

Characteristics

Onset: within 30 sec (IV). Duration: dissipation within 10 min. Protein binding: insignificant. Metabolism: rapidly by plasma pseudocholinesterase. Excretion: up to 10% unchanged in urine, metabolites eventually excreted in urine.

Administration and dosage

NOTE: There is wide patient variation in response to neuromuscular blocking agents. Dosages must be individualized based on the length of surgery, the anesthetics used, and the clinical condition of the patient. The following dosages are to be used as guidelines only.

Adult

IV—Short procedures (2 to 4 min): 40 to 60 mg (0.75 to 1 mg/kg). Supplemental doses of 20 to 30 mg may be given as required.

IV INFUSION—Prolonged procedures: 0.5 to 5 mg/min, depending on the response and requirements of the patient. Dilute 500 to 1000 mg in 500 ml of dextrose 5%, saline solution, or lactated Ringer's solution.

Pediatric
Neonates

IV—Initially, 1 to 2 mg/kg, followed by supplementary doses of 0.25 to 0.5 mg as required. The total dosage should not exceed 50 mg.

Children

IV—Initially, 1 mg/kg, followed by supplemental doses of 0.3 mg/kg.

Nurse and patient considerations

* Vagal activity and secretory effects of succinylcholine may be blocked by premedication with atropine.

* An idiosyncratic response of prolonged neuromuscular blockade is occasionally seen after normal dosages of succinylcholine. About 1 person in 2800 has a genetic abnormality that causes the production of an atypical pseudocholinesterase that only slowly metabolizes succinylcholine. Prolonged muscle relaxation results when succinylcholine is administered to these patients. Plasma pseudocholinesterase levels may also be decreased in patients with hepatocellular disease, malnutrition, severe anemia, or severe dehydration.
* Administration of succinylcholine causes an abrupt rise in intraocular pressure that may be hazardous to patients with glaucoma or penetrating wounds of the eye. A small dose of a competitive neuromuscular blocking agent before the use of succinylcholine can prevent the rise in intraocular pressure.
* Succinylcholine should be used with caution in patients with bone fractures. Initial muscle fasciculations may cause additional trauma. Small doses of a competitive neuromuscular blocking agent may be used to abolish the initial fasciculations.
* Succinylcholine may cause release of intracellular potassium into the plasma. Patients most susceptible to developing hyperkalemia are those with burns, trauma, spinal cord injuries, and degenerative muscle diseases and those with cardiac arrhythmias that may result from potassium ion shift in digitalized patients.
* See also General information on neuromuscular blocking agents (p. 532).

Drug interactions

Patients with glaucoma who are treated with echothiophate iodide (Phospholine iodide) may develop lower levels of pseudocholinesterase. These patients are susceptible to prolonged muscle relaxation if succinylcholine is administered.

Caution should be used in administering succinylcholine to patients also receiving cyclophosphamide (Cytoxan) or promazine (Sparine). Case reports suggest that these agents may reduce cholinesterase levels, prolonging the action of succinylcholine.

See also General information on neuromuscular blocking agents (p. 532).

Tubocurarine chloride

AHFS 12:20
CATEGORY Skeletal muscle relaxant

Action and use

Tubocurarine chloride is the oldest skeletal muscle relaxant in clinical use. It was first used as a muscle relaxant with anesthesia in 1942. Tubocurarine is classified as a competitive (nondepolarizing) neuromuscular blocking agent. Other pharmocologic actions include varying degrees of sympathetic blockade, resulting in hypotension and mild tachycardia, and occasional bronchospasm secondary to histamine release. It is also occasionally used to aid in the diagnosis of myasthenia gravis. See also General information on neuromuscular blocking agents (p. 532).

Characteristics

Onset: maximum within 5 min (IV). Duration: dependent on the total dosage and the number of doses administered, the anesthetic used, and the depth of anesthesia; single doses usually begin to subside in 20 to 30 min. Protein binding: 40% to 45%. Metabolism: hepatic. Excretion: 33% to 75% unchanged in urine, up to 11% in bile, in 24 hr.

Administration and dosage

NOTE: There is wide patient variation in response to neuromuscular blocking agents. Dosage must be individualized based on the length of surgery, anesthetics used, and the clinical condition of the patient. The following dosages are to be used as guidelines only.

Adult

IV—Initially, 15 to 30 mg (or 100 to 300 µg/kg) with supplementary doses of 5 to 10 mg at 45 to 60 min intervals. Administer each injection over 60 to 90 sec.

Pediatric

IV—Initially, 0.1 mg/lb (0.45 mg/kg).

Nurse and patient considerations

* If severe hypotension occurs, treat with IV fluids and sympathomimetic agents such as dopamine.
* Patients with liver disease often require higher dosages of tubocurarine.
* See General information on neuromuscular blocking agents (p. 532).

Drug interactions

See General information on neuromuscular blocking agents (p. 532).

Baclofen
(Lioresal)

AHFS 12:20
CATEGORY Skeletal muscle relaxant

Action and use

Baclofen is a skeletal muscle relaxant that acts on spinal and supraspinal sites to decrease the frequency and amplitude of muscle spasms. The exact mechanism of action is unknown. Baclofen is used to reduce the spasticity associated with severe chronic spinal disorders such as multiple sclerosis. It decreases the number and severity of flexor spasms, alleviating associated pain, clonus, and muscle rigidity.

Patients must have a degree of reversible spasticity so that baclofen can restore residual function. Baclofen has not been shown to be effective in spastic disorders associated with rheumatic disease.

Characteristics

Absorption: rapid, but with interpatient variability (PO); GI absorption is decreased as dosage is increased. Peak levels: 2 to 3 hr. Serum half-life: 2.5 to 4 hr. Metabolism: 15% in liver. Excretion: 70% to 80% unchanged or as metabolites in urine, remainder in feces. Breast milk: unknown.

Administration and dosage
Adult

PO 1. Initially, 5 mg 3 times daily. Daily dosage may be increased by 15 mg at 72 hr intervals until an optimum effect is observed, usually at 40 to 80 mg daily.
 2. Some patients receive a smoother antispastic activity if the drug is administered 4 times daily.
 3. One to 2 months of therapy may be necessary to determine whether full benefits of therapy have been achieved.
 4. When baclofen is discontinued, daily therapy must be gradually reduced. Abrupt withdrawal may precipitate hallucinations and aggravate spasticity.

Pediatric

Baclofen is not recommended in children under 12 years of age.

Nurse and patient considerations

* Common side effects of baclofen include drowsiness, fatigue, nausea, dizziness, hypotonia, muscle weakness, mental depression, and headache. The severity of side effects can be minimized by slowly increasing the dosage to maintenance levels.
* Elderly patients, patients with psychiatric disorders, and patients with brain lesions, including those with strokes, must have dosage adjustments made very slowly. These patients are more susceptible to episodes of euphoria, mental excitation, depression, confusion, and hallucinations.
* Use with caution in patients with seizure disorders such as epilepsy, since there may be a deterioration in seizure control. The epileptic patient's clinical state should be monitored closely while baclofen therapy is initiated.
* Allergic manifestations such as urticaria, pruritus, rash, and conjunctivitis with nasal congestion may occur in patients receiving baclofen. Such reactions are successfully treated by discontinuation of baclofen and, if necessary, with administration of antihistamines, epinephrine, and corticosteroids.
* Hyperglycemia, increased SGOT, and elevated alkaline phosphatase levels have been reported in patients receiving baclofen therapy.
* Other side effects that occur much less frequently include genitourinary effects of frequency or retention, cardiovascular effects of hypotension, dyspnea, and palpitations, and gastrointestinal effects of constipation, vomiting, anorexia, and taste disorders. Many of these side effects may be associated more with the underlying disease and not baclofen therapy.
* The safety of baclofen in pregnancy is not known. It should not be used in nursing mothers.

Drug interactions

Other drugs that may cause sedation may enhance the drowsiness and sedation occasionally seen in patients receiving baclofen.

Chlorzoxazone
(Paraflex)

AHFS 12:20
CATEGORY Skeletal muscle relaxant

Action and use

Chlorzoxazone is a skeletal muscle relaxant that acts by CNS depression. Its exact mechanism of action is not known; however, it does not directly relax skeletal muscle and does not depress neuronal conduction, neuromuscular conduction, neuromuscular transmission, or muscle excitability. Most authorities attribute its beneficial effects to its sedative properties. It is used, in addition to physical therapy, rest, and analgesics, for the relief of muscle spasm associated with acute, painful musculoskeletal conditions. It should not be used in muscle spasticity associated with cerebral or spinal cord disease.

Characteristics

Onset: within 1 hr. Duration: 3 to 4 hr. Half-life: 66 min. Metabolism: liver, inactive metabolites. Excretion: urine, as inactive glucuronide. Breast milk: unknown.

Administration and dosage
Adult

PO—Usual dose: 250 mg 3 to 4 times daily. Range: 250 to 750 mg 3 to 4 times daily. Tablets may be administered with food if nausea occurs.

Pediatric

Dosage range: 125 to 500 mg 3 to 4 times daily according to age and weight.

Nurse and patient considerations

* The most frequent side effects are drowsiness and dizziness. Gastrointestinal side effects including nausea, vomiting, heartburn, constipation, and diarrhea occur occasionally.
* Allergic reactions manifested by rash, petechiae, urticaria, and pruritus have rarely occurred.
* Patients should be warned against engaging in activities requiring mental alertness or physical coordination because of the sedative properties of chlorzoxazone.

* Chlorzoxazone should not be administered to patients with a history of liver disease or hypersensitivity to this agent.
* Patients should be informed that a metabolite of chlorzoxazone may produce an orange or purple-red color in the urine upon standing and that this discoloration is harmless.
* The safety of chlorzoxazone in pregnancy is not known and should therefore be used only on a risk to benefit basis. It should not be administered to nursing mothers.

Drug interactions

Ethanol, narcotics, barbiturates, anticonvulsants, sedative-hypnotics, tranquilizers, phenothiazines, and tricyclic antidepressants may enhance the CNS depressant effects of chlorzoxazone.

Cyclobenzaprine
(Flexeril)

AHFS 12:20
CATEGORY Skeletal muscle relaxant

Action and use

Cyclobenzaprine is a skeletal muscle relaxant that acts as a CNS depressant, primarily at the level of the brainstem. It is chemically related to the tricyclic antidepressants. Its exact mechanism of action is not known; however, it does not directly relax skeletal muscle and does not depress neuronal conduction, neuromuscular transmission, or muscle excitability. It is used, in addition to physical therapy and rest, for the relief of muscle spasm associated with acute, painful musculoskeletal conditions. It should not be used in muscle spasticity associated with cerebral or spinal cord disease.

Characteristics

Onset: within 1 hr (PO). Peak levels: 3 to 8 hr. Duration: 12 to 24 hr. Protein binding: 93%. Half-life: 1 to 3 days. Metabolism: liver, enterohepatic recycling inactive metabolites. Excretion: urine, primarily inactive; feces, primarily unchanged via the bile. Breast milk: high probability.

Administration and dosage
Adult

PO
1. Usual dose: 10 mg 3 times daily. Range: 20 to 40 mg daily, not to exceed 60 mg daily.
2. Cyclobenzaprine therapy should not be continued for more than 2 to 3 weeks without reevaluation of the patient.

NOTE: Cyclobenzaprine is contraindicated in patients with hyperthyroidism, congestive heart failure, arrhythmias, or hypersensitivity to the drug.

Pediatric

Cyclobenzaprine is not recommended in patients under 15 years of age.

Nurse and patient considerations

* The most frequent side effects include drowsiness, dry mouth, and dizziness. Tachycardia, nausea, dyspepsia, blurred vision, and unpleasant taste occur occasionally.
* Cyclobenzaprine should be used with caution in patients with a history of urinary retention, narrow-angle glaucoma, increased intraocular pressure, or cardiac disorders, which may be affected by tachycardia.
* The safety of cyclobenzaprine in pregnancy is not known. It should not be used in nursing mothers.

Drug interactions

Severe reactions (convulsions, hyperpyrexia, and fatalities) have been observed with the concomitant administration of an MAO inhibitor (isocarboxazid [Marplan], pargyline hydrochloride [Eutonyl], tranylcypromine sulfate [Parnate]). It is recommended that 2 weeks lapse between discontinuing an MAO inhibitor and starting tricyclic antidepressants.

The antihypertensive effect of guanethidine (Ismelin) is blocked by tricyclic antidepressants because of the inhibition of uptake of guanethidine into the adrenergic neuron.

Tricyclic antidepressants may display additive anticholinergic effects (dry mouth, constipation, urinary retention, acute glaucoma, blurred vision) when administered with antihistamines (Benadryl), phenothiazines, trihexiphenidyl (Artane), benzotropine (Congentin), meperidine (Demerol), and other agents with anticholinergic activity. Usually, however, the side effects are not serious enough to require discontinuance of therapy.

Tricyclic antidepressants may enhance meperidine-induced respiratory depression. This reaction may be particularly significant in those patients with lung disease.

Dantrolene sodium
(Dantrium)

AHFS 12:20
CATEGORY Skeletal muscle relaxant

Action and use

Dantrolene is a muscle relaxant that acts directly on the skeletal muscle. It is thought that dantrolene decreases the release of calcium from the sarcoplasmic reticulum, causing a decreased response of the muscle to electrical stimulation, thus diminishing the force of muscle contraction. The drug has no effect on electrical activity and does not affect the rate of acetylcholine production or release. Dantrolene is used to control the spasticity of chronic disorders such as cerebral palsy, multiple sclerosis, spinal cord injury, and stroke syndrome. It has also been used investigationally in the treatment of malignant hyperthermia associated with the use of general anesthesia.

Characteristics

Absorption: 35% (PO). Plasma half-life: 7 to 9 hr. Metabolism: liver by microsomal enzymes. Excretion: primarily in urine as metabolites.

Administration and dosage
Adult

PO—Initially, 25 mg daily. Dosage may be increased in increments of 25 mg every 4 to 7 days until therapeutic response is attained or side effects demand dosage reduction or discontinuation. The manufacturer suggests incremental changes of 25 to 100 mg 2 to 4 times daily. Some patients may require up to 200 mg 4 times daily; however, doses over 400 mg daily are rarely necessary.

Pediatric

NOTE: Not recommended in children under 5 years of age.
PO—0.5 mg/kg 3 to 4 times daily, then by increments of 0.5 mg/kg up to 3.0 mg/kg 2, 3, or 4 times daily. Do not exceed 400 mg daily.

NOTE: Dantrolene may cause hepatotoxicity as evidenced by abnormal liver function tests and symptomatic hepatitis. The incidence of hepatic disease appears to be greater in those patients taking over 400 mg daily, those taking other medications, those with previous liver disease, those over 35 years of age, and women. Hepatitis occurs most frequently between the third and twelfth months of therapy. Therapy should be discontinued if no significant benefit is derived after 45 days of therapy.

Nurse and patient considerations

* Common side effects of dantrolene include muscle weakness, drowsiness, dizziness, light-headedness, nausea, diarrhea, malaise, and fatigue. These adverse effects are generally transient and often dose related. Dantrolene is a drug with a wide variety of possible side effects. Its use must be weighed against the clinical improvement of and the toleration of adverse effects by the patient.
* As a muscle relaxant, dantrolene must be used with caution in patients with obstructive lung disease or severely impaired cardiac function due to myocardial disease.
* Counseling must include warning the patient of possible photosensitivity. Patients should avoid unnecessary exposure to sunlight.
* The safety of dantrolene in pregnancy is not known. It should not be used in nursing mothers.

Drug interactions

Other drugs that may cause sedation may enhance the drowsiness and sedation occasionally seen in patients receiving dantrolene.

Although no direct cause and effect relationship has been established, hepatoxicity has occurred more frequently in women over 35 years of age receiving concomitant estrogen therapy.

Methocarbamol
(Robaxin)

AHFS 12:20
CATEGORY Skeletal muscle relaxant

Action and use

Methocarbamol is a CNS depressant traditionally suggested for use in acute, painful musculoskeletal conditions such as muscle tension and pains associated with anxiety states. The mechanism of action is not known, although research studies indicate that methocarbamol does not directly relax skeletal muscle. Many clinicians conclude that muscle relaxation is due to the sedative properties of the drug.

Characteristics

Onset: 30 min (PO), immediate (IV). Half-life: 1 to 2⅕ hr. Metabolism: liver. Excretion: unknown.

Administration and dosage
Adult

PO—Initially, 1.5 g 4 times daily for the first 48 to 72 hrs. The maintenance dosage is 4 g daily in 3 to 6 divided doses.

SC—Not recommended.

IM—Initially, up to 1 g every 8 hr. Do not exceed 3 g daily for more than 3 consecutive days. Do not infuse more than 500 mg/gluteal region.

IV—As for IM administration. Administer undiluted at a rate no faster than 300 mg/min to minimize side effects. The patient should be recumbent during and for 10 to 15 min following the injection. Methocarbamol may be diluted to not more than 1 g in 250 ml of dextrose 5% for infusion.

NOTE: Avoid extravasation; observe patient closely for phlebitis and pain at the injection site. Do not administer IV for more than 3 consecutive days. Do not administer parenterally to patients with impaired renal function, since the diluent, polyethylene glycol-300, may be nephrotoxic.

Pediatric

Not recommended in children under 12 years of age.

Nurse and patient considerations

* As with most CNS depressants, common side effects include drowsiness, dizziness and light-headedness. Patients should be warned against engaging in activities requiring mental alertness.
* Allergic manifestations such as urticaria, pruritis, rash, and conjunctivitis with nasal congestion may occur in patients receiving methocarbamol. Such reactions may be successfully treated with antihistamines, epinephrine, and corticosteroids.

* Use with caution in patients with seizure disorders such as epilepsy. Seizure activity has been reported during IV administration.
* Patients taking methocarbamol should be told that their urine may turn brown, black, or green on standing.
* Safe use of methocarbamol in pregnancy and lactation has not been proven, and its use is not recommended in these conditions.

Drug interactions

The CNS depressant effects of antihistamines, analgesics, anesthetics, tranquilizers, and sedative-hypnotic agents may potentiate the sedative effects of methocarbamol.

CHAPTER TWENTY-TWO

Agents used in the treatment of parkinsonism

Amantadine
Bromocriptine mesylate

Carbidopa
Levodopa
General information on
*   anticholinergic agents*

Amantadine
(Symmetrel)

AHFS 92:00
CATEGORY Antiparkinsonian agent

Action and use

Amantadine is a synthetic compound developed for the treatment of certain strains of influenza virus. It was found, serendipitously, to also reduce the clinical manifestations of parkinsonism. It is not structurally related to any other antiparkinsonian agents. The exact mechanism of action is unknown but appears to be unrelated to its antiviral activity. It is hypothesized that amantadine may exert its antiparkinsonian effects by blocking the reuptake of dopamine, allowing accumulation of dopamine in the presynaptic cleft of neurons in the basal ganglia. It may also directly stimulate postsynaptic receptors and, in higher doses, may cause the release of dopamine into the synaptic clefts.

Amantadine does not treat the underlying disease but can be very beneficial in treating the symptoms associated with parkinsonism and drug-induced extrapyramidal reactions.

Characteristics

Improvement in extrapyramidal symptoms: 4 to 48 hr. Optimum therapy: 2 weeks to 3 months. Duration: improvement may last for over 2 years; however, many patients become refractory after 2 to 3 months. Half-life: 9 to 37 hr, average of 24 hr. Metabolism: none. Excretion: renal, unchanged, acidification of urine enhances excretion; accumulates in renal failure. Dialysis: unknown. Breast milk: yes.

Administration and dosage
Adults

PO 1. When used alone: 100 mg 2 times daily.
   2. In conjunction with other antiparkinsonian agents: 100 mg daily, increased to 100 mg 2 times daily after 1 to 3 weeks. Maximum dose: 400 mg daily.

NOTE: Sudden discontinuation of amantadine (even in those patients without therapeutic benefit) may cause an exacerbation of parkinsonian symptoms 1 to 3 days after discontinuation. Gradually decrease the dosage over a few weeks.

Nurse and patient considerations

* More than half of the patients who derive therapeutic benefit from amantadine will begin to experience a reduction in benefit after 2 to 3 months of therapy. Temporary discontinuation with a reinitiation of therapy several weeks later may restore the therapeutic benefits.

* Patients receiving therapeutic benefit should resume normal activities gradually, especially if other underlying medical conditions such as osteoporosis are present.

* Most of the adverse effects of amantadine therapy are dose related and reversible. Common side effects include confusion, disorientation, mental depression, dizziness and light-headedness, nervousness, insomnia, and gastrointestinal complaints (nausea, anorexia, abdominal discomfort, constipation). Hallucinations are frequently observed when high doses are used. Less frequent side effects include visual disturbances, ataxia, dryness of mouth, lethargy, and drowsiness.

* Amantadine should be used cautiously in patients with a history of seizure disorders, liver disease, recurrent eczmatoid dermatitis, uncontrolled psychosis, and congestive heart failure. Amantadine therapy may cause an exacerbation of these disorders.

* A dermatologic condition known as livido reticularis is frequently observed in conjunction wtih amantadine therapy. It is characterized by a diffuse, rose-colored mottling of the skin, often accompanied by pedal edema, predominantly in the extremities. It is

more noticeable when the patient is standing or exposed to cold. It is reversible within 2 to 6 weeks after discontinuation of amantadine but generally does not require discontinuation of therapy.

* Amantadine therapy is not recommended in pregnant patients. Teratogenicity has been reported in laboratory animals.

Drug interactions

Amantadine may exacerbate the side effects of anticholinergic agents (trihexyphenidyl, benztropine, procyclidine, diphenhydramine) that may also be used to control the symptoms of parkinsonism. Confusion and hallucinations may gradually develop. The dosage of either or both amantadine and the anticholinergic agent should be reduced.

Bromocriptine mesylate
(Parlodel)

AHFS 92:00
CATEGORY Antiparkinsonian agent

Action and use

Bromocriptine is a dopamine receptor stimulant and an inhibitor of prolactin secretion. It has many neuroendocrinologic effects. It restores ovarian function and ovulation in certain amenorrheic women, suppresses galactorrhea, postpartum lactation, growth hormone in patients with acromegaly, and stimulates dopaminergic receptors in the basal ganglia to treat the signs and symptoms of parkinsonism. It has also been used investigationally to treat Cushing's disease, chronic hepatic encephalopathy, premenstrual symptoms of breast discomfort, edema, weight gain, migraine headache, and mood changes, and to increase sperm counts in certain infertile men.

Before bromocriptine therapy is initiated, patients must have a complete diagnostic workup to determine underlying causes for the neuroendocrinologic dysfunction. In some cases, bromocriptine therapy may mask tumor activity.

Characteristics

Therapeutic response to bromocriptine is dependent on the disorder being treated. Antiparkinsonian effects may be observed within 1 to 2 hr of initiating therapy. Alleviation of amenorrhea may take 6 months, although the average time is 6 weeks. Galactorrhea usually subsides to a significant extent within 7 to 12 weeks, but some patients require longer therapy for complete cessation. Postpartum lactation is inhibited if bromocriptine is administered within 12 hr of delivery.

Absorption: 28% from GI tract. Protein binding: 90% to 96% to albumin. Half-life: alpha phase—4 to 4.5 hr; beta phase—45 to 50 hr. Metabolism: liver, extensive first-pass effect, to inactive metabolites. Excretion: renal—2% to 5%, feces—remainder. Dialysis: unknown.

Administration and dosage

PO   1. Administer with food. Initial daily dose: 1.25 to 2.5 mg. Initiate therapy in the evening to reduce adverse effects.
2. Amenorrhea/galactorrhea: 2.5 mg 2 to 3 times daily.
3. Postpartum lactation: start at least 4 hr after delivery and only if the patient's vital signs are stable. Usual dose: 2.5 mg every 12 hr for 14 to 21 days.

NOTE: Be observant for signs of hypotension with initial doses. After discontinuation of therapy, there is a 20% to 40% incidence of rebound breast secretion, congestion, or engorgement of mild to moderate severity.

4. Female infertility: initial dosage: 2.5 mg daily, increasing to 2.5 mg 2 to 3 times daily by the end of the first week.

NOTE: To reduce the possibility of fetal exposure in an unsuspected pregnancy, a mechanical contraceptive should be used until normal ovulatory menstrual cycles have been restored. Contraceptives should then be discontinued. If menstruation does not occur within 3 days of the expected date, bromocriptine therapy should be discontinued and a pregnancy test performed.

5. Parkinsonism: initial dosage: 1.25 mg 2 times daily with meals. Increase the dosage by 2.5 mg/day every 2 to 4 weeks. Dosage of bromocriptine must be adjusted according to the patient's response and tolerance. During initial bromocriptine therapy, maintain the levodopa therapy. Dosages in the 50 to 100 mg daily range are not uncommon for maximal therapeutic benefit. Levodopa dosages must frequently be reduced to minimize adverse reactions.

Nurse and patient considerations

* Although the incidence of side effects is quite high, especially for those patients receiving over 15 to 20 mg daily, the severity of adverse effects can be minimized by starting with small doses, increasing dosage gradually to effective levels, and administering the drug in the evening with food. Side effects can also be decreased if the dosage is reduced and then increased more gradually.
* Adverse effects based on organ system are:

  Gastrointestinal:

  Nausea, vomiting, anorexia, abdominal cramps, and constipation on long-term use are very common. Most of these effects can be minimized by temporary reduction in dosage, administration with food, and use of stool softeners for constipation.

  Neurologic:

  Involuntary movements, headache, migraine, dizziness, light-headedness and sedation have been reported. Patients taking doses greater than 100 mg daily suffer a high incidence of delusions, confusion, hallucinations, and erythromelalgia (paroxysmal throbbing and painful burning of the skin, usually of the feet or hands, often accompanied by a mottled redness of the affected areas). These adverse effects dissipate within 2 to 3 weeks of discontinuing therapy.

  Cardiovascular:

  Hypotension commonly occurs. Palpitations, angina and cold-induced vasospasm of the extremities have been reported.

  Other side effects include dryness of the mouth, diplopia, nasal congestion, urticaria, and metallic taste.

* Abnormality of laboratory tests include elevations of BUN, SGOT, SGPT, GGPT, CPK, alkaline phosphatase, and uric acid. Most elevations are transient and of no clinical significance.
* Since bromocriptine inhibits lactation, it should not be administered to nursing mothers.

Drug interactions

Drugs that increase prolactin levels are tricyclic antidepressants (amitriptyline, imipramine, doxepin), reserpine, haloperidol, methyldopa, and the phenothiazines (chlorpromazine, thioridazine). Therefore the dosage of bromocriptine may have to be increased for therapeutic activity.

Patients being treated for acromegaly report a decreased tolerance to alcohol. These patients should be warned to limit their intake while receiving bromocriptine therapy.

Bromocriptine and levodopa have additive neurologic effects. This may be advantageous in the patient with parkinsonism because it often allows a reduction in dosage of the levodopa.

Bromocriptine and antihypertensive agents (methyldopa, clonidine, guanethidine, hydralazine) have additive hypotensive effects. Dosage adjustment of the antihypertensive agent is frequently necessary when combined therapy is used.

Carbidopa
(Sinemet)

AHFS 92:00
CATEGORY Antiparkinsonian agent

Action and use

Carbidopa is an enzyme inhibitor that diminishes the peripheral metabolism of levodopa. It does not cross the blood-brain barrier into the central nervous system. When carbidopa is administered in conjunction with levodopa, the metabolic enzymes, the dopa decarboxylases, are inhibited, allowing a greater portion of the administered levodopa to reach the desired receptor sites in the basal ganglia. Advantages of combined therapy include (1) an acceptable therapeutic response is achieved with a much smaller dose of levodopa; (2) nausea, vomiting, and cardiac stimulation are minimized; (3) full therapeutic activity of levodopa is achieved much more quickly, since tolerance does not have to be developed to the peripheral side effects of levodopa; (4) pyridoxine does not antagonize therapeutic activity when combination therapy is used; and (5) patients manifest less diurnal variation in the control of the symptoms of parkinsonism.

Sinemet is a combination product that contains carbidopa and levodopa (p. 556) in a 1:10 ratio (Sinemet 10/100 and Sinemet 25/250) and a 1:4 ratio (Sinemet 25/100). Physicians can obtain carbidopa as a single agent (Lodosyn) on request from the manufacturer for those patients who do not receive optimal benefit from the combination product.

Characteristics

Absorption: 40% to 70%. Half-life: 1 to 2 hr. Protein binding: 36%. Daily doses of 70 to 100 mg of carbidopa saturate peripheral dopa decarboxylase. When carbidopa and levodopa are administered concurrently, the half-life of levodopa is extended to 2 hr. Excretion: renal, 30% unchanged in 24 hr.

Administration and dosage

Patients receiving levodopa:

NOTE: When Sinemet is to be given to patients who are being treated with levodopa, levodopa must be discontinued at least 8 hr before Sinemet is started. Start Sinemet therapy with the morning dose after a night (at least 8 hr) when the patient has not received any levodopa.

NOTE: A daily dosage of Sinemet should be chosen that will provide approximately 25% of the previous levodopa daily dosage.

PO—Start at 1 tablet of Sinemet 25/250 3 to 4 times daily. Patients who require less than 1500 mg of levodopa daily should start with 1 tablet of Sinemet 10/100 or Sinemet 25/100 3 to 4 times daily.

Patients not currently receiving levodopa:

PO 1. Initially, Sinemet 10/100 or 25/100 3 times daily, increasing by 1 tablet every other day until a dosage of 6 tablets daily is attained.

2. If nausea and vomiting occur with Sinemet 10/100, substitute Sinemet 25/100, tablet for tablet.

3. As therapy progresses and patients show indications of needing more levodopa, substitute Sinemet 25/250, 1 tablet 3 to 4 times daily. Increase by 1 tablet every other day to a maximum of 8 tablets daily.

Nurse and patient considerations

* Carbidopa has no effect when used alone, but must be used in combination with levodopa. The side effects seen with combination therapy are actually an enhancement of the effects of levodopa, since the carbidopa is allowing more intact levodopa to reach the brain. Side effects such as involuntary movements and mental disturbances may occur at

lower dosages and sooner with Sinemet than with levodopa, thus requiring a reduction in dosage.
* See also Levodopa, p. 556.

Drug interactions

Sinemet may be used to treat parkinsonism in conjunction with amantadine or anticholinergic agents (Congentin, Artane, Kemadrin, others). The dosages of all medications may need to be reduced due to combined therapy.

See also Levodopa, p. 556.

Levodopa
(Dopar, Larodopa)

AHFS 92:00
CATEGORY Antiparkinsonian agent

Action and use

It is hypothesized that parkinsonism is induced by an imbalance of neurotransmitters in the basal ganglia of the brain. The primary imbalance is an excess of acetylcholine and a deficiency of dopamine; however, other neurotransmitters such as norepinephrine, histamine, GABA, and serotonin appear to play a role in the progression of this complex disease.

Dopamine, when administered systemically, does not cross the blood-brain barrier; however, its precursor, levodopa, does. Large doses of levodopa must be administered orally, since about 95% of the drug is rapidly metabolized. It is hypothesized that less than 1% of an administered dose of levodopa reaches the basal ganglia where it is metabolized to the active compound, dopamine. Levodopa is thus indicated for the symptomatic treatment of parkinsonism. About 75% of patients with parkinsonism respond favorably to levodopa therapy, but, after a period of 2 to 3 years, the response diminishes, becomes more uneven, and is accompanied by many more side effects. This loss of effect is secondary to progression of the underlying disease process. Levodopa is frequently used in combination with anticholinergic agents (benztropine, trihexyphenidyl, procyclidine), antihistamines (diphenhydramine), amantadine, and carbidopa to help control various side effects of drug therapy and the underlying disease process.

Characteristics

Onset: about 1 hr. Duration: 3 to 5 hr. Metabolism: extensive degradation in stomach, intestines, and the first pass through liver to over 30 active and inactive metabolites. Excretion: renal, 1% as unchanged levodopa. Dialysis: unknown. Breast milk: unknown.

Administration and dosage
Adult

PO 1. Dosages must carefully be titrated to each patient.
2. Initially, 0.5 to 1 g daily, divided into 2 or more doses administered with food. If patients are unable to swallow the capsules, the capsules may be emptied and mixed with food or liquid.
3. The total daily dosage is increased gradually in increments of not more than 750 mg every 3 to 7 days as tolerated.
4. Do not exceed 8 g daily.
5. In some patients, optimal therapeutic response may not be obtained until 6 months of treatment.

Pediatric

Levodopa therapy is not recommended for children under 12 years of age.

Nurse and patient considerations

∗ Levodopa causes numerous side effects, most of which are more troublesome than serious. The intensity and type vary greatly at different stages of therapy. Side effects are usually dose dependent and reversible. Adverse effects, listed according to organ systems, include:

Cardiovascular:
Arrhythmias such as sinus tachycardia, atrial flutter, and premature ventricular contractions occur. These are readily controlled by beta-blocking agents (propranolol). Low blood pressure is frequently observed in patients with parkinsonism. Levodopa may aggravate this by causing orthostatic hypotension. Tolerance to hypotension frequently develops after a few weeks of therapy.

Central nervous system:
Abnormal involuntary movements occur in over half the patients taking levodopa for

over 6 months. These movements present as chewing motions, bobbing of the head and neck, facial grimacing, active tongue movement, and rocking movements of the trunk. As the disease progresses, patients will complain of an "on-off" phenomena, which is characterized by a sudden inability to move (akinesia) that may last for several minutes to hours, followed by an abrupt return to mobility that is often accompanied by abnormal involuntary movements. The "on-off" effect may be particularly noticeable near the end of a dosing interval. The duration of therapeutic effect diminishes from about 4 hr to 2 to 3 hr.

Gastrointestinal:

Anorexia, nausea, and vomiting are frequently reported at the initiation of therapy. These effects can be minimized by slowly increasing the dose, dividing the total daily dose into 4 to 6 doses, and administering with food or antacids.

Psychiatric:

Drug-induced mental changes are somewhat difficult to assess due to the age of the patient and parkinsonism itself. Levodopa may cause nightmares, restlessness, anxiety, insomnia, depression, dementia, loss of memory, paranoia, delusions, and hallucinations. Reduction of the total daily dosage may control these adverse effects.

Ophthalmic:

All patients should be screened for the presence of narrow-angle glaucoma. Levodopa may precipitate an acute attack of angle-closure glaucoma. Patients with open-angle glaucoma can safely use levodopa in conjunction with miotic therapy.

* *Abnormalities of laboratory tests:* Urinary metabolites of levodopa cause false-positive tests for urinary ketones with Ketostix and Labstix. Acetest tablets are generally not affected.

Levodopa may cause a false-negative reading in the presence of glycosuria when the glucose oxidase method (Tes-Tape, Clinistix) is used, and a false-positive "trace" reading with the copper reduction method (Clinitest).

Urinary metabolites may color the urine red to black on exposure to air or alkaline substances (bowl cleaners). Patients should be told not to be alarmed.

Levodopa may cause a false-positive elevation of serum and urinary uric acid when the colorimetric method is used. When the uricase method is used, there is no interference with test results.

Elevations of BUN, SGOT, SGPT, LDH, bilirubin, and alkaline phosphatase have been reported. The significance is not known.

Occasional reductions in WBC, hemoglobin, and hematocrit have been reported. Leukopenia may require temporary cessation of levodopa therapy.

The Coombs' test becomes positive during extended therapy.

* Use in pregnancy is not recommended unless the benefits significantly outweigh the risk of therapy.
* Levodopa should not be used in nursing mothers.

Drug interactions

Pyridoxine (vitamin B_6) in oral doses of 5 to 10 mg reverses the toxic and therapeutic effects of levodopa. Normal diets contain less than 1 mg of pyridoxine, so dietary restrictions are not necessary. The ingredients of multiple vitamin products should be considered, however. There is a pyridoxine-free multiple vitamin (Larobec) made specifically for patients taking levodopa.

Phenothiazines, reserpine, haloperidol (Haldol), and methyldopa (Aldomet) can produce a parkinsonism-like syndrome. Since these drugs nullify the effects of levodopa, they should not be used.

Monoamine oxidase inhibitors (MAOI) such as phenelzine (Nardil) and isocarboxazid (Marplan) interfere with the metabolism of dopamine. They unpredictably exaggerate the effects of levodopa and its metabolites. The MAOI should be discontinued at least 14 days before the administration of levodopa.

Diazepam (Valium), chlordiazepoxide (Librium), papaverine (Pavabid), phenylbutazone (Butazolidin), clonidine (Catapres), and phenytoin (Dilantin) appear to cause a deterioration in the therapeutic effects of levodopa. These agents should be used with caution in patients with parkinsonism and should be discontinued if there is deterioration in the patient's clinical status.

Isoniazid should be used with caution in patients taking levodopa. Isoniazid has some properties resembling inhibition of monoamine oxidase (MAO). Discontinue isoniazid if patients taking levodopa develop hypertension flushing, palpitations, and tremor.

GENERAL INFORMATION ON ANTICHOLINERGIC AGENTS

It is hypothesized that parkinsonism is induced by an imbalance of neurotransmitters in the basal ganglia of the brain. The primary imbalance is a relative excess of acetylcholine and a deficiency of dopamine; however, other neurotransmitters such as norepinephrine, histamine, GABA, and serotonin appear to play a role in the progression of this complex disease. The two primary modes of treatment are the use of levodopa, which helps correct the dopamine deficiency, and centrally acting anticholinergic agents, which attempt to reduce hyperstimulation secondary to a relative excess of acetylcholine. Antihistamines with anticholinergic activity are also occasionally used for patients with mild symptoms of parkinsonism. The anticholinergic agents reduce the incidence and severity of the akinesia, rigidity, and tremor that characterizes parkinsonism and the secondary symptoms such as hyperhidrosis, drooling, and depressed mood.

Even though levodopa and carbidopa are now the cornerstones of antiparkinsonian therapy, the anticholinergic agents are still quite useful as adjunctive therapy. Anticholinergic agents may be useful for patients with minimal symptoms, for those unable to tolerate the side effects of levodopa, and for those who have not benefited from levodopa therapy. Combination therapy with levodopa and anticholinergic agents is also successful in more completely controlling symptoms of the disease in about half of the patients already stabilized on levodopa therapy.

Administration and dosage

Dosage should be initiated at a low level and increased gradually, particularly in elderly or debilitated patients. Increases in dosage should be made in the evening, since increased sedation is often present.

Tolerance to therapy may develop, necessitating a change in dosage or the use of combination therapy.

The anticholinergic agents may be taken with food to reduce any nausea.

See Tables 22-1 and 22-2 for generic and brand names and recommended dosages.

Nurse and patient considerations

Although there are essentially no pharmacologic differences between the anticholinergic agents used to treat parkinsonism, certain patients often tolerate one preparation better than another.

Do not use in patients with narrow-angle glaucoma. An acute attack may be precipitated. Anticholinergic agents may, however, be used in open-angle glaucoma. Gonioscopy and monitoring of intraocular pressures should be performed on a regular basis.

Most side effects observed with anticholinergic agents are direct extensions of their pharmacologic properties. Frequently seen adverse effects that usually dissipate with therapy are dryness and soreness of mouth and tongue, blurring

Table 22-1. Anticholinergic agents used to treat parkinsonism
AHFS 12:08

Generic name	Brand name	Initial dose (PO)	Maximum daily dosage (mg)
Benztropine mesylate	Cogentin	0.5 to 1 mg at bedtime	1-6
Biperiden hydrochloride	Akineton	2 mg 1 to 3 times daily	2-10
Ethopropazine hydrochloride	Parsidol	50 mg 1 to 2 times daily	600
Procyclidine hydrochloride	Kemadrin	2 mg 3 times daily	15-20
Trihexyphenidyl hydrochloride	Artane, Tremin	1 mg daily	12-15

Table 22-2. Antihistamines used to treat parkinsonism

AHFS 4:00

Generic name	Brand name	Initial dose (PO)	Maximum daily dosage (mg)
Diphenhydramine hydrochloride	Benadryl	25 to 50 mg 3 to 4 times daily	400
Orphenadrine hydrochloride	Disipal	50 mg 3 times daily	150-250

of vision, dizziness, mild nausea, and nervousness. Psychiatric disturbances such as mental confusion, delusions, euphoria, paranoia, and hallucinations may be indications of overdosage. The drug should be discontinued for a few days and then restarted at a lower dose, allowing tolerance to the adverse effects to develop.

Other side effects include constipation, urinary hesitancy or retention, tachycardia, palpitations, mydriasis, muscle cramping, paresthesias, mental dullness, loss of memory, and mild, transient postural hypotension.

Patients should be counseled that anticholinergic agents may impair mental and physical capabilities and to use caution when performing tasks requiring alertness.

Drug interactions

Amantadine, tricyclic antidepressants (Elavil, Tofranil, Aventyl, others) and phenothiazines (Thorazine, Compazine, Mellaril, others) may potentiate the anticholinergic side effects. Developing confusion and hallucinations are characteristic of excessive anticholinergic activity.

Extrapyramidal symptoms have been reported in patients taking methotrimeprazine (Levoprome) and anticholinergic agents concomitantly.

Large doses of anticholinergic agents may delay gastric emptying, allowing a significant decrease in absorption of levodopa and chlorpromazine (Thorazine). Adjustment in dosages may be required.

CHAPTER TWENTY-THREE

Biologic agents

GENERAL INFORMATION

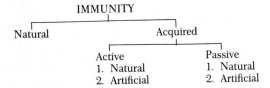

Definitions

A. Natural immunity: immunity present at birth. It does not include any mechanisms to develop immunity during the life of the individual.

B. Acquired: immunity derived from an exogenous source.

  1. Active: immunity developed by an individual in response to the introduction of antigenic substances into the body. Immunity develops slowly, but is long lasting.

    a. Natural: immunity developed secondary to an infection (for example, measles).

    b. Artificial: immunity produced by stimulating body defense mechanisms to produce antibodies to specific antigens injected into the body (for example, influenza virus or mumps vaccines).

  2. Passive: immunity developed by introducing specific

antibodies produced from another source into the body. Immunity is produced quickly, but is not long lasting.

   a. Natural: an example is antibodies passed to a neonate from the blood of the mother.
   b. Artificial: injection of biologics (for example, tetanus antitoxin, tetanus immune globulin) that contain antibodies to a specific organism.
C. Antibody: protein substance developed by the body as a protective mechanism in response to the presence of an antigen.
D. Antigen: a foreign substance that includes the formation of antibodies.
E. Antitoxins: a specific antibody harvested from animals that have been injected repeatedly with a toxin (that is, diphtheria antitoxin, tetanus antitoxin, botulism antitoxin).
F. Human immune globulin: solution of globulins derived from human blood that contains many antibodies normally present in adult human blood (measles, pertussis, tetanus, poliomyelitis).
G. Toxoids: modification of a toxin to reduce or eliminate the poisonous properties while retaining the antigenic properties that are capable of producing antibodies (that is, diphtheria toxoid, tetanus toxoid).
H. Toxins: bacterial waste products considered poisonous. When injected, they act as antigens, resulting in the production of antibodies called antitoxins (that is, diagnostic diphtheria toxin).
 I. Vaccines: living, attenuated, or killed viruses, killed rickettsiae, or killed bacteria that are used to stimulate the production of antibodies (that is, smallpox, rabies, influenza virus, poliomyelitis, measles, mumps vaccines).

Administration and dosage

NOTE: If immune globulin (such as immune serum globulin [human], USP; hepatitis immune globulin [human], USP; tetanus immune globulin [human], USP) has been given before a scheduled administration of a parenterally administered *live*, attenuated vaccine, the administration of the vaccine should be delayed for 6 weeks to 3 months after the immune globulin was administered. The antibodies contained in the immune globulin may inhibit replication of the vaccine virus and, therefore, the patient's antibody response to the vaccine. If the vaccine is administered orally (such as trivalent oral polio vaccine) or if the vaccine is an inactivated vaccine (such as influenza virus vaccine), the immune globulin will not interfere with developing immunity.

See individual monographs on biologic agents.

See Tables 23-1, 23-2, and 23-3 for pediatric immunization schedules.

Nurse and patient considerations

Before administration of any biologic agent, histories of allergies and tests for sensitivity should be completed. Since biologic agents are protein and foreign to the body, sensitivity ranging from erythema and fever to urticaria, angioedema, respiratory distress (including dyspnea and bronchospasm), and anaphylaxis have occurred.

Biologic agents should not be administered IV because of the potential for serious hypersensitivity reactions. Epinephrine 1:1000 and other emergency drugs and equipment should be readily available in the event that severe systemic reactions should develop.

Vaccines should not be administered to patients taking corticosteroids. Steroids may interfere with the antibody response to the vaccine, inhibiting the production of active immunity by the vaccine.

Patients with immune deficiency disease, or patients with diseases such as leukemia, lymphoma, or generalized malignancy, or those under treatment with corticosteroids, alkylating agents, antimetabolites, or radiation should be given live vaccines only after serious consideration of their clinical status. Patients who are immunosuppressed may have an enhanced response to viral replication after administration of live, attenuated virus vaccines.

Immunizations should usually be deferred during acute febrile illness.

Patients should be informed about what type of biologic agent is being administered. They should be informed of the reasons for use and the associated reactions that might occur. Patients should be encouraged to report any adverse response to immunizations. A record of immunization should also be completed and given to the patient, indicating the date, the biologic agent used, the site of injection, and the dosage.

Interruptions in the schedule of immunizations of infants and children, with a delay between doses, does not interfere with the final immunity achieved. The series need not be started over, regardless of the length of time elapsed.

Observe expiration dates of the agents and store at proper temperature.

Table 23-1. Recommended schedule for active immunization of normal infants and children

Recommended age*	Vaccine(s)†	Comments
2 months	DTP-1,‡ OPV-1§	Can be given earlier in areas of high endemicity
4 months	DTP-2, OPV-2	6-week to 2-month interval desired between OPV doses to avoid interference
6 months	DTP-3	An additional dose of OPV at this time is optional for use in areas with a high risk of polio exposure
15 months‖	MMR¶	
18 months‖	DTP-4, OPV-3	Completion of primary series
4-6 years**	DTP-5, OPV-4	Preferably at or before school entry
14-16 years	Td††	Repeat every 10 years throughout life

From Centers For Disease Control: Morbid. Mortal. Week. Rep. **32:**2-16, Jan. 14, 1983.

*These recommended ages should not be construed as absolute; that is, 2 months can be 6-10 weeks, etc.

†For all products used, consult manufacturer's package enclosure for instructions for storage, handling, and administration. Immunobiologics prepared by different manufacturers may vary, and those of the same manufacturer may change from time to time. The package insert should be followed for a specific product.

‡DTP—Diphtheria and tetanus toxoids and pertussis vaccine.

§OPV—Oral, attenuated poliovirus vaccine contains poliovirus types 1, 2, and 3.

‖Simultaneous administration of MMR, DTP, and OPV is appropriate for patients whose compliance with medical care recommendations cannot be assured.

¶MMR—Live measles, mumps, and rubella viruses in a combined vaccine.

**Up to the seventh birthday.

††Td—Adult tetanus toxoid and diphtheria toxoid in combination, which contains the same dose of tetanus toxoid as DTP or DT and a reduced dose of diphtheria toxoid.

Table 23-2. Recommended immunization schedule for infants and children up to seventh birthday not immunized at the recommended time in early infancy*

Timing	Vaccine(s)	Comments
First visit	DTP-1,† OPV-1,‡ (If child is ≥ 15 months of age, MMR§)	DTP, OPV, and MMR can be administered simultaneously to children ≥ 15 months of age
2 months after first DTP, OPV	DTP-2, OPV-2	
2 months after second DTP	DTP-3	An additional dose of OPV at this time is optional for use in areas with a high risk of polio exposure
6-12 months after third DTP	DTP-4, OPV-3	
Preschool‖ (4-6 years)	DTP-5, OPV-4	Preferably at or before school entry
14-16 years	Td¶	Repeat every 10 years throughout life

From Centers For Disease Control: Morbid. Mortal. Week. Rep. **32**:2-16, Jan. 14, 1983.

*If initiated in the first year of life, give DTP-1, 2, and 3, OPV-1 and 2 according to this schedule and give MMR when the child becomes 15 months old.

†DTP—Diphtheria and tetanus toxoids with pertussis vaccine. DTP may be used up to the seventh birthday.

‡OPV—Oral, attenuated poliovirus vaccine contains poliovirus types 1, 2, and 3.

§MMR—Live measles, mumps, and rubella viruses in a combined vaccine.

‖The preschool dose is not necessary if the fourth dose of DTP and third dose of OPV are administered after the fourth birthday.

¶Td—Adult tetanus toxoid and diphtheria toxoid in combination, which contains the same dose of tetanus toxoid as DTP or DT and a reduced dose of diphtheria toxoid.

Table 23-3. Recommended immunization schedule for persons 7 years of age or older

Timing	Vaccine(s)	Comments
First visit	Td-1,* OPV-1,† and MMR‡	OPV not routinely administered to those ≥ 18 years of age
2 months after first Td, OPV	Td-2, OPV-2	
6-12 months after second Td, OPV	Td-3, OPV-3	OPV-3 may be given as soon as 6 weeks after OPV-2
10 years after Td-3	Td	Repeat every 10 years throughout life

From Centers For Disease Control: Morbid. Mortal. Week. Rep. **32**:2-16, Jan. 14, 1983.

*Td—Tetanus and diphtheria toxoids (adult type) are used after the seventh birthday. The DTP doses given to children under 7 who remain incompletely immunized at age 7 or older should be counted as prior exposure to tetanus and diphtheria toxoids (for example, a child who previously received 2 doses of DTP needs only 1 dose of Td to complete a primary series).

†OPV—Oral, attenuated poliovirus vaccine contains poliovirus types 1, 2, and 3. When polio vaccine is to be given to individuals 18 years or older, IPV is preferred.

‡MMR—Live measles, mumps, and rubella viruses in a combined vaccine. Persons born before 1957 can generally be considered immune to measles and mumps and need not be immunized. Rubella vaccine may be given to persons of any age, particularly to women of childbearing age. MMR may be used, since administration of vaccine to persons already immune is not deleterious.

Hepatitis B immune globulin (human), USP

AHFS 80:04

(Hep-B-Gammagee, HyperHep, H-BIG)

Hepatitis B immune globulin is a solution of immuno-globulin obtained from pooled plasma drawn from individuals with high titers of antibody to the hepatitis B surface antigen. Human antihepatitis B globulin is used to provide immediate passive immunity for patients exposed to the risk of hepatitis B.

Administration and dosage
Adult

IM—0.06 ml/kg (3 to 5 ml for most adults).

Pediatric

IM—0.06 ml/kg.

NOTE: Administer as soon after exposure as possible (within 7 days) and repeat 28 to 30 days after exposure. Use a separate needle and syringe for each patient inoculated to prevent transmission of hepatitis B. See General information on biologic agents (p. 564).

Nurse and patient considerations

* Persons with isolated immunoglobulin A deficiency have the potential for developing antibodies to immunoglobulin A (contained in hepatitis B immune globulin) and could have anaphylactic reactions to subsequent administration of blood products that contain immunoglobulin A. Therefore hepatitis B immune globulin should be administered to patients with an immunoglobulin A deficiency on a risk to benefit basis.
* The effects of hepatitis B immune globulin on pregnant patients, the fetus, or on nursing mothers are unknown. Administration should be on a risk to benefit basis.
* See General information on biologic agents (p. 564).

Drug interactions

Antibodies present in immune globulin solutions may interfere with the immune response to live virus vaccines such as measles, mumps, and rubella. Therefore vaccination with live virus vaccines should be deferred until approximately 3 months after administration of hepatitis B immune globulin. It may be necessary to revaccinate persons who received hepatitis B immune globulin shortly after live virus vaccination.

Hepatitis B vaccine
(Heptavax-B)

AHFS 80:12

Hepatitis B vaccine represents a significant advance in the science of preventive medicine. It is a noninfectious, inactivated, subunit vaccine derived from hepatitis B surface antigen. The vaccine is produced from the plasma of chronic hepatitis B virus carriers. When administered according to schedule, it provides active immunity against hepatitis B virus. The vaccine is recommended for people who are at high risk for developing the disease. These include (but are not limited to) dentists, oral surgeons, dental hygienists, medical personnel who have frequent contact with blood or blood products, hemodialysis patients, homosexually active males, and family contacts of chronic hepatitis B virus carriers. The effectiveness of the vaccine for postexposure prophylaxis is not known. For those patients with known exposure to hepatitis B, hepatitis B immune globulin should be administered in conjunction with the vaccine.

Administration and dosage
Adults and children over 10 years of age

IM—Three 1 ml injections initially and at 1 and 6 months.

For dialysis patients and immunosuppressed patients:
IM—Three 2 ml injections initially and at 1 and 6 months.

Pediatric (3 months to 10 years of age)

IM—1. 3 0.5 ml injections at 0, 1 month, and 6 months.
2. A booster injection may be necessary in 5 years.
NOTE: Store the vaccine at 2° to 8° C (35° to 46° F).

Nurse and patient considerations

∗ The most commonly reported adverse effects include mild local tenderness at the site of injection (10% in adults, 4% in children) and slight elevations in temperature (less than 38° C [101° F]) in 3% of adults and 10% in children within 48 hr of vaccination.

∗ Other minor side effects include malaise, fatigue, headaches, nausea, dizziness, myalgias, arthralgias, and skin rashes.

∗ Pregnancy should not be considered a contraindication to vaccination for persons who are otherwise eligible.

∗ See General information on biologic agents (p. 564).

Immune serum globulin (human), USP
AHFS 80:04

Immune serum globulin (human) contains the antibodies present in normal blood. It is indicated for the modification or prevention of measles (rubeola), german measles, chickenpox (varicella), and infectious hepatitis (hepatitis A) and for patients deficient in gamma globulin or specific immunoglobulins.

Administration and dosage

IM   1. Measles (rubeola):
   Modification: 0.02 ml/lb (0.009 ml/kg).
   Prevention: 0.1 ml/lb (0.045 ml/kg).
   With vaccine: 0.01 ml/lb (0.0045 ml/kg).
2. German measles (rubella):
   Prevention in pregnant women in first trimester: 20 to 30 ml.
3. Chickenpox (varicella):
   Modification: 0.1 to 0.6 ml/lb (0.045 to 0.27 ml/kg) up to 20 to 30 ml.
4. Infectious hepatitis:
   Prevention: 0.01 to 0.05 ml/lb (0.0045 to 0.0225 ml/kg) to be repeated at 4- to 6-month intervals when there is repeated or continued exposure.

Store at 2° C to 8° C (36° F to 46° F). Do not freeze.

NOTE: See General information on biologic agents (p. 564).

Immune globulin intravenous, 5%

AHFS 80:04

(Gammimune)

Immune globulin intravenous is derived from large pools of human venous plasma. It supplies the IgG antibodies present in normal blood. Immune globulin intravenous is used for the maintenance treatment of patients who are unable to produce adequate amounts of IgG antibodies. It is particularly useful in patients who need an immediate increase in intravascular immunoglobulin levels and in patients who should not receive IM injections, such as those with bleeding tendencies or small muscle mass.

Characteristics

The half-life is approximately 3 weeks, but individual patient variation has been observed.

Administration and dosage

IV 1. 100 mg/kg of body weight (2 ml/kg) administered monthly. Dosages of 200 mg/kg or more frequent administration may be used in patients showing an inadequate level of IgG. Infuse at a rate of 0.01 to 0.02 ml/kg/min. If after 30 min the patient is showing no adverse effects, the infusion rate may be increased to 0.02 to 0.04 ml/kg/min. If adverse effects occur, reduce the rate of infusion or discontinue until the adverse effects subside.

2. Store at 2° to 8° C (35° to 46° F). Do not use a solution that has been frozen. Discard partially used vials. Do not use if turbid.

NOTE: IV administration of this agent can cause sudden hypotension and a clinical picture resembling anaphylaxis even when the patient is not known to be sensitive to immune globulin products. These reactions appear to be related to the rate of infusion. Therefore follow the above guidelines closely and monitor the patient's vital signs continuously. Epinephrine should be available for treatment of any acute anaphylactoid reaction.

Nurse and patient considerations

* Persons with isolated immunoglobulin A deficiency have the potential for developing antibodies to immunoglobulin A (contained in immune globulin intravenous) and could have anaphylactic reactions to subsequent administration of blood products that contain immunoglobulin A.

* The incidence of adverse effects associated with the administration of intravenous immune globulin is about 10%. Side effects reported, in addition to the hypotension noted above, are mild back pain, flushing, and nausea.

* The effects of immune globulin intravenous on pregnant patients, the fetus, or on nursing mothers are unknown. Administration should be on a risk to benefit basis.

* See General information on biologic agents (p. 564).

Drug interactions

It is recommended that the infusion of immune globulin intravenous be given through a separate line, by itself, without mixing with other IV fluids (other than dextrose 5%) or medications the patient might be receiving.

Pneumococcal vaccine, polyvalent
(Pneumovax)

AHFS 80:12

Polyvalent pneumococcal vaccine is a solution containing antigenic capsular polysaccharides from 23 types of pneumococcal microorganisms. The vaccine provides active immunity against the 23 most common pneumococcal organisms that currently cause over 80% of pneumococcal infections. No protection is provided against other types of pneumococcal disease or other bacterial infections.

Pneumococcal vaccine is recommended for patients over the age of 2 who are at high risk from pneumococcal infection. Patients who should be considered for immunization are those with chronic debilitating diseases, institutionalized patients, those convalescing from severe illness, and those over 50 years of age. Revaccination should be no more frequent than every 3 years.

Administration and dosage
Adult and pediatric (over 2 years of age)

SC or IM—0.5 ml.

Nurse and patient considerations

* Use in pregnancy is not recommended because the effects on the fetus are unknown.
* See General information on biologic agents (p. 564).

Rabies immune globulin (human)
(Hyperab)

AHFS 80:04

Rabies immune globulin is a solution of immunoglobulin obtained from the pooled plasma of individuals with high titers of antibody to the rabies virus. It is used to provide short-term, passive immunity to rabies in the initial prophylactic treatment of those exposed to rabies virus. It should be administered as promptly as possible, followed by a course of rabies vaccine (human diploid cell culture) therapy.

Characteristics

The plasma half-life of rabies immune globulin (human) is 21 days.

Administration and dosage

NOTE: If the patient was suspected to be exposed to rabies virus via a bite or other type of wound, infiltrate the lacerated area with half of the dosage. Administer the remainder intramuscularly.

IM—20 IU/kg or 9.09 IU/lb. Not more than 5 ml should be administered IM at one injection site. Divide doses exceeding 5 ml and administer at different sites. Do not administer to patients who are allergic to gamma globulin or thimerosal.

Nurse and patient considerations

* Rabies immune globulin may partially suppress the antibody-formation response to rabies vaccine. This interference can be minimized by administering the

immune globulin in a single dose, followed by a course of rabies vaccine (human diploid cell culture) therapy using postexposure dosages. Do not repeat the dose of rabies immune globulin.

∗ Slight soreness at the site of injection and slight temperature elevation may occur. In very rare instances cases of angioneurotic edema, nephrotic syndrome, and anaphylactic shock have been reported.

∗ There is no evidence of fetal abnormalities developing from rabies immune globulin. If a pregnant patient is exposed to rabies, treatment should follow the same guidelines as for nonpregnant patients.

∗ See General information on biologic agents (p. 564).

Drug interactions

Corticosteroids should not be administered to patients following exposure to rabies virus; the corticosteroids may interfere with the antibody-formation response to rabies vaccine.

Rabies vaccine (human diploid cell cultures)

AHFS 80:12

(Imovax rabies vaccine)

Action and use

Rabies vaccine is a stable, freeze-dried suspension of inactivated rabies virus that has been cultured on human diploid cells. The vaccine produces active immunity in 10 to 15 days after vaccination has started. It is recommended for persons (physicians, veterinarians, hospital personnel) who treat rabid patients or animals or those who work with rabies virus. It is also indicated for persons who may be potentially exposed to rabid animals while living or visiting regions where animal rabies occurs. Hunters, forest rangers, taxidermists, stock breeders, and slaughterhouse workers should be included in this category.

Administration and dosage

Preexposure dosage:

PRIMARY VACCINATION—3 IM injections of 1.0 ml each, given initially, on day 7, and on either day 21 or 28. Alternative: 0.1 ml intradermally (ID) in the lateral aspect of the upper arm over the deltoid initially, on day 7, and on either day 21 or 28.

BOOSTER DOSE—Persons working with live rabies virus should have rabies antibody titers checked every 6 months and boosters given as needed to maintain an adequate titer. Persons with continuing risk of exposure should have rabies antibody titers checked every 2 years, with boosters given as needed. The dosage is 1.0 ml either IM or ID.

Postexposure dosage:

1. 6 IM injections of 1.0 ml each, given initially and on days 3, 7, 14, 30, and 90. The first dose should be accompanied by an IM injection of rabies immune globulin (human).

2. For patients who have already been vaccinated, do *not* administer immune globulin. The number of doses of vaccine indicated is dependent on the level of rabies antibody titer present.

3. Before reconstitution, store at 2° to 8° C (35° to 46° F). Do not freeze. Use only the diluent supplied by the manufacturer to reconstitute the vaccine. Use immediately after reconstitution.

Nurse and patient considerations

∗ Soreness, swelling, and erythema at the site of injection (3% to 15%) and mild systemic reactions (1% to 4%) such as elevation in temperature and hives have been reported. No reactions have been reported to date that would necessitate discontinuation of the immunization schedule. Reactions may be treated with antiinflammatory and antipyretic agents (aspirin, diphenhydramine). If an anaphylactic reaction should occur, epinephrine should be administered.

∗ There is no evidence of fetal anomalies developing from rabies vaccine. If a pregnant patient is exposed

to rabies, treatment should follow the same guidelines as for nonpregnant patients.
* See General information on biologic agents (p. 564).

Drug interactions

Corticosteroids should not be administered to patients following exposure to rabies virus; the corticosteroids may interfere with the antibody-formation response to rabies vaccine.

Rh$_o$ (D) immune globulin (human)

AHFS 80:04

(RhoGAM, HypRho-D, Gamulin Rh)

Rh$_o$ (D) immune globulin (human) is used to prevent isoimmunization in the Rh$_o$ (D)-negative, D^u-negative patient exposed to Rh$_o$ (D)-positive or D^u-positive blood as the result of a transfusion accident, during a termination of a pregnancy, or as the result of a delivery of a Rh$_o$ (D)-positive or D^u-positive infant.

Rh hemolytic disease of the newborn can be prevented in subsequent pregnancies by administering Rh$_o$ (D) immune globulin (Rh$_o$ [D] antibody) to the Rh$_o$ (D)-negative, D^u-negative mother shortly after delivery of a Rh$_o$ (D)-positive or D^u-positive child. Rh$_o$ (D) immune globulin suppresses the stimulation of active immunity by Rh$_o$ (D)-positive or D^u-positive foreign red blood cells that enter the maternal circulation either at the time of delivery, termination of pregnancy, or during a transfusion reaction.

Administration and dosage

1. *Never* administer intravenously.
2. *Never* administer to to a neonate.
3. *Never* administer to an Rh$_o$ (D)-negative or D^u-negative patient who has been previously sensitized to the Rh$_o$ (D) or D^u antigen.
4. *Administer within 72 hr* only to postpartum mother, postmiscarriage woman, or the recipient in a transfusion accident.

One vial of Rh$_o$ (D) immune globulin will completely suppress the immune response to 15 ml of Rh-positive packed red blood cells.

Pregnancy

1. Postpartum prophylaxis: 1 vial IM. Additional vials may be necessary if there was unusually large fetal-maternal hemorrhage.
2. Antepartum prophylaxis: 1 vial IM at about 28 weeks gestational age. This *must* be followed by another vial administered within 72 hr of delivery.
3. Following miscarriage, abortion, or ectopic pregnancy: 1 vial IM.

Transfusion

Rh-negative, premenopausal women who receive Rh-positive red cells by transfusion: 1 vial IM for each 15 ml of transfused packed red cells.

Nurse and patient considerations

* Adverse effects are infrequent, but an occasional patient may respond with a slight elevation in temperature. Patients who receive several vials as the result of a mismatched transfusion may report fever, myalgia, and lethargy with mild jaundice.
* There is no evidence to indicate that there is any danger to the fetus when Rh_o (D) immune globulin is administered to the mother ante partum.

Rubella virus vaccine, live　　AHFS 80:12
(Various)

Rubella virus vaccine is administered to provide active immunity against rubella (German measles). The vaccine is not effective in the prevention of rubeola (measles), nor is it of any benefit when administered to patients after they have been exposed to rubella virus.

Administration and dosage

sc—0.5 ml.

Before reconstitution, store at 2° to 8° C (35° to 46° F). Protect from light.

Use only the diluent supplied by the manufacturer to reconstitute the vaccine.

Use the reconstituted vaccine as soon as possible. Protect from light and store at 2° to 8° C (35° to 46° F). Discard if not used within 8 hr of reconstitution.

The color of the reconstituted solution may vary from red to pink to yellow. It may be administered if crystal clear.

Nurse and patient considerations

* Rubella virus vaccine *must not* be administered to pregnant women or those who may become pregnant within the following 3 months. Multiple teratogenic effects are associated with naturally acquired rubella virus infections, although the possible effects of the vaccine on fetal development are unknown at this time.

* Rubella virus vaccine should be administered with caution in patients who have shown previous allergic reactions to neomycin, chicken or duck feathers or eggs, dogs, or rabbits. Epinephrine should be available for immediate use should an anaphylactoid reaction occur.

* It is not uncommon for patients, especially older women, to experience symptoms of joint and muscle stiffness and pain and peripheral numbness and tingling within 4 weeks after administration of the vaccine. Patients may be assured that the symptoms are transient and that there are no long-term complications.

* See General information on biologic agents (p. 564).

Tetanus immune globulin (human), USP

AHFS 80:04

Tetanus immune globulin is a solution of gamma globulin pooled from venous plasma of individuals hyperimmunized to tetanus. Each vial (and prefilled syringe) contains 250 units of tetanus antibody.

Human antitetanus globulin is used to provide immediate passive immunization for patients exposed to the risk of tetanus. The administration of 250 units provides protective levels of antibody for several weeks. Tetanus toxoid may be administered concurrently to allow the patient to develop active immunity to tetanus while deriving short-term protection from tetanus immune globulin.

Administration and dosage
Adult

IM—250 units.

Pediatric

IM—4 units/kg.
    Store at 2° to 8° C (36° to 46° F). Do not freeze.
NOTE: See General information on biologic agents (p. 564).

Tetanus antitoxin, USP   AHFS 80:04

Tetanus antitoxin is a sterile solution of the refined and concentrated proteins, primarily globulins, containing antibodies obtained from the blood plasma of a healthy animal, usually the horse, that has been immunized with tetanus toxin or toxoid, thus producing antitoxin antibodies.

Tetanus antitoxin may be used in the treatment and prophylaxis of tetanus, creating passive immunity. It is recommended for use, however, only if tetanus immune globulin (human) is not available. Antitoxins are derived from animal sources and contain foreign proteins that may initiate an allergic reaction.

Tetanus toxoid, USP   AHFS 80:08

Tetanus toxoid is a sterile solution of the formaldehyde-treated products of growth of the tetanus bacillus *(Clostridium tetani)*. Treatment with formaldehyde and heat causes modification of the toxins, resulting in loss of toxic effects but with retention of the property for inducing active immunity. Adequate dosages provide active immunity against tetanus.

Administration and dosage

IM—0.5 ml of tetanus toxoid, USP 4 weeks apart, with a
    booster at 9 months and subsequent boosters every 10
    years.
NOTE: *Shake well before administration*. See General information on biologic agents (p. 564).

DTP (diphtheria and tetanus AHFS 80:08 toxoids and pertussis vaccine)

DTP is used for simultaneous active immunization against diphtheria, tetanus, and pertussis. (It is not recommended for use in children over 6 years of age.) The combination product reduces the number of necessary injections and does not impair the resultant immunity.

Primary immunization may be started as early as 2 months of age.

Administration and dosage

IM
1. Primary immunization: 3 doses of 0.5 ml each, 4 to 6 weeks apart.
2. Reinforcing dose; 0.5 ml, 1 year after third primary immunization dose.
3. A second reinforcing dose is recommended upon entering school.

Store at 2° to 8° C. (36° to 46° F). Do not freeze.

NOTE: *Shake thoroughly*. See General information on biologic agents (p. 564).

CHAPTER TWENTY-FOUR

Antihyperlipidemic agents

Cholestyramine
Clofibrate
Colestipol hydrochloride

Gemfibrozil
Probucol

Cholestyramine
(Questran)

AHFS 24:06
CATEGORY Adsorbant resin

Action and use

Cholestyramine is an insoluble anion-exchange resin that interrupts enterohepatic recirculation by binding to bile acids in the intestine. The insoluble complex formed is then excreted in the feces.

The primary use of cholestyramine is treatment of patients with elevated cholesterol levels. In conjunction with diet control, cholestyramine reduces cholesterol by binding to and enhancing the excretion of low-density lipoproteins (LDL). Cholestyramine is usually used only in patients with excesses of LDL (familial hypercholesterolemia, type II). It has no activity on chylomicrons or intermediate density lipoproteins (IDL) and may elevate very low–density lipoproteins (VLDL). Thus it should not be used to treat hyperlipoproteinemias of types I, III, IV, or V.

Because of its binding capacities, cholestyramine may also be used to treat severe diarrhea secondary to diabetes mellitus, vagotomy, or antibiotic associated colitis, and to decrease digitoxin levels or hyperbilirubinemia by inhibiting its enterohepatic circulation.

Characteristics

Type II hyperlipidemia: LDL start falling within 4 to 7 days, with maximal effects within about 2 weeks. Total reduction in LDL is 25% to 35%.

Administration and dosage
Adult

PO—1 tsp (about 4 g of resin) 3 or 4 times daily with meals. The resin must be mixed with 2 to 6 ounces of water, fruit juices, soups, or applesauce and should be allowed to stand in the liquid for a few minutes to allow complete absorption and dispersion. Never attempt to swallow in the dry form. Follow administration with another glass of water.

NOTE: Cholestyramine should be administered at least 1 to 2 hr after other medications to prevent adsorption and binding of these medications to the resin. Patients must restrict their dietary intake of cholesterol and saturated fats and limit ingestion of sugar and alcohol.

Nurse and patient considerations

* The most frequent adverse effect is constipation. This problem is usually transient but may be aleviated by increasing fluid intake, especially when the resin is mixed, or by reducing the dosage. If the patient becomes constipated, add roughage to the diet, increase fluids, add a stool softener (docusate sodium [Colace]), and/or decrease the dosage.

* Other adverse effects include abdominal discomfort, heartburn, anorexia, diarrhea, and rash and irritation of the skin, tongue, and perianal area. Since cholestyramine is in the chloride form of the exchange resin, it may produce hyperchloremic acidosis. Younger and smaller patients may be more prone to this because the relative dosage may be higher.

* When cholestyramine is administered for long periods of time, deficiencies of the lipid-soluble vitamins A, D, and K may develop. Hypoprothrombinemia, with and without bleeding, has been reported. These rare reports occur most frequently in elderly, debilitated, or otherwise compromised patients with a borderline deficiency of vitamin K. Folate deficiency has also been reported. Supplementation with water-miscible or parenteral vitamins should be considered.

* Cholestyramine contains FD & C Yellow no. 5 dye (tartrazine). This dye rarely causes allergy, but patients most susceptible are those who are prone to allergy and those who have aspirin hypersensitivity.

* Check serum cholesterol and serum triglycerides along with CBC, electrolytes, and glucose levels periodically during drug therapy.

> * Since cholestyramine is not absorbed, it is not
> expected that there would be problems with use in
> pregnant or nursing patients. Therapy, however,
> should be on a risk to benefit basis.

Drug interactions

Cholestyramine may reduce the absorption of concomitant oral medication such as phenylbutazone, warfarin, chlorothiazide, tetracycline, penicillin G, phenobarbital, thyroid and thyroxine preparations, and digitalis glycosides. Use extreme caution with close observation in initiating or discontinuing cholestyramine therapy in patients receiving other medications. Patients should take other drugs at least 1 hr before or 4 to 6 hr after colestipol to avoid impeding absorption.

Clofibrate
(Atromid S)

AHFS 24:06
CATEGORY Antilipemic agent

Action and use

Clofibrate is an antilipemic agent structurally related to gemfibrozil. It is particularly effective in reducing elevated serum triglyceride levels and is therefore used to treat types III, IV, and V hyperlipoproteinemias. Clofibrate appears to have several sites of action; its mechanisms of action are largely unknown.

Characteristics

Primary activity is due to a metabolite, chlorophenoxyisobutyric acid (CPIB). Onset: 2 to 5 days. Protein binding (CPIB): 95%. Half-life (CPIB): 54 hr. Excretion: in urine, 60% as glucuronide. Dialysis: unknown.

Administration and dosage

PO—2 g daily divided into 2 to 4 doses. Administer with meals to reduce stomach upset.

NOTE: Before initiating therapy, attempts should be made to control serum triglycerides by weight reduction and dietary control. Serum cholesterol and triglyceride levels should be measured before and every 2 weeks during initial therapy. After 3 months of therapy, the patient should be fully reevaluated to determine whether further therapy is justified.

Nurse and patient considerations

∗ Two large clinical studies with clofibrate have shown that there was no difference in mortality between clofibrate- and placebo-treated patients with previous myocardial infarction; there was a significantly higher incidence of gallstone formation and cholecystitis requiring surgery in the clofibrate-treated group; and there was a 36% higher mortality from noncardiovascular causes (malignancy, postcholecystectomy complications, pancreatitis) in the group treated with clofibrate. One of the studies also reported an increase in cardiac arrhythmias, intermittent claudication, angina, and thromboembolic activity in the clofibrate-treated group.

∗ Gastrointestinal complaints of nausea, vomiting, flatulence, and abdominal cramping and diarrhea occur most frequently. Most symptoms are mild and diminish with continued therapy.

∗ Other rare adverse effects include drowsiness, weakness, skin reactions, cardiac arrhythmias, decreased libido in men, and "flulike symptoms" (muscle aches, soreness, and cramping).

∗ Check serum cholesterol and triglycerides along with CBC, electrolytes, and glucose levels periodically during drug therapy.

∗ Use clofibrate with caution in patients with hepatic and renal disease. Dosage adjustment may be required if the decision is made to continue therapy.

∗ Do not use in pregnant or lactating women. Animal studies indicate that fetal enzyme immaturity inhibits metabolism of clofibrate. In patients who plan to become pregnant, clofibrate should be withdrawn several months before conception.

Drug interactions

Clofibrate displaces warfarin (Coumadin) from protein-binding sites. If concomitant therapy is indicated, start warfarin at half the normal dosage and adjust the dosage according to the prothrombin time.

Clofibrate may induce hypoglycemic episodes by blocking the renal excretion of the oral hypoglycemic agent chlorpropamide (Diabinese).

Furosemide (Lasix) and clofibrate may compete for similar protein-binding sites. Observe patients receiving both agents for increased clinical response and/or toxicity from either agent.

Probenecid inhibits the metabolism of clofibrate. Patients complaining of the development of muscle pain and weakness while taking clofibrate and probenecid concomitantly should be evaluated with the possibility of reducing the clofibrate dosage.

Colestipol hydrochloride
(Colestid)

AHFS 24:06
CATEGORY Adsorbant resin

Action and use

Colestipol is an insoluble anion-exchange resin structurally unrelated to other binding resins. Contrary to cholestyramine, it is odorless and tasteless. It is used in conjunction with diet control to reduce elevated serum cholesterol in primary hypercholesterolemia (type IIa hyperlipidemia).

Administration and dosage
Adults

PO—15 to 30 g daily divided into 2 to 4 doses. The granular resin must be mixed with 2 to 6 ounces of water, fruit juices, soups, or applesauce and should be allowed to stand in the liquid for a few minutes to allow complete absorption and dispersion. Never attempt to swallow in the dry form. Follow administration with another glass of water.

NOTE: Colestipol should be administered at least 1 to 2 hr after other medications to prevent adsorption and binding of the medication to the resin.

Nurse and patient considerations

* The most frequent adverse effect is constipation (10%). This problem is usually transient but may be alleviated by increasing fluid intake, especially when the resin is mixed, or by reducing the dosage.
* Other adverse effects include abdominal discomfort, heartburn, belching, anorexia, flatulence, diarrhea, and rash and irritation of the skin, tongue, and perianal area.

* When colestipol is administered for long periods of time, deficiencies of the lipid-soluble vitamins A, D, and K may develop. Hypoprothrombinemia, with and without bleeding, has been reported. These rare reports occur most frequently in elderly, debilitated, or otherwise compromised patients with borderline deficiency of vitamin K. Supplementation with water-miscible or parenteral vitamins should be considered.
* Check serum cholesterol and triglycerides along with CBC, electrolytes, and glucose levels periodically during drug therapy.
* Since colestipol is not absorbed, it is not expected that there would be problems with use in pregnant or nursing patients. Therapy, however, should be on a risk to benefit basis.

Drug interactions

Colestipol may reduce the absorption of concomitant oral medication such as phenylbutazone, warfarin, chlorothiazide, tetracycline, penicillin G, phenobarbital, thyroid and thyroxine preparations, and digitalis glycosides. Use extreme caution with close observation in initiating or discontinuing colestipol therapy in patients receiving other medications. Patients should take other drugs at least 1 hr before or 4 to 6 hr after colestipol to avoid impeding absorption.

Gemfibrozil
(Lopid)

AHFS 24:06
CATEGORY Antilipemic agent

Action and use

Gemfibrozil is a lipid-regulating agent that acts by inhibiting peripheral lipolysis and hepatic triglyceride synthesis. The net result is a reduction in the very low–density lipoprotein (VDL) fraction, occasionally a reduction of the low-density lipoprotein (LDL) fraction, and an elevation of the high-density lipoprotein (HDL) cholesterol fraction. Gemfibrozil, in conjunction with diet control, is indicated in the treatment of type IV hyperlipidemia when diet alone has not been effective in reducing serum triglyceride levels.

Characteristics

Peak serum levels: 1 to 2 hr. Half-life: 1.3 hr. Metabolism: liver. Excretion: 70% in urine as unchanged drug, 6% in feces. Dialysis: unknown. Breast milk: unknown.

Administration and dosage

NOTE: Gemfibrozil is contraindicated in patients with gallbladder disease, hepatic or biliary cirrhosis, or severe renal dysfunction. Serum lipid levels should be measured before the initiation of therapy and 3 months later. If there is no significant improvement in triglyceride levels, therapy should be discontinued.

Adult

PO—600 mg 30 min before morning and evening meals. Dosage range: 900 to 1500 mg daily.

Nurse and patient considerations

* Because of structural and pharmacologic similarities between gemfibrozil and clofibrate, the adverse findings of two large clinical studies may also apply to gemfibrozil. The studies showed that there was no difference in mortality between the clofibrate- and placebo-treated patients with a previous myocardial infarction; there was a significantly higher incidence of gallstone formation and cholecystitis requiring surgery in the clofibrate-treated group; and there was a 36% higher mortality from noncardiovascular causes (malignancy, postcholecystectomy complications, pancreatitis) in the group treated with clofibrate.
* Adverse effects observed with gemfibrozil therapy are abdominal pain (6%), epigastric pain (5%), diarrhea (4.8%), nausea (4%), vomiting (1.6%), and flatulence (1.1%). Other adverse effects reported include rash, pruritus, headache, dizziness, and painful extremities. Patients also reported a higher incidence of colds, coughs, and urinary tract infections than placebo-treated patients.
* Abnormalities in laboratory tests that have developed during gemfibrozil therapy are mild decreases in hemoglobin and hematocrit levels and white blood cells and elevations of SGOT, SGPT, LDH, and alkaline phosphatase levels. These laboratory

tests should be repeated periodically. Therapy should be discontinued if abnormalities persist.
* High doses of gemfibrozil have been found to be tumorigenic in laboratory animals. No teratogenic effects have been reported, but gemfibrozil therapy is not recommended in pregnant or nursing mothers because of the potential for tumorigenicity.

Drug interactions

Gemfibrozil interacts with warfarin to enhance the anticoagulant activity. Prothrombin times should be closely monitored to prevent excessive anticoagulation and bleeding.

Probucol
(Lorelco)

AHFS 24:06
CATEGORY Antilipemic agent

Action and use

Probucol is used to reduce elevated serum cholesterol levels in patients with primary type II hyperlipoproteinemia. Effects on serum triglyceride levels are variable. The mechanism of action is unknown, and therapy should be instituted only after dietary therapy has failed to reduce elevated cholesterol levels adequately.

Characteristics

Probucol is poorly absorbed from the gastrointestinal tract, and 3 months of therapy may be required before significant reduction in serum cholesterol levels is noted. Elimination is biphasic; initial phase half-life is 24 hr, second phase half-life is about 20 days. Metabolic fate is unknown.

Administration and dosage

PO—500 mg twice daily administered *with* meals.

Nurse and patient considerations

* Diarrhea may occur in about 10% of patients. Flatulence, nausea, and vomiting may also occur, but they are usually mild and subside with continued administration. Hyperhydrosis (excessive perspira-

tion) and foul-smelling sweat have also been reported. Of patients in clinical trials, 2% discontinued therapy because of side effects.

* Before initiation of therapy, hypercholesterolemia must first be treated by weight reduction and dietary control. Serum cholesterol and triglyceride levels should be measured prior to and during therapy. After 6 months of therapy, the patient must be reevaluated to determine whether further therapy is justified.

* Safe use of probucol in pregnant or lactating patients has not been established.

Drug interactions

No specific drug interactions have been reported.

CHAPTER TWENTY-FIVE

Miscellaneous agents

Atropine sulfate

AHFS 12:08
CATEGORY Anticholinergic

Action and use

Atropine blocks the cholinergic response by competitively binding to the acetylcholine receptor site. This reduces vagal tone, enhances atrioventricular conduction, and accelerates the cardiac rate. It also suppresses perspiration, saliva, bronchial mucus and gastric secretion and produces mydriasis. Atropine is indicated for the treatment of sinus bradycardia with a pulse of less than 60 beats/min when accompanied by PVCs or a systolic blood pressure of less than 90 mm Hg. It is also used in AV block with bradycardia. Other uses of atropine include control of secretions and spasm of smooth muscle during surgery and the symptomatic treatment of organophosphate insecticide poisoning.

Administration and dosage
Adult

IM—0.3 to 1.2 mg.

IV—0.3 to 1.2 mg (usual dose: 0.5 mg) bolus; may be repeated in 4 to 5 min if pulse rate is less than 60 beats/min.

Pediatric

PO—0.01 mg/kg; may repeat every 2 hours as needed. The maximum single dose is 0.4 mg.

SC or IM—As for PO administration.

Nurse and patient considerations

∗ The total dosage of atropine sulfate should not exceed 2 mg except in cases of third degree AV block and the treatment of organophosphate insecticide poisoning, when larger dosages may be required.

∗ Side effects often include dry mouth with thirst and dysphagia, flushing, dizziness, blurred vision and photophobia, tachycardia, and urinary retention.

∗ Indications of atropine toxicity include anxiety, delirium, disorientation, hallucinations, hyperactivity, convulsions, and respiratory depression.

Drug interactions

Enhanced anticholinergic effects may occur with tricyclic antidepressants (amitriptyline [Elavil], imipramine [Tofranil], doxepin [Sinequan]), haloperidol (Haldol), procainamide (Pronestyl), quinidine, antihistamines, and meperidine (Demerol).

Benztropine
(Cogentin)

AHFS 12:08
CATEGORY Anticholinergic

Action and use

Benztropine is an anticholinergic, antihistaminic agent used to help control the symptoms of parkinsonism (tremor; drooling, rigidity in gait, posture, and balance; and masklike facies). It may also be effective in controlling extrapyramidal effects caused by other drugs such as phenothiazines.

Administration and dosage

PO 1. Parkinsonism: usual dosage is 1 to 2 mg daily, with a range of 0.5 to 6 mg/day. Therapy should be initiated at low doses, 0.5 to 1 mg daily, and increased in increments of 0.5 mg every 5 to 6 days because of its accumulative activity.

2. Drug-induced extrapyramidal disorders: 1 to 4 mg 1 to 2 times daily usually provides relief in 1 to 2 days.

IM—Acute drug-induced extrapyramidal disorders: 1 to 2 mg. If the symptoms return, repeat the dosage. After parenteral doses, PO administration 1 to 2 mg 2 times daily usually prevents recurrence.

iv—As for IM administration.

Nurse and patient considerations

* Dry mouth, blurred vision, nausea, and nervousness may develop and become severe enough to require dosage adjustment. Patients may also complain of constipation, numbness of the fingers, listlessness, and depression.

* With higher dosages mental confusion and visual hallucinations may occur. In patients being treated for mental disorders with phenothiazines or reserpine, psychiatric symptoms may be exacerbated, and antiparkinsonian drugs can precipitate a toxic psychosis.

* After long-term therapy with phenothiazines, patients may develop tardive dyskinesia. Benztropine is usually not effective against these symptoms (involuntary movement of the mouth and face with frequent smacking of the lips with thrusting tongue movement) and in some instances may aggravate this adverse effect.

* Benztropine may produce anhidrosis, a decrease or absence of secretion of sweat. This adverse effect may be seen in hot weather, in older, chronically ill patients, in alcoholics, and in those patients who have CNS disorders. Dosage may have to be diminished to allow body heat equilibration.

* Benztropine may aggravate narrow-angle glaucoma and is not recommended for use in patients with this disease.

* Benztropine probably should not be used in pregnancy and may diminish lactation in the nursing mother.

Drug interactions

Benztropine may display additive anticholinergic effects (dry mouth, constipation, urinary retention, blurred vision) when administered with antihistamines, phenothiazines, trihexiphenidyl (Artane), meperidine (Demerol), and other agents with anticholinergic activity.

Calcium chloride

AHFS 68:24

Action and use

Calcium chloride increases myocardial contractility, prolongs systole, and enhances ventricular excitability. It is useful in profound cardiovascular collapse (for example, electromechanical dissociation where QRS complexes are observed without an adequate pulse). It may be useful in restoring an electrical rhythm in instances of asystole and may enhance electrical defibrillation.

Administration and dosage

NOTE: Do not administer IM. It is extremely irritating to tissues.

IV—2.5 to 5 ml of 10% calcium chloride (3.4 to 6.8 mEq Ca^{2+}). Rate is 1 to 2 ml/min. When required, calcium chloride boluses may be repeated every 10 min.

Nurse and patient considerations

* Digitalis and calcium ions are synergistic in their inotropic and toxic effects. Use with extreme caution in digitalized patients.
* Calcium gluconate provides less ionizable calcium per unit volume. If it is used the dose should be 10 ml of a 10% solution (4.8 mEq Ca^{2+}). Calcium gluceptate, 5 ml (4.5 mEq Ca^{2+}) may also be used.

Drug interactions

Beware of injecting calcium chloride and sodium bicarbonate concurrently or immediately following each other. Rinse the line briefly to avoid precipitation.

Cimetidine
(Tagamet)

AHFS 56:40
CATEGORY H_2 receptor antagonist

Action and use

Cimetidine is the first histamine H_2 receptor antagonist approved by the Food and Drug Administration for use in the United States. Cimetidine inhibits the action of histamine on specific H_2 receptors of parietal cells of the stomach, reducing gastric acid output. It has no apparent effect on gastric motility, emptying time, or biliary or pancreatic secretion. Cimetidine is now being extensively used in the management of duodenal ulcers and pathologic hypersecretory conditions such as Zollinger-Ellison syndrome and for the prevention and treatment of stress ulcers.

Characteristics

Onset: 20 to 30 min (PO). Peak activity: (fasting PO): biphasic, 1 to 2 hr, 3 to 5 hr. Duration: 4 to 5 hr. Protein binding: 13% to 25%. Metabolism: hepatic to two inactive metabolites. Half-life: 2 hr (normal renal function), 2$\frac{9}{10}$ hr (CCR = 20 to 50 ml/min), 3$\frac{7}{10}$ hr (CCR = less than 20 ml/min), 5 to 10 hr (anephric patients). Excretion: 60% to 75% unchanged in urine, 20% to 40% as metabolites in urine, 10% in feces. Dialysis: yes, H. Breast milk: yes.

Administration and dosage
Adult

PO—300 mg 4 times daily with meals and at bedtime. Dosage increases should be made by increasing the frequency of administration. Do not exceed 2.4 g daily. Antacid therapy may be continued for relief of symptoms but should be administered 1 to 2 hr before or after the cimetidine dosage.

IV—300 mg every 6 hr. Dilute in 20 ml of saline solution or dextrose 5% and administer over 1 to 2 min *or* dilute in 100 ml of IV fluid and infuse over 15 to 20 min.

NOTE: Initial recommended dosage for patients with impaired renal function is 300 mg every 12 hr.

Pediatric

Cimetidine is not recommended in patients under 16 years of age.

Nurse and patient considerations

* Adverse reactions reported with use of cimetidine are usually quite mild. Mental confusion, slurred speech, and disorientation are associated with the use of high dosages in patients with hepatic dysfunction renal dysfunction and patients over 50 years of age. Mild bilateral gynecomastia and breast soreness may occur on long-term use (greater than 1 month) but resolves after discontinuation of therapy. Other adverse effects include transient hyperthermia, maculopapular rashes, urticaria, muscular pain, transient neutropenia, hypotension, and bradycardia.

＊ Safe use in pregnancy has not been established.

Drug interactions

Limited evidence indicates that cimetidine may inhibit the metabolism of quinidine. Observe patients for evidence of quinidine toxicity and reduce the dosage if necessary.

Cimetidine significantly inhibits the metabolism of chlordiazepoxide (Librium), diazepam (Valium), and possibly clorazepate (Tranxene), flurazepam (Dalmane), halazepam (Paxipam), and prazepam (Centrax). The metabolism of temazepam (Restoril), oxazepam (Serax), and lorazepam (Ativan) does not appear to be affected. Patients taking cimetidine and a benzodiazepine concurrently should be observed for increased sedation and may require a reduction in dosage of the benzodiazepine.

Cimetidine enhances the hypoprothrombinemic effects of warfarin (Coumadin). A reduction in the dosage of warfarin will usually be necessary to prevent excessive anticoagulation.

It significantly impairs the hepatic metabolism of theophylline derivatives, causing an increase in serum levels with potential for toxicity. Patients at greater risk include those receiving large doses of theophylline and/or those with diseases that impair theophylline metabolism. Patients should be monitored closely for signs of toxicity.

Cimetidine impairs the elimination of phenytoin (Dilantin) in some patients. Patients should be monitored closely for signs of phenytoin toxicity.

Cimetidine significantly inhibits the metabolism of propranolol (Inderal) and probably certain other beta-adrenergic blocking agents that are metabolized by the liver. The patient's cardiovascular status should be monitored closely. Nadolol (Corgard) and atenolol (Tenormin) are excreted by the kidneys unchanged and do not interact with cimetidine.

Cimetidine prolongs the activity of lidocaine. Monitor patients closely for toxicity to lidocaine infusion.

Antacids appear to affect the absorption of cimetidine. Antacid and cimetidine doses should be separated by 1 to 2 hr.

Cimetidine inhibits the metabolism and excretion of

procainamide and its metabolite, N-acetylprocainamide. Observe patients closely for an altered procainamide response if cimetidine therapy is started or stopped.

Diphenoxylate hydrochloride
(Lomotil)

<small>AHFS 56:08; C-V</small>
<small>CATEGORY Antidiarrheal agent</small>

Action and use

Diphenoxylate is a synthetic narcotic derivative that diminishes intestinal smooth muscle spasm, thus inhibiting gastrointestinal motility. Lomotil is a combination product containing diphenoxylate, 2.5 mg, and atropine, 0.025 mg. The atropine is added in subtherapeutic dosages to prevent deliberate abuse. Lomotil is used for the symptomatic relief of acute nonspecific diarrhea.

Characteristics

Onset of action: 45 to 60 min. Peak activity: 2 hr. Duration: 3 to 4 hr. Half-life: 2½ hr. Metabolism: to diphenoxylic acid (active) and hydroxydiphenoxylic acid. Excretion: primarily fecal.

Administration and dosage
Adult

PO—Initially, 2 tablets or 10 ml of Lomotil liquid 4 times daily. After control is achieved, reduce the dosage as needed to maintain control (usually 1 tablet 4 times daily).

Pediatric (2 to 12 years of age)

NOTE: Do not use in patients under 2 years of age. Pediatric patients are more susceptible to atropine overdosage.
1. Initial dosage (Lomotil liquid):

Ages 2 to 5 years

PO—4 ml 3 times daily.

Ages 5 to 8 years

PO—4 ml 4 times daily.

Ages 8 to 12 years

PO—4 ml 5 times daily.
2. After control is achieved, reduce the dosage to half the initial dosage.

Nurse and patient considerations

∗ Overdosage of Lomotil results in symptoms related to narcotic analgesic overdosage (diphenoxylate) and atropine toxicity. The full effects of overdosage may not be apparent until 24 to 30 hr after the agent was taken. Early manifestations may include symptoms of atropism such as tachycardia, dry mouth, nose, and throat, flushing, and hyperthermia. Symptoms progress to include drowsiness, hypotonia, hyperreflexia, nystagmus, miosis, and convulsions followed by respiratory depression and total apnea.

∗ All cases of diarrhea should be investigated fully, and specific treatment instituted as soon as possible. Lomotil, an antimotility drug, is indicated only for *symptomatic* control of diarrhea. Do not use in (1) acute diarrhea when bacterial pathogens are suspected, since medications that slow intestinal motility may delay clearance of infecting organisms from the bowel; (2) antibiotic-induced colitis, since it may prolong the disorder; and (3) severe, acute attacks of ulcerative colitis, since antimotility drugs may cause a paralytic ileus with overdilatation of the bowel (toxic megacolon).

∗ Treatment consists of gastric lavage, close observation for at least 48 hr, use of naloxone (Narcan) to reverse respiratory depression, and mechanical ventilatory assistance. Patients may require multiple doses of naloxone because of its short duration of activity. Urinary bladder catheterization may also be necessary because of urinary retention.

∗ Side effects reported during diphenoxylate therapy are usually gastrointestinal in nature and may be related to the condition being treated. Nausea, vomiting, and abdominal distention are common side effects. Other side effects reported include sedation, dizziness, tachycardia, numbness of extremities, blurred vision, weakness, and mental depression.

∗ Allergic manifestations including pruritus, urticaria, and angioneurotic edema have been reported.

∗ Use with caution in patients with cirrhosis or other liver disease. Hepatic coma has been reported following administration of Lomotil to these patients.

∗ Repeated use may lead to tolerance, dependence, and addiction. Evaluate the *patient's* response to this antidiarrheal product and suggest a change to another form of antidiarrheal product when indicated. Observe patients for dehydration and electrolyte imbalance (see Table 4-1).

* Lomotil should be used with caution in pregnant and lactating women. Effects on the fetus are unknown. Diphenoxylate and atropine are excreted in breast milk.

Drug interactions

The depressant effects of diphenoxylate are additive with those of general anesthetics, phenothiazines, tranquilizers, sedative-hypnotics, tricyclic depressants, antihistamines, and other CNS depressants, including alcohol.

Disulfiram
(Antabuse)

AHFS 92:00
CATEGORY Antialcohol agent

Action and use

Disulfiram is an agent that, when ingested before any form of alcohol, produces a very unpleasant reaction to the alcohol. Disulfiram acts by inhibiting the metabolic pathway of alcohol, allowing an intermediate by-product, acetaldehyde, to accumulate to 5 to 10 times its normal concentration. The "Antabuse reaction" is actually the body's physiologic response to toxic amounts of acetaldehyde.

Disulfiram therapy is not a cure for alcoholism but is strictly an aid to patients abstaining from alcohol while receiving appropriate psychiatric support. Patients must truly want to discontinue drinking for disulfiram therapy to be anything but a short-term benefit.

Administration and dosage

NOTE: Disulfiram must never be administered to patients when they are in a state of intoxication or when they are unaware of receiving therapy. Family members should also be knowledgeable of the treatment to help provide motivation and support and to help avoid accidental disulfiram-alcohol reactions.

Do not administer disulfiram until the patient has abstained from alcohol for at least 12 hr.

PO 1. Initially, a maximum of 500 mg 1 time daily for 1 to 2 weeks. It may be administered at bedtime to avoid sedative side effects.

2. Maintenance dosage is usually 250 mg daily (range: 125 to 500 mg). Do not exceed 500 mg daily.
3. Therapy is continued for weeks to months until a patient has shown strong evidence of social rehabilitation and self-control. The longer patients are on therapy, the more sensitive they are to alcohol.

For treatment of disulfiram-alcohol reaction:

Generally, therapy is only supportive, consisting of monitoring the patient's vital signs and maintaining electrolytes and hydration. If severe hypotension or shock develops, treat with pressor agents such as dopamine. Other recommendations include oxygen, carbogen (95% oxygen and 5% carbon dioxide), vitamin C in 1 g IV doses, and ephedrine sulfate.

Nurse and patient considerations

* Patients must be fully informed of the consequences of drinking alcohol while receiving disulfiram therapy. Ten to 15 ml of alcohol ingested by a patient receiving therapeutic doses of disulfiram produces a reaction (usually within 5 to 10 min) that is initially characterized by a sensation of facial warmth. The face soon becomes flushed and scarlet. Vasodilatation spreads throughout the body, producing intense throbbing in the head and neck with a pulsating headache. Respiratory difficulties, nausea, copious vomiting, sweating, thirst, chest pain, palpitations, dyspnea, tachycardia, hypotension, weakness, marked uneasiness, vertigo, blurred vision, and mental confusion may develop. Very severe reactions may produce respiratory depression, cardiovascular collapse, arrhythmias, myocardial infarction, acute congestive heart failure, unconsciousness, convulsions, and/or death. The intensity of the reaction is somewhat dependent on the sensitivity of the individual and the amount of alcohol consumed. The duration of the reaction depends on the presence of alcohol in the blood. Mild reactions may last from 30 to 60 min, whereas more severe reactions may last for several hours. Disulfiram does not appear to inhibit the rate of metabolism of alcohol.
* Patients must be fully informed of dietary and drug restrictions necessary to prevent accidental reactions. Patients must not ingest alcohol in any form.

This restriction applies to over-the-counter products containing alcohol such as sleep aids, cough and cold products, aftershave lotions, topicals, mouthwashes, and rubbing lotions and dietary supplements such as sauces and vinegars. A disulfiram-alcohol reaction may occur with the ingestion of any alcohol for 1 to 2 weeks after the discontinuation of disulfiram therapy.

* Disulfiram generally does not induce many side effects; however, some patients have reported drowsiness, fatigability, impotence, headache, acne and allergic dermatitis, or a metallic or garlic taste associated with disulfiram therapy. These side effects are generally mild and transient.

* Because of the consequences of a disulfiram-alcohol reaction on other disease states, use disulfiram therapy very cautiously in patients with diabetes mellitus, hypothyroidism, epilepsy, cerebral damage, chronic and acute nephritis, hepatic cirrhosis, or hepatic insufficiency.

* Baseline transaminase levels are recommended, with follow-up levels in 10 to 14 days, to detect hepatic dysfunction that has been rarely reported. Routine liver and kidney function tests, as well as measurement of electrolytes, are recommended every 6 months.

* Safety in pregnancy has not been established. Use only when the benefits of therapy significantly outweigh the risk of toxicity to the fetus.

Drug interactions

Coagulation studies must be monitored closely when disulfiram is administered concurrently with warfarin. Disulfiram probably inhibits the metabolism of warfarin.

Disulfiram inhibits the metabolism of phenytoin, resulting in signs of phenytoin toxicity (nystagmus, ataxia, lethargy, and confusion). The dosage of phenytoin may need to be reduced.

Disulfiram alters the metabolism of isoniazid, causing changes in behavior, mental status, and physical coordination. Discontinue disulfiram if these adverse effects develop.

Combined therapy of disulfiram and metronidazole may result in psychotic episodes and confusional states. Combined therapy is not recommended.

Hetastarch
(Hespan)

AHFS 40:12
CATEGORY Plasma expander

Action and use

Hetastarch is an artificial colloid suitable for use as a plasma expander. Its plasma-expanding capabilities are somewhat similar to those of human albumin. Hetastarch is not a substitute for blood or plasma but is used to expand plasma volume in the treatment of shock associated with hemorrhage, burns, surgery, infection, and other trauma.

Characteristics

IV infusion of hetastarch expands plasma volume slightly in excess of the volume infused. The plasma expansion activity then diminishes over the next 24 to 36 hr. Approximately 40% of a given total dose is excreted via the urine within 24 hr. Less than 1% of the total infused dose remains in the vascular compartment after 2 weeks. Solution osmolarity: 310 m0sm/L. Concentration of electrolytes (mEq/L): sodium 154, chloride 154.

Administration and dosage
Adult

IV 1. Plasma volume expansion: 500 to 1000 ml/24 hr, not to exceed 1500 ml/day or approximately 20 ml/kg/24 hr.

2. The total dosage and rate of infusion is dependent on the amount of blood lost and the amount of hemoconcentration. In acute hemorrhagic shock, a rate of 20 ml/kg/hr may be used. Burn or septic shock usually requires slower rates.

NOTE: Hetastarch must be used with extreme caution in patients with severe bleeding disorders, congestive heart failure, and renal failure with oliguria or anuria.

Nurse and patient considerations

* Large volumes of hetastarch may alter the coagulation mechanism, resulting in transient prolongation of the prothrombin, partial thromboplastin, and clotting times.
* Hemodilution manifested by a drop in hematocrit and plasma protein values should be expected.

* Circulatory overload resulting in congestive heart failure and pulmonary edema may develop if patients are not closely observed. Monitor fluid input and all sources of fluid loss, breath sounds, and central venous pressure or pulmonary wedge pressure and cardiac output if available.
* Hypersensitivity reactions manifested by urticaria, wheezing, and periorbital edema have been reported. Treat by immediate discontinuation of the hetastarch infusion, and, if necessary, administration of an antihistamine such as diphenhydramine.
* Other side effects reported include chills, flulike symptoms, vomiting, itching, headaches, muscle pains, and submaxillary and parotid glandular enlargement.
* Use of hetastarch in pregnant women must be used only on a risk versus benefit basis.

Drug interactions

No significant drug interactions have been reported.

The safety and compatibility of additives to the infusion have not been established.

Ipecac

AHFS 56:20

CATEGORY Emetic

Action and use

Syrup of ipecac is used to induce vomiting in cases of poisoning by orally ingested drugs and other chemicals.

Characteristics

Onset: 15 to 45 min.

Administration and dosage

PO—15 to 30 ml syrup of ipecac. Administer with copious amounts of fluid.

NOTE: Do *not* use fluid extract of ipecac. It is as much as 14 times more potent than the syrup.

Nurse and patient considerations

* Do not use emetics in deeply sedated or unconscious patients. Emetics are not active when medullary centers are depressed. Patients may also aspirate gastric contents.

* Emetics should not be used in patients who are convulsing or who have ingested a convulsant or corrosives such as alkali (lye), strong acids, strychnine, and strong petroleum distillates (kerosene, gasoline, paint thinner, cleaning fluid).

* Toxic effects include sweating, tachycardia, hypotension, dyspnea, and weakness.

Drug interactions

No specific interactions have been reported.

Lactulose
(Cephulac, Chronulac)

AHFS 40:10
CATEGORY Laxative, ammonia detoxicant

Action and use

Lactulose is a dissacharide sugar that when ingested is metabolized in the colon by lactobacilli, *Bacteroides* species, *Escherichia coli,* and *Clostridia* species to lactic acetic and formic acids and carbon dioxide. These acids promote bowel evacuation by increasing osmotic pressure and by slightly acidifying colonic contents, resulting in an increase in stool water content and stool softening.

Lactulose may also be used (in conjunction with low-protein diets) to reduce serum ammonia concentrations in patients with portal-systemic encephalopathy. The acids generated from lactulose degradation acidify colonic contents, causing serum ammonia to migrate from the blood into the colon. In the acidic environment of the colon, ammonia is converted to ammonium ion, which is unresorbable. The laxative action of the lactulose metabolites then expells the trapped ammonium ion from the colon.

Characteristics

Less than 3% of an oral dose of lactulose is absorbed. That which is absorbed is not metabolized and is excreted in the urine within 24 hr. Lactulose that is not absorbed reaches the colon intact, where it is metabolized to acids by colonic bacteria. Essentially no lactulose or its metabolites is absorbed from the colon. Onset of action may require 24 to 48 hr when administered orally.

Administration and dosage
Adult

Laxative (Chronulac):

PO—Initial dose: 15 to 30 ml daily. May increase to 60 ml daily. Twenty-four to 48 hr may be required to produce a normal bowel movement. Chronulac is more palatable when mixed with fruit juice, water, or milk.

Portal-systemic encephalopathy (Cephulac):

PO—Initial doses: 30 to 45 ml every hour may be used to product rapid laxation in the initial treatment of portal-systemic encephalopathy. Once the laxative effect is achieved, the dosage is reduced to 30 to 45 ml 3 to 4 times daily. The dosage should be titrated to produce 2 or 3 soft, formed stools daily.

RECTAL
1. Mix 300 ml of Cephulac with 700 ml of water or normal saline. Instill rectally every 4 to 6 hr via a rectal balloon catheter. Attempt to retain for 30 to 60 min.
2. Do not use soapsuds or cleansing enemas.
3. The goal of rectal therapy is to reverse the coma so that patients may take the medication orally. Oral administration of lactulose should be started before rectal treatment is completely stopped.

Pediatric
Infants

PO—2.5 to 10 ml daily in divided doses.

Older children and adolescents

PO—40 to 90 ml daily in divided doses. The goal of treatment is to produce 2 to 3 soft, yet formed stools daily.

NOTE: Under normal conditions, a gradual darkening of lactulose will occur. Store in light-resistant containers. On long-term exposure to light or temperatures above 30° C (86° F), extreme darkening and turbidity may develop. Do not use. If the lactulose solution is exposed to freezing temperatures, it will become a semisolid. Viscosity will return to normal on warming to room temperature.

Nurse and patient considerations

* Common adverse effects frequently observed in the early stages of therapy are belching, gaseous distention, flatulence, and cramping. These side effects resolve with continued therapy, but dosage reduction may also be necessary. Diarrhea is a sign of overdosage and responds to dosage reduction.

* Use with caution in patients with diabetes mellitus. Lactulose syrup contains small amounts of free lactose (less than 1.2 g/15 ml), galactose (less than 2.2 g) and other sugars (less than 1.2 g/15 ml).

* Patients who use lactulose chronically for 6 months or longer should have serum potassium and chloride levels measured periodically.

* Safe use in pregnancy has not been established. Use only if the benefits significantly outweigh the risks of therapy.

Drug interactions

Do not administer other laxatives with lactulose therapy. Diarrhea that may be produced makes it difficult to titrate a proper dosage of lactulose.

Although neomycin and lactulose are frequently used concurrently in the initial treatment of portal-systemic encephalopathy, the neomycin may reduce effectiveness of lactulose by destroying too much of the saccharolytic bacteria in the colon. Monitor patients closely for reduced lactulose activity when concomitant antibiotic therapy is prescribed.

Loperamide hydrochloride

AHFS 56:08; C-V
CATEGORY Antidiarrheal agent

(Imodium)

Action and use

Loperamide hydrochloride is a new synthetic orally active antidiarrheal agent. Loperamide slows peristalsis of the gastrointestinal tract by acting directly on cholinergic and noncholinergic nerve receptors in the intestinal wall. The intestinal transit time is prolonged, resulting in greater fecal viscosity and bulk density with reduced loss of fluids and electrolytes. It has been effective in providing symptomatic relief of acute, nonspecific diarrhea and chronic diarrhea associated with inflammatory bowel disease, and in reducing the volume of discharge from ileostomies.

Characteristics

Peak serum levels: 4 hr (PO). There are no published studies on the relationship between plasma levels and clinical response or on whether the delayed transit time caused by loperamide affects its own absorption. Half-life: 7 to 15 hr. Excretion: unchanged in feces, 10% unchanged in urine (PO). The metabolic pathways in humans for the remainder of the drug have not been delineated.

Administration and dosage
Adult

PO 1. Acute diarrhea: initially, 2 capsules (4 mg), followed by 1 capsule (2 mg) after each unformed stool. Daily dosage should not exceed 8 capsules (16 mg). If clinical improvement does not occur within 48 hr, loperamide should be discontinued.

2. Chronic diarrhea: initially, 2 capsules (4 mg), followed by 1 capsule (2 mg) after each unformed stool until diarrhea is controlled. The average daily maintenance dosage is 2 to 4 capsules (4 to 8 mg)/day.

Pediatric

Safe use in children under 12 years of age has not been established.

NOTE: Observe patients for dehydration and electrolyte imbalance (see Table 4-1).

Nurse and patient considerations

* Side effects reported during loperamide therapy have usually been gastrointestinal in nature and may be related to the condition being treated. Constipation is the most frequent adverse effect. Nausea, abdominal pain, dizziness, and dry mouth have occasionally occurred.
* All cases of diarrhea should be investigated fully, and specific treatment instituted as soon as possible. Loperamide, an antimotility drug is indicated only for *symptomatic* control of diarrhea. Do not use in (1) acute diarrhea when bacterial pathogens are

suspected, since medications that slow intestinal motility may delay clearance of infecting organisms from the bowel; (2) antibiotic-induced colitis, since loperamide may prolong the disorder; and (3) severe, acute attacks of ulcerative colitis, since antimotility drugs may cause a paralytic ileus with overdilatation of the bowel (toxic megacolon).

* Physical dependence has not been observed in humans; however, it has developed in laboratory animals.

* Safe use during pregnancy and lactation has not been established.

Drug interactions

No specific drug interactions with loperamide have been reported.

Metoclopramide hydrochloride
(Reglan)

AHFS unlisted
CATEGORY GI Stimulant,
antiemetic

Action and use

Metoclopramide stimulates motility of the upper gastrointestinal tract without stimulating gastric, biliary, or pancreatic secretions. It increases gastric contractions, relaxes the pyloric sphincter, and increases peristalsis of the duodenum and jejunum, resulting in an increased rate of gastric emptying and intestinal transit. The mechanism of action is unknown.

Metoclopramide is used to relieve the symptoms of diabetic gastroparesis, as an antiemetic for vomiting associated with cancer chemotherapy, as an aid in small bowel intubation, and to stimulate gastric emptying and intestinal transit of barium after radiologic examination of the upper GI tract.

Characteristics

Onset: 1 to 3 min (IV), 10 to 15 min (IM), 30 to 60 min (PO). Duration: 1 to 2 hr. Half-life: 1.5 to 2 hr. Protein binding: 13% to 22%. Metabolism: liver, extensive first-pass effect. Excretion: 85% in urine in 72 hr as free and conjugated drug. Dialysis: unknown. Breast milk: unknown.

Administration and dosage

Diabetic gastroparesis:

PO—10 mg 30 min before each meal and at bedtime. Duration of therapy is dependent on response and continued well-being after discontinuation of therapy.

Antiemesis:

IV   1. Initial 2 doses: 2 mg/kg. If vomiting is suppressed, follow with 1 mg/kg.
  2. Dilute the dose in 50 ml of parenteral solution (D_5W, sodium chloride 0.9%, D_5/.45 normal saline, Ringer's solution, or lactated Ringer's solution).
  3. Infuse over at least 15 min, 30 min before beginning chemotherapy, and repeating every 2 hr for 2 doses, followed by 1 dose every 3 hr for 3 doses.

NOTE: Rapid IV infusion may cause sudden, intense anxiety and restlessness, followed by drowsiness.

Small bowel intubation and radiologic examination:

Adult

IV—10 mg (2 ml)

Pediatric

Under 6 years of age

IV—0.1 mg/Kg.

6 to 14 years of age

IV—2.5 to 5 mg (0.5 to 1 ml).

Inject as a single dose undiluted slowly over 1 to 2 min.

NOTE: If extrapyramidal symptoms should develop, inject diphenhydramine (Benadryl), 50 mg IM.

Dilutions may be stored for up to 48 hr after dilution if protected from light. Dilutions should be protected from light during infusion.

Nurse and patient considerations

* Extrapyramidal symptoms manifested by restlessness, involuntary movements, facial grimacing, and possibly oculogyric crisis, torticollis, or rhythmic protrusion of the tongue occurs in about 1 in 500 patients. Patients most susceptible are children and young adults and those receiving higher doses of metoclopramide for prophylaxis against vomiting. Metoclopramide should not be used in patients with epilepsy or in patients receiving the drugs (phenothiazines) that are likely to cause extrapyramidal reactions, since the frequency and severity of seizures or extrapyramidal reactions may be increased.

* Metoclopramide must not be used in patients when increased gastric motility may be dangerous, such as gastrointestinal perforation, mechanical obstruction, or hemorrhage.

* Common side effects of metoclopramide are drowsiness, fatigue, and lassitude. Patients should be cautioned about doing tasks that require mental alertness. Other less frequent adverse effects include insomnia, headache, dizziness, nausea, and bowel disturbances.

* Because of lack of evidence supporting the use of metoclopramide in pregnant women, it should be used only when the benefits gained significantly outweigh the risks associated with use in these patients.

Drug interactions

Metoclopramide will antagonize the prolactin inhibitory action of bromocriptine.

Anticholinergic drugs (atropine, Cogentin, Bentyl, antihistamines) and narcotic analgesics (meperidine, morphine, oxycodone) antagonize the gastrointestinal stimulatory effects of metoclopramide.

Alcohol, sedative-hypnotics, tranquilizers, and narcotics may enhance the sedative effects of metoclopramide.

The gastrointestinal stimulatory effects may alter the absorption of food and drugs: absorption of digoxin may be diminished; absorption of alcohol, levodopa, tetracycline, and acetaminophen may be enhanced; and absorption of food may be altered, requiring an adjustment in timing or dosage of insulin in patients with diabetes mellitus.

Naloxone hydrochloride
(Narcan)

AHFS 28:10
CATEGORY Narcotic antagonist

Action and use

Naloxone is a semisynthetic narcotic antagonist. It antagonizes respiratory depression induced by natural and synthetic narcotics, pentazocine (Talwin), and propoxyphene (Darvon). When administered to patients who have not recently received narcotics, there is no further respiratory depression, psychomimetic effects, circulatory changes, or other pharmacologic activity. Naloxone is a drug of choice for treatment of respiratory depression when the causative agent is unknown.

Characteristics

Onset: 1 to 2 min (IV), 3 to 5 min (IM or SC). Duration: 3 to 5 hr (dose dependent). Metabolic fate: unknown.

Administration and dosage
Adult

IM—0.4 mg (1 ml). If immediate response is not obtained, the dose may be repeated every 2 to 3 min for 2 to 3 doses.

IV or SC—As for IM administration.

Pediatric

IM—10 μg/kg. The dosage may be repeated every 2 to 3 min for 2 or 3 times.

IV or SC—As for IM administration.

Nurse and patient considerations

* Because of a relatively short duration of action, naloxone may have to be readministered as the effects of the antagonist subside and those of the narcotic return.
* Naloxone is not effective in the treatment of respiratory depression caused by sedatives, hypnotics, anesthetics, or other nonnarcotic CNS depressants.
* In patients dependent on opiates, naloxone may precipitate a withdrawal syndrome, the severity of which depends on the dose of the naloxone and the degree of dependence.

> * Safe use of naloxone during pregnancy has not been determined.

Drug interactions

There are no drug interactions other than that of the antagonist activity toward opiates, pentazocine, and propoxyphene.

Oxybutynin chloride
(Ditropan)

AHFS 86:00
CATEGORY Urinary antispasmodic

Action and use

Oxybutynin is an anticholinergic agent that has direct antispasmodic activity on the detrusor muscle of the bladder and the smooth muscle of the small intestine and colon. It is used as an antispasmodic agent in patients with uninhibited neurogenic or reflex neurogenic bladders to increase vesical capacity, diminish the frequency of uninhibited contractions of the detrusor muscle, and delay the initial desire to void. These actions decrease the symptoms of urgency, frequency, incontinence, and nocturia associated with neurogenic bladder.

Characteristics

Onset: 30 to 60 min (PO). Peak activity: 3 to 6 hr. Duration: 6 to 10 hr. Metabolism: liver. Excretion: primarily renal.

Administration and dosage
Adult

PO—5 mg 2 to 3 times daily to a maximum of 20 mg daily.

Pediatric (5 years of age and older)

PO—5 mg 1 to 2 times daily to a maximum of 15 mg daily.

Nurse and patient considerations

* The side effects of oxybutynin are those associated with all anticholinergic agents: dry mouth, decreased sweating, hot flashes, tachycardia, palpitations, transient blurred vision, mydriasis, cycloplegia, drowsiness, weakness, dizziness, and constipation. The side effects are rarely severe enough to require discontinuation of therapy. Sugarless hard candy or gum may help the dry mouth. The use of stool softeners such as docusate (Colace) and occasionally a potent laxative such as bisacodyl (Dulcolax) may be required for constipation. Drowsiness may be circumvented by initiating therapy at bedtime. Patients should also be cautioned not to perform tasks that require mental alertness or physical coordination.

* Oxybutynin must not be used in patients with glaucoma, myasthenia gravis, obstruction of the gastrointestinal tract, adynamic ileus, severe colitis, intestinal atony, obstructive uropathy, or hemorrhage with unstable cardiovascular status.

* Oxybutynin must be used with caution during hot weather. It may induce fever and heat stroke due to suppression of sweating. Oxybutynin may also aggravate the symptoms of hyperthyroidism, arrhythmias, congestive heart failure, tachycardia, hypertension, prostatic hypertrophy, and reflux esophagitis.

* The safety of the use of oxybutynin during pregnancy has not been established. It should be used in pregnant patients only when the benefits significantly outweigh the risks of therapy. It is not known whether oxybutynin is secreted into breast milk.

Drug interactions

Amantadine, tricyclic antidepressants (Thorazine, Compazine, Mellaril), other anticholinergic agents (Cogentin, Akineton, Pagitane, Parsidol, Kemadrin, Artane), and antihistamines (Benadryl, Disipal, Phenoxene) may potentiate the anticholinergic action and side effects of oxybutynin.

Physostigmine salicylate
(Antilirium)

<small>AHFS 12:08</small>
<small>CATEGORY Anticholinesterase agent</small>

Action and use

Physostigmine enhances cholinergic activity by inhibiting cholinesterase, the enzyme that destroys acetylcholine. Consequently parasympathetic activity is sustained by physostigmine administration. Physostigmine is used as an antidote for reversing most of the cardiovascular (tachycardia, arrhythmias) and CNS effects (delirium, coma) of overdosage with tricyclic antidepressants (amitriptyline [Elavil], imipramine [Tofranil], doxepin [Sinequan], others) and belladonna alkaloids (atropine, scopolamine).

Characteristics

Onset: 3 to 8 min. Duration: 30 to 60 min.

Administration and dosage
Adult

IV 1. Therapeutic trial: 2 mg slowly at a rate of 1 mg/min. A second dose of 1 to 2 mg may be repeated in 20 min if there is no response.
2. Therapeutic dose: 1 to 4 mg slowly as life-threatening symptoms recur.

IM—As for IV administration.

Pediatric

IV 1. Therapeutic trial: 0.5 mg slowly over 1 min. Repeat at 5 min intervals if no cholinergic effects are produced and there are no therapeutic effects. Maximum dosage is 2 mg.
2. Therapeutic dose: the lowest effective trial dose.

NOTE: Physostigmine overdosage may result in cholinergic crisis. Overdosage may be manifested by excessive salivation and sweating, pupil constriction, nausea, vomiting, bradycardia, tachycardia, hypertension, hypotension, confusion, convulsions, coma, and paralysis. Treat with mechanical respiration, frequent bronchial aspiration, and atropine, 2 to 4 mg IV every 3 to 10 min until symptoms reverse. Atropine, however, will not reverse muscular weakness and respiratory depression. Pralidoxime chloride (Protopam) may be useful in treating this adverse effect.

Nurse and patient considerations

＊ Side effects of physostigmine usually result from enhanced parasympathetic activity caused by the blockade of acetylcholine's metabolic enzyme. They include salivation, sweating, lacrimation, nausea, vomiting, diarrhea, irregular pulse, and palpitations. The dosage should be reduced if they become prominent.

＊ Physostigmine should be used with caution in patients with epilepsy, parkinsonism, or bradycardia.

＊ Physostigmine should be used with extreme caution in patients with asthma, diabetes, cardiovascular disease, or mechanical obstruction of the intestinal or urogenital tract.

＊ Physostigmine crosses the placental barrier. It should only be used in pregnant women when the benefit of therapy outweighs the risk to the mother and the fetus.

Drug interactions

Physostigmine exaggerates the activity of other cholinergic agents such as bethanechol (Urecholine), methacholine (Mecholyl), and edrophonium (Tensilon).

Physostigmine may potentiate muscular paralysis induced by depolarizing neuromuscular blocking agents (decamethonium [Syncurine] and succinylcholine [Anectine]).

Physostigmine may antagonize muscular paralysis induced by nondepolarizing neuromuscular blocking agents (gallamine [Flaxedil], pancuronium [Pavulon], and tubocurarine).

Sodium bicarbonate
Action and use

AHFS 40:08
CATEGORY Alkalinizing agent

As an alkalinizing agent, sodium bicarbonate increases plasma bicarbonate, buffers excess hydrogen ion, and increases blood pH. It is used to treat metabolic acidosis as a result of a variety of conditions including renal disease, diabetes, circulatory insufficiency caused by shock or dehydration, and cardiac arrest. It is also indicated in barbiturate intoxication and salicylate or methyl alcohol poisoning.

Administration and dosage

IV—Initial dose: 1 mEq/kg bolus, followed by 1 ampule (50 ml = 1 mEq/ml) every 5 to 10 min as dictated by the patient's condition.

Nurse and patient considerations

* It is recommended that, in hospitalized patients, further administration of sodium bicarbonate be governed by arterial blood gas and pH measurement.
* Be aware of other drugs running in the same IV line. Many drugs used in critical medicine are unstable in alkaline media (for example, calcium chloride, calcium gluconate, dopamine hydrochloride, and penicillin G).

Sucralfate
(Carafate)

AHFS unlisted
CATEGORY Antiulcer agent

Action and use

Sucralfate is a chemical complex of aluminum hydroxide and sulfated sucrose. It is used for the treatment of duodenal ulcer. When swallowed, sucralfate forms an adherent, protective complex with proteinaceous material over the ulcer itself, preventing acid, pepsin, and bile salts from aggravating the lesion. Sucralfate does not stimulate or inhibit gastric secretory rates, nor does it alter gastric pH. It compares favorably with intensive antacid therapy and cimetidine in terms of safety and efficacy for the short-term (up to 8 weeks) treatment of duodenal ulcers.

Characteristics

Absorption: only 3% to 5% is absorbed, the remaining 95% to 97% remains in the gastrointestinal tract. Duration: dependent on time of contact at ulcer site. Binding to ulcer site may last up to 6 hr. Excretion: renal—absorbed fraction; fecal—unabsorbed fraction. Breast milk: unknown.

Administration and dosage
Adult

PO 1. 1 g 1 hr before each meal and at bedtime, all on an empty stomach.

2. Antacids may also be used but should not be administered within half an hour before or after sucralfate.
3. Treatment is usually continued for 4 to 8 weeks unless complete healing has been demonstrated by x-ray or endoscopic examination.

Pediatric

Safety and use in children have not been established.

Nurse and patient considerations

* Sucralfate is minimally absorbed, so it is not surprising that there are no major systemic reactions reported. The overall incidence of adverse effects is 3.5%. Most common complaints are constipation (2.2%) and xerostomia (<1%). Other reported effects include nausea, increased upper gastrointestinal complaints, stomach discomfort, and dizziness.

* There have been no studies of sucralfate in pregnant or nursing patients. Therapy with sucralfate in these patients should be only on a risk to benefit basis.

Drug interactions

Sucralfate is an aluminum salt that may interfere with the absorption of tetracycline.

GENERAL INFORMATION ON LAXATIVES
Classification

Saline: hypertonicity of the saline cathartic increases liquid in the colon.

Irritants or stimulants: increase intestinal tract motor activity.

Bulk-producing products: absorb imbibed water, adding bulk and moisture to the feces, thus causing distention and elimination.

Emollients: lubricate the intestinal tract and soften feces.

Fecal softeners: penetrate and soften fecal masses through the action of the contained wetting agents.

Miscellaneous agents 619

Table 25-1. Laxative active ingredients

Product	Stimulant	Saline	Bulk-forming	Emollient	Fecal softener
Agoral	Phenolphthalein	—	Agar, tragacanth, acacia	Mineral oil	—
Colace	—	—	—	—	Docusate sodium
Dialose	—	—	—	—	Docusate potassium
Dialose Plus	Casanthranol	—	—	—	Docusate sodium
Doxidan	Danthron	—	—	—	Docusate sodium
Dulcolax	Bisacodyl	—	—	—	—
Haley's M-O	—	Milk of magnesia	—	Mineral oil	—
Peri-Colace	Casanthranol	—	—	—	Docusate sodium
Phillip's Milk of Magnesia	—	Milk of magnesia	—	—	—
Surfak	—	—	—	—	Docusate calcium
X-Prep	Standardized senna concentrate	—	—	—	—

Contraindications

Do not administer when nausea, vomiting, abdominal pain, or other symptoms of appendicitis are present.

Do not administer when fecal impaction exists or when there is intestinal obstruction, hemorrhage, severe spasm, diarrhea, or intestinal perforation.

Warnings and precautions

Use laxatives with caution in presence of inflamed or irritable colon.

Rectal bleeding or failure to respond to enema therapy may indicate a serious condition that may have to be treated surgically.

Persons with a hernia, severe hypertension, or cardio-vascular disease and those who are about to undergo or who have undergone surgery for hemorrhoids or other anorectal disorders should not strain at the stool. In such cases an emollient fecal-softening laxative is indicated.

Administration techniques for eye, ear, nose, rectal, and parenteral products

INSTRUCTIONS FOR INSTILLING EYE DROPS AND OINTMENT

1. Place the patient's head on a suitable support, such as a firm pillow, and direct his face toward the ceiling.
2. Instruct the patient to fix his gaze on a point above his head.
3. With clean fingertips, apply gentle traction to the lid bases at the bony rim of the orbit; do not apply pressure to the eyeball (Fig. A-1).
4. Approach the eye from below with the dropper or the ointment tube, outside the patient's field of vision; do not touch the eye with the dropper or the tube (Fig. A-2).
5. Release the dose; drops should not fall more than 1 inch before striking the eye.
6. Apply gentle pressure inward and downward against the bones of the nose for about 2 min to the lacrimal canaliculi at the inner corner of the eyelids. This prevents the eye medication from entering the nasal cavity and being absorbed through the nasal cavity's highly vascular mucosa. Many eye medications are very powerful; take care to prevent their systemic absorption.

ADMINISTRATION OF EAR DROPS

1. Allow drops to warm to body temperature by having the patient hold the bottle in his hand for a few minutes.
2. Look into the external ear canal to determine whether significant ear wax has accumulated. If the canal appears to be impacted, the canal should be cleaned before drops are instilled. If the eardrum is intact and if the physician approves, irrigate the ear canal with 3% saline (2 tablespoons of salt per quart of warm water), using an ear syringe.

From Squire, J.E., and Clayton, B.D.: Basic pharmocology for nurses, ed 7, St. Louis, 1981, The C.V. Mosby Co.

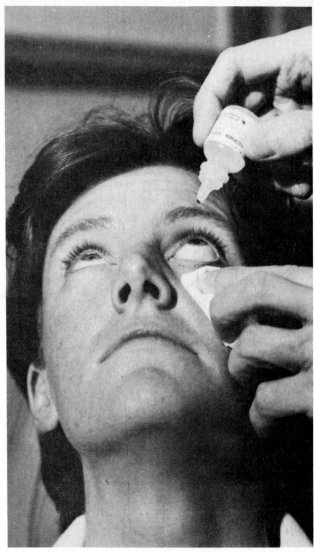

Fig. A-1. The patient should tilt his face upward to receive an eye drop. Use an absorbent tissue to prevent excess drops and tears from flowing down the patient's face. (From Saunders, W.H., et al.: Nursing care in eye, ear, nose, and throat disorders, ed. 4, St. Louis, 1979, the C.V. Mosby Co.)

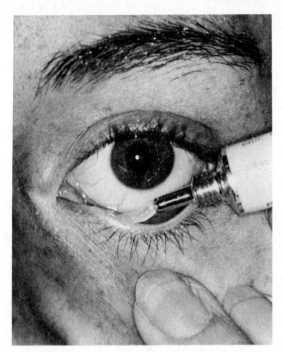

Fig. A-2. To instill ointment, pull down the lower eyelid as the patient looks upward. Squeeze the ointment into the lower conjunctival sac. Avoid touching the tube to the eye or lid. (From Saunders, W.H., et al.: Nursing care in eye, ear, nose, and throat disorders, ed. 4, St. Louis, 1979, the C.V. Mosby Co.)

3. Have the patient lie on his side with the ear to be treated upward.
4. Shake the medicine if required and draw up into the dropper.
5. To allow the drops to run in (Fig. A-3):
   a. Adults—pull the pinna (earlobe) back and up and allow the drops to fall in the external canal.
   b. Children—pull the pinna (earlobe) back and down and allow the drops to fall in the external canal.
6. Do not insert the dropper into the ear and do not allow the dropper to come into contact with any portion of the ear.

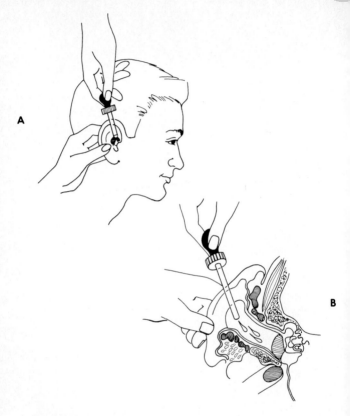

Fig. A-3. Ear drops. **A,** Ask patient to turn his head to the side so that the ear being treated faces upward. Manipulate the external ear gently to expose the external canal. **B,** Direct medication toward the internal wall of the canal. (From Dison, N.: Clinical nursing techniques, ed. 4, St. Louis, 1979, The C.V. Mosby Co.)

7. Have the patient remain on his side for a few minutes to allow the medication to reach the eardrum.
8. Insert a soft cotton plug if ordered. Never pack the plug tightly into the ear.

ADMINISTRATION OF NOSE DROPS

1. Instruct the patient to gently blow his nose.
2. Draw the medicine into the dropper (Fig. A-4). To properly regulate dosage, draw only what should be instilled.

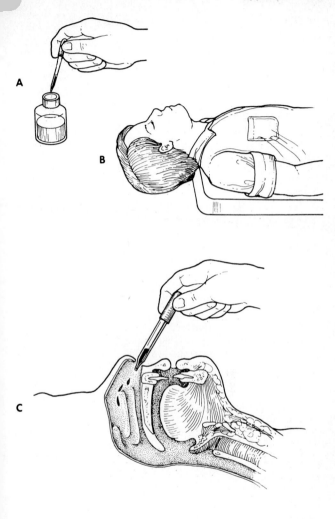

Fig. A-4. Nose drops. **A,** Draw proper dose into dropper. **B,** Tilt patient's head backward. **C,** Cross section showing instillation of drops. (From Squire, J.E., and Clayton, B.D.: Basic pharmacology for nurses, ed. 7, St. Louis, 1981, The C.V. Mosby Co.)

3. Have the patient lie down and tilt his head backward over the edge of the bed.
4. Insert the dropper ⅓ to ½ inch into the nasal passage and instill the medicine.
5. Have the patient remain in this position for several minutes to allow the medication to be absorbed.
6. Instruct the patient not to blow his nose unless absolutely necessary.
7. Each patient should have his own bottles of nasal solutions to prevent cross-contamination of patients.

INSERTION OF RECTAL SUPPOSITORIES

1. When possible, have the bowel evacuated before insertion of the suppository.
2. If suppositories are soft and unmanageable, hold the foil-wrapped suppository under cold water to harden before insertion.
3. Put on a disposable glove or a finger cot to protect the finger used for insertion (index finger for adults, fourth finger for infants).
4. Ask the patient to lie on his side and draw his upper leg up toward his waist (Fig. A-5).
5. Unwrap the suppository.
6. Lubricate the suppository with a water-soluble lubricant such as K-Y Jelly (do not use mineral oil or Vaseline). If a lubricant is not available, wet the rectal orifice with tap water.
7. Place the tip of the suppository at the rectal entrance and ask the patient to take a deep breath and exhale through his mouth (many patients will have an involuntary rectal gripping when the suppository is pressed against the rectum). Gently insert the suppository about an inch beyond the orifice past the internal sphincter.
8. Ask the patient to remain lying on his side for 15 to 20 min to allow melting and absorption of the medication.
9. Discard used materials and wash hands thoroughly.

ADMINISTRATION OF RECTAL RETENTION ENEMAS

1. For maximum absorption, the bowel should be evacuated before the enema.
2. Collect all of the apparatus and mix the solution before preparing the patient.
3. Ask the patient to lie on his side and draw his upper leg up toward his waist (Fig. A-6).
4. Remove the protective cap and lubricate the catheter tip with tap water.

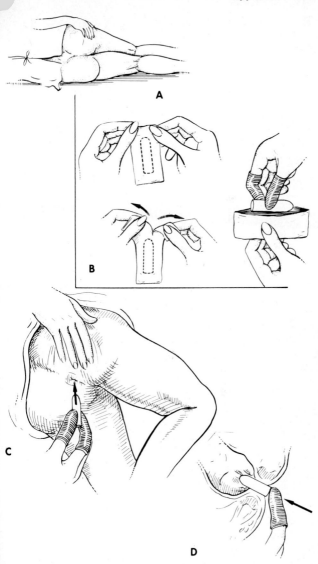

Fig. A-5. Rectal suppositories. **A,** Position of patient. **B,** Open wrapper and remove suppository. **C,** Insert suppository. **D,** Cross section showing insertion of suppository. Advance suppository beyond anal sphincter. (From Dison, N.: Clinical nursing techniques, ed. 4, St. Louis, 1979, The C.V. Mosby Co.)

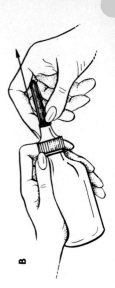

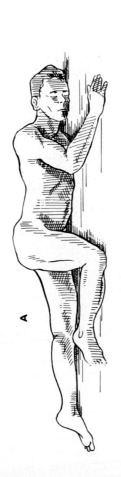

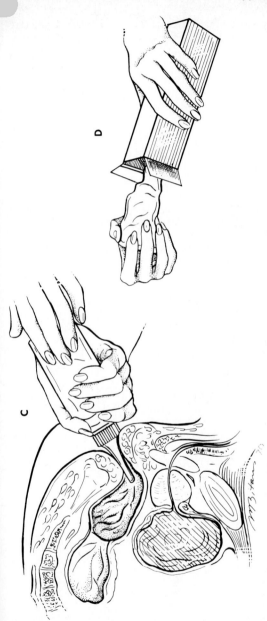

Fig. A-6. Administration of disposable enema (Fleet enema). **A,** Place patient in left lateral position, unless knee-chest position has been specified. **B,** Remove protective covering from rectal tube and lubricate tube with lubricant contained in this cover. **C,** Insert lubricated rectal tube into rectum and insert solution by compressing plastic container. **D,** Replace used container in its original container for disposal. (Courtesy C.B. Fleet Co., Lynchburg, Va. From Dison, N.: Clinical nursing techniques, ed. 4, St. Louis, 1979, The C.V. Mosby Co.)

5. Place the tip of the catheter at the rectal entrance and ask the patient to take a deep breath and exhale through his mouth. This maneuver will help relax the rectal sphincter.
6. Gently insert the catheter tip past the internal sphincter and administer the enema slowly, using no more than 120 ml of solution, to prevent peristaltic activity from expelling the solution.
7. After instillation, remove the catheter and ask the patient to lie flat for 30 min.
8. Discard used materials and wash hands thoroughly.

SUBCUTANEOUS INJECTIONS

1. Subcutaneous (subq; sc; hypodermic) injections are given by means of a 3 cc or tuberculin (1 cc) syringe with a ⅝-inch 25-gauge, needle. Trajectory of the needle is at a 45-degree angle to the outer skin surface (Fig. A-7). **(NOTE**: A tuberculin syringe has a total volume of 1 cc and is calibrated in 0.01 ml.)
2. Needle should be inserted through the skin with a quick, even movement.
3. Plunger of syringe should be withdrawn slightly to determine and prevent penetration into a blood vessel.
4. Outer surface of upper arm, anterior surface of thigh, and lower abdomen are common sites.
5. Injection is made slowly and steadily.

INTRADERMAL INJECTIONS

1. Intradermal (intracutaneous) injections are given by means of a tuberculin syringe with ⅝-inch, 26-gauge needle. A minute amount of solution is injected just under the outer layers of skin. The trajectory of the needle is parallel to the outer skin surface, between the epidermis and the dermis and avoiding subcutaneous tissue (Fig. A-7).

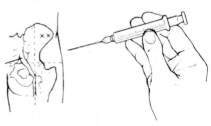

Fig. A-7. Injection sites.   Posterior gluteal

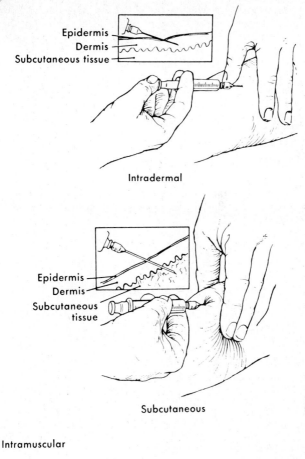

Intradermal

Subcutaneous

Intramuscular

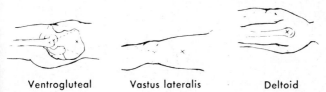

Ventrogluteal   Vastus lateralis   Deltoid

Fig. A-7. Injection sites. (From Squire, J.E., and Clayton, B.D.: Basic pharmacology for nurses, ed. 7, St. Louis, 1981, The C.V. Mosby Co.)

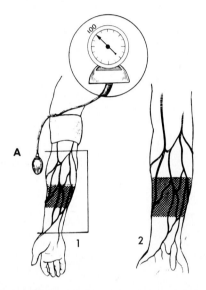

Fig. A-8. Venipuncture. **A,** Preparation for venipuncture. *1,* A sphygmomanometer or tourniquet is applied to the upper arm and inflated to distend the veins. *2,* An average pattern of superficial veins. The preferred area for fluid therapy is shaded. **B,** Venipuncture with steel needle. *1,* Tension of the thumb, distal to the site of venipuncture, stretches the skin and stabilizes the vein. The needle, attached to a syringe, is inserted through the skin adjacent to the vein. *2,* The needle is held at little less than a 45-degree angle for penetration of the skin. When the needle enters the vein, the bevel is rotated to prevent puncture of the posterior wall of the vessel. *3,* The needle and syringe are lowered nearly parallel to the skin for advancement into the vein. **C,** Venipuncture with plastic needle. *1,* Formation of skin wheal with local anesthetic agent. *2,* A pathway for the plastic needle is formed by puncturing the skin with large-bore steel needle. *3,* Plastic needle, Jelco IV catheter placement unit. *4,* The plastic needle is attached to syringe for introduction through the preformed channel. *5,* Cross section showing needle being introduced through the channel. (From Squire, J.E., and Clayton, B.D.: Basic Pharmacology for Nurses, ed. 7, St. Louis, 1981, The C.V. Mosby Co.)

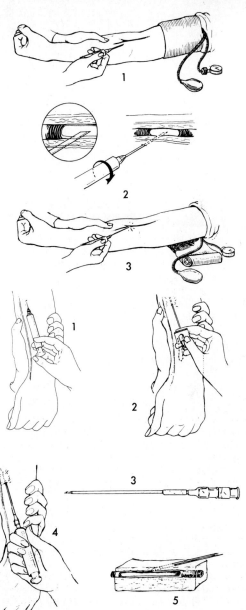

B

C

Continued.

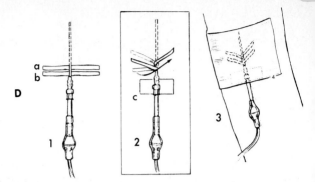

Fig. A-8, cont'd. D, Securing plastic needle. *1,* Approximate placement of narrow strips of tape. The first tape, *a,* is anchored before the second one, *b,* is placed. The tape must adhere to the distal end of the plastic needle. *2,* Method of fastening tape to needle and skin. Tape beneath hub is placed with its adhesive side up, *c.* Its adherence to overlying tape prevents movement of the needle, which may contribute to separation and loss of the plastic tube. *3,* A large piece of tape completes stabilization of the needle. It is labeled to show the date of insertion and that plastic needle is in place.

INTRAMUSCULAR INJECTIONS

1. Tuberculin (1 cc) or 3 cc syringe.
2. Needles from 1 to 3 inches and 19 to 22 gauge, depending on the site of injection.
3. Trajectory of needle is at a 90-degree angle.
4. Usual sites are the buttocks.
   a. Posterior gluteal. Divide buttocks into four quadrants and insert needle at 90-degree angle into upper, outer quadrant.
   b. Ventrogluteal. Using your left hand, place the index finger on right iliac spine of the patient and the middle finger stretched back and slipped to a point just below the crest of the ilium, with your palm resting on the patient's hip. The injection site is the apex of the triangle between the index and middle finger. Insert needle at a 90-degree angle.
   c. Vastus lateralis. Spot injection site a handbreadth above the knee and an equal distance below the greater trochanter. Insert needle at a 90-degree angle.
   d. Deltoid. Cover the head of the humerus. Insert below acromion and lateral to the axilla.

Common medical abbreviations

A

A	Assessment (POMR)	ANA	Antinuclear antibodies
A_2	Aortic second sound		
$A_2 > P_2$	Aortic sound larger than second pulmonary sound	AODM	Adult-onset diabetes mellitus
		A & P	Anterior and posterior; auscultation and percussion
AAL	Anterior axillary line		
Ab	Abortion		
Abd	Abdomen, abdominal	ASAP	As soon as possible
ABE	Acute bacterial endocarditis	AP	Apical pulse, anteroposterior
ABG	Arterial blood gases	APB	Atrial premature beats
ACD	Anterior chest diameter	AS	Anal sphincter; arteriosclerosis
ADH	Antidiuretic hormone		
ADT	Alternate day therapy	ASCVD	Arteriosclerotic cardiovascular disease
AF	Atrial fibrillation; acid fast	ASHD	Arteriosclerotic heart disease
AFB	Acid-fast bacteria; acid-fast bacilli	ASO	Antistreptolysin titer; arteriosclerosis obliterans
A/G	Albumin to globulin ratio		
AGN	Acute glomerular nephritis	ATN	Acute tubular necrosis
AHF	Antihemophilic factor	AV	Arteriovenous; atrioventricular
AHFS	American Hospital Formulary Service		
		A & W	Alive and well
AHG	Antihemophilic globulin		

B

AI	Aortic insufficiency	BAL	British anti-lewisite (dimercaprol)
AJ	Ankle jerk		
AK	Above knee (amputation)	bands	Banded neutrophils
		BBB	Bundle branch block; blood brain barrier
ALD	Alcoholic liver disease	BBT	Basal body temperature
ALL	Acute lymphocytic leukemia	BE	Barium enema; base excess
ALS	Amyotrophic lateral sclerosis	BEI	Butanol-extractable iodine
AMA	Against medical advice	bili	Bilirubin
AMI	Acute myocardial infarction	BJ	Biceps jerk; bone and joint

BK	Below knee (amputation)	CHO	Carbohydrate
		Chol	Cholesterol
BLB	A type of oxygen mask	CI	Color index; contra-indication
BLOBS	Bladder observation	CK	Check
BM	Bowel movement; basal metabolism	CLL	Chronic lymphocytic leukemia
BMR	Basal metabolic rate	CNS	Central nervous system
B & O	Belladonna and opium	COAP	Cyclophosphamide, Oncovin, Ara-C, Prednisone
BP	Blood pressure; British Pharmacopoeia		
		C/O	Complains of
BPH	Benign prostatic hypertrophy	Cong	Congenital
		COP	Cyclophosphamide, Oncovin, Prednisone
BRP	Bathroom privileges		
BS	Bowel sounds; breath sounds	COPD	Chronic obstructive pulmonary disease
BSO	Bilateral salpingoophorectomy	CPK	Creatine phosphokinase
BSP	Bromsulphalein	C & P	Cystoscopy and pyelography
BT	Breast tumor; brain tumor		
		CP	Cerebral palsy; cleft plate
BTL	Bilateral tubal ligation	CPR	Cardiopulmonary resuscitation
BTFS	Breast tumor frozen section		
		CR	Cardiorespiratory
BU	Bodansky unit	CRF	Chronic renal failure
BUN	Blood urea nitrogen	CRP	C-reactive protein
BVL	Bilateral vas ligation	CS	Coronary sclerosis
BW	Body weight	C & S	Culture and sensitivity
Bx	Biopsy		
		CSF	Cerebrospinal fluid
C		C sect	Cesarean section
C	Centigrade, Celsius	CT	Circulation time
C_2	Second cervical vertebra	CV	Cardiovascular; costovertebral angle
CA	Carbonic anhydrase	CVA	Cerebrovascular accident
Ca	Cancer, calcium		
C & A	Clinitest and Acetest	CVP	Central venous pressure
CAD	Coronary artery disease		
		CX	Cervix, cervical
CBC	Complete blood count	CXR	Chest x-ray
CC	Chief complaint	**D**	
CCR	Creatinine clearance	DC (D/C)	Discontinue
CCU	Coronary Care Unit	D & C	Dilatation and curettage
Ceph floc	Cephalin flocculation		
CF	Complement fixation	DD	Differential diagnosis
CHF	Congestive heart failure	DDD	Degenerative disc disease

DIC	Disseminated intravascular coagulation
Diff	Differential blood count
DJD	Degenerative joint disease
DM	Diabetes mellitus
DOA	Dead on arrival
DOE	Dyspnea on exertion
DPT	Diphtheria, pertussis, and tetanus
DSD	Dry sterile dressing
DT	Delirium tremens
DTR	Deep tendon reflex
Dx	Diagnosis
D_5W	Dextrose 5% in water

E

E	Enema
EBL	Estimated blood loss
ECF	Extracellular fluid
ECG	Electrocardiogram
ECT	Electroconvulsive therapy
ECW	Extracellular water
EDC	Expected date of confinement (obstetrics)
EEG	Electroencephalogram
EENT	Eyes, ears, nose, throat
EFA	Essential fatty acids
EH	Enlarged heart
EKG	Electrocardiogram
EM	Electron microscope
EMG	Electromyography
ENT	Ears, nose and throat
ER	Emergency room
ESR	Erythroctye sedimentation rate (sed rate)
EST	Electroshock therapy
EUA	Examine under anesthesia

F

F	Fahrenheit
FB	Finger breadths; foreign bodies
FBS	Fasting blood sugar
FEV_1	Forced expiratory volume in one second
FF	Filtration fraction
FFA	Free fatty acids
FH	Family history
FLK	Funny looking kid
FP	Family practice; family planning
FSH	Follicle-stimulating hormone
FTA	Fluorescent treponemal antibody
FUO	Fever of undetermined origin
Fx	Fracture; fraction

G

G	Gravida
GA	General appearance
GB	Gallbladder
GC	Gonococcus; gonorrhea
GFR	Glomerular filtration rate
GI	Gastrointestinal
G6PD	Glucose-6-phosphate dehydrogenase
G-P-	Gravida-; para-
GU	Genitourinary
GYN	Gynecology

H

H	Hypodermic; heroin
HA	Headache
HAA	Hepatitis-associated antigen
HBP	High blood pressure
Hct	Hematocrit
HCVD	Hypertensive cardiovascular disease
HEENT	Head, eyes, ears, nose, throat
Hgb	Hemoglobin
HHD	Hypertensive heart disease

HO	House officer
HOB	Head of bed
HPF	High power field
HPI	History of present illness
HSA	Human serum albumin
HTN	Hypertension
HTVD	Hypertensive vascular disease
Hx	History

I

IASD	Intraatrial septal defect
IBC	Iron-binding capacity
IBI	Intermittent bladder irrigation
ICF	Intracellular fluid volume
ICM	Intracostal margin
ICS	Intercostal space
ICU	Intensive Care Unit
ICW	Intracellular water
ID	Initial dose; intradermal
I & D	Incision and drainage
IDU	Idoxuridine
I & O	Intake and output
IHSS	Idiopathic hypertrophic subaortic stenosis
IM	Intramuscular
Imp	Impression
Int	Internal
IP	Intraperitoneal
IPPB	Intermittent positive pressure breathing
ISW	Interstitial water
ITh	Intrathecal
IU	International unit
IUD	Intrauterine device (contraceptive)
IVP	Intravenous pyelogram
IVPB	Intravenous piggyback
IVSD	Intraventricular septal defect

J

JRA	Juvenile rheumatoid arthritis
JVD	Jugular venous distention

K

K^+	Potassium
KO	Keep open
17-KS	17-Ketosteroids
KUB	Kidney, ureter, and bladder
K.W.	Keith Wagner (ophthalmoscopic findings)

L

L_2	Second lumbar vertebra
LA	Left atrium
Lap	Laparotomy
LATS	Long-acting thyroid stimulator
LBBB	Left bundle branch block
LCM	Left costal margin
LD	Longitudinal diameter (of heart)
LDH	Lactic dehydrogenase
LDL	Low density lipoproteins
LE	Lupus erythematosus
LFT's	Liver function tests
LHF	Left heart failure
LKS	Liver, kidneys, and spleen
LLE	Left lower extremity
LLL	Left lower lobe
LLQ	Left lower quadrant (abdomen)
LMD	Local medical doctor
LML	Left middle lobe (lung)
LMP	Last menstrual period
LOA	Left occipital anterior
LOM	Limitation of motion
LOP	Left occipital posterior

LP	Lumbar puncture		NSR	Normal sinus rhythm
lpf	Low power field		NTG	Nitroglycerin
LUQ	Left upper quadrant		NVD	Nausea, vomiting, di-arrhea; neck vein distention
LVH	Left ventricular hy-pertrophy			
L & W	Living and well		NYD	Not yet diagnosed
LWCT	Lee-White clotting time			
			O	
lytes	Electrolytes			
M			Oz	Oxygen
			O	Objective data (POMR)
M	Murmur		OB	Obstetrics; occult blood
M²	Square meters of body surface			
			OOB	Out of bed
M₁	First mitral sound		OOBBRP	Out of bed with bathroom privi-leges
MCH	Mean corpuscular hemoglobin			
MCHC	Mean corpuscular hemoglobin con-centraton		OD	Overdose
			OR	Operating room
			OT	Occupational therapy
MCL	Midclavicular line		**P**	
MCV	Mean corpuscular volume			
			P	Plan (POMR), pulse
MF	Myocardial fibrosis		P & A	Palpation and auscul-tation
MH	Marital history; men-strual history			
			PA	Posteroanterior
MI	Myocardial infarc-tion; mitral insuffi-ciency		PAT	Paroxysmal atrial tachycardia
			PBI	Protein-bound iodine
MIC	Minimum inhibitory concentration		PC	After meals
			PCN	Penicillin
MJT	Mead Johnson tube		PCV	Packed cell volume (hematocrit)
ML	Midline			
MOM	Milk of Magnesia		PE	Physical examination
MS	Morphine sulfate; multiple sclerosis; mitral stenosis		PEEP	Positive and expirato-ry pressure
			PEG	Pneumoencephalo-gram
MSL	Midsternal line			
N			PERRLA	Pupils equal, round, react to light and accommodation
N	Normal; Negro			
NAD	No acute distress; no apparent distress		PH	Past history
			PI	Present illness
NG	Nasogastric		PID	Pelvic inflammatory disease
NM	Neuromuscular			
NPN	Nonprotein nitrogen		PIE	Pulmonary infiltra-tion with eosino-philia
NPO	Nothing by mouth			
NR	No refill			
NS	Normal saline		PKU	Phenylketonuria
NSFTD	Normal spontaneous full-term delivery		PMH	Past medical history

PMI	Point of maximal impulse or maximum intensity	RQ	Respiratory quotient
PMN	Polymorphonuclear neutrophil	RR	Recovery room; respiratory rate
PMT	Premenstrual tension	RSR	Regular sinus rhythm
PND	Paroxysmal nocturnal dyspnea	RTA	Renal tubular acidosis
PNX	Pneumothorax	RTN	Renal tubular necrosis
POMR	Problem-oriented medical record	RUL	Right upper lobe
Postop	After surgery	RUQ	Right upper quadrant
PO	By mouth	RV	Right ventricle
PP	Postpartum; postprandial	RVH	Right ventricular hypertrophy
PPD	Purified protein derivative		
PPL	Penicilloyl-polylysine conjugate	**S**	
P & R	Pulse and respiration	S	Subjective data (POMR)
Preop	Before surgery	S_1	First heart sound
PT	Physical therapy; prothrombin time	S_2	Second heart sound
		SA	Sinotrial
PTA	Prior to admission	SBE	Subacute bacterial endocarditis
PUD	Peptic ulcer disease	SC	Subclavian, subcutaneous
PVC	Premature ventricular contraction	Sed rate	Erythrocyte sedimentation rate
PZI	Protamine zinc insulin	Segs	Segmented neutrophils
		SGOT	Serum glutamic oxaloacetic transaminase
R			
R	Respiration	SGPT	Serum glutamic pyruvic transaminase
RA	Rheumatoid arthritis; right atrium	SH	Social history; serum hepatitis
RBC	Red blood cell	SID	Sudden infant death
RBF	Renal blood flow	SL	Sublingual
RCM	Right costal margin	SLE	Systemic lupus erythematosus
RF	Rheumatoid factor		
RHD	Rheumatic heart disease; renal hypertensive disease	SLDH	Serum lactic dehydrogenase
RISA	Radioactive iodine serum albumin	SMA	Serial multiple analysis
RLL	Right lower lobe	SOAP	Subjective, objective, assessment plan (POMR)
RLQ	Right lower quadrant		
RO	Rule out		
ROM	Range of motion	SOB	Shortness of breath
ROS	Review of systems; review of symptoms	S/P	Status post
		SR	Sedimentation rate (ESR)
RPF	Renal plasma flow; relaxed pelvic floor		

SSE	Saline solution enema; soapsuds enema
SSPE	Subacute sclerosing panencephalitis
STD	Skin test dose
STS	Serologic test for syphilis
SVC	Superior vena cava

T

T	Temperature
T_3	Triiodothyronine
T_4	Thyroxin
T & A	Tonsillectomy and adenoidectomy
TAH	Total abdominal hysterectomy
TAO	Thromboangitis obliterans
TB	Tuberculosis
TBW	Total body water
TD	Transverse diameter (of heart)
TEDS	Elastic stockings
TIA	Transient ischemic attack
TIBC	Total iron-binding capacity
TKO	To keep open
TLC	Tender loving care
TM	Tympanic membrane
TP	Total protein; thrombophlebitis
TPI	*Treponema pallidum* immobilization
TPN	Total parenteral nutrition
TPR	Temperature, pulse, and respiration
TRA	To run at
T-set	Tracheotomy set
TSH	Thyroid-stimulating hormone
TUR	Transurethral resection
TV	*Trichomonas vaginalis*

U

UA (U/A)	Urinalysis
U & C	Urethral and cervical
UCHD	Unusual childhood diseases
UGI	Upper gastrointestinal
URI	Upper respiratory infection
UTI	Urinary tract infection

V

V	Vein
Vag hyst	Vaginal hysterectomy
VAH	Veteran's Administration Hospital
VC	Vena cava
VCU	Voiding cystourethrogram
VDRL	Venereal Disease Research Laboratories (for syphilis)
VF	Ventricular fibrillation
VMA	Vanillylmandelic acid
VP	Venous pressure
VPC	Ventricular premature contraction
VS	Vital signs
VSD	Ventricular septal defect
VT	Ventricular tachycardia

W

W	White; widow
WBC	White blood cell; white blood count
WDWN-WF	Well-developed, well-nourished, white female
WDWN-WM	Well-developed, well-nourished, white male
WNL	Within normal limits
Wt	Weight

Derivatives of medical terminology

adeno-	gland	*lympho-*	lymph
adreno-	adrenal gland	*macro-*	large
-algia	pain	*masto-*	breast
angio-	vessel	*medius*	middle
arterio-	artery	*megalo-*	huge
arthro-	joint	*meningo-*	meninges
auto-	self	*metra-, metro-*	uterus
broncho-	bronchus	*micro-*	small
brachy-	short	*myco-*	fungus
brady-	slow	*myelo-*	bone marrow; spinal cord
carcino-	cancer		
cardio-	heart		
cele-	herniation	*myo-*	muscle
-centesis	puncture	*necro-*	death
chole-	bile	*neo-*	new
chondro-	cartilage	*nephro-*	kidney
costo-	ribs	*neuro-*	nerve
cranio-	head	*oculo-*	eye
cysto-	bladder	*oligo-*	few
cyto-	cell	*-oma*	tumor
derma-	skin	*oophoro-*	ovary
diplo-	double	*orchio-, orchido-*	testes
-ectomy	out	*os*	mouth; bone
edem-	swell	*-osis*	condition
entero-	intestines	*osteo-*	bone
erythro-	red	*-ostomy*	opening
gastro-	stomach	*-otomy*	into
glomerulo-	glomerulus	*patho-*	disease
glyco-	sweet	*phago-*	eat
hem-, hemato-	blood	*phlebo-*	vein
hepato-	liver	*-phobia*	fear
-hesion	join together	*pilo-*	hair
hetero-	different	*-plegia*	paralysis
homo-	same	*pneumo-*	lungs; air
hydro-	wet, water	*procto-*	rectum
hystero-	uterus	*ptosis*	fall
ileo-	ileum	*pyelo-*	pelvis of kidney
-itis	inflammation		
jejuno-	jejunum	*pyo-*	pus
laparo-	loin or flank	*rhino-*	nose
laryngo-	larynx	*-rrhagia*	burst forth
leuko-	white	*-rrhaphy*	suture
lipo-	fat	*rrhea*	flow; discharge
litho-	stone		

sero-	serum	*tom-*	cut
splanchno-	viscera	*tricho-*	hair
spleno-	spleen	*uretero-*	ureter
-stasis	stop	*urethro-*	urethra
stoma-	mouth	*uro-*	urine
tachy-	fast; swift	*vaso-*	vessel
thrombo-	clot	*veno-*	vein
thyro-	thyroid		

Prescription abbreviations

aa, $\overline{aa}$	of each (equal parts)
a.c.	before meals
ad	to; up to
ad lib	as much as desired
b.i.d.	twice daily
$\bar{c}$, c	with
caps	capsules
d	day
et	and
ext	an extract
fl	fluid
gtt	a drop
h.s.	at bedtime
o.d.	right eye
o.s.	left eye
o.u.	both eyes
p.c.	after meals
p.r.n.	as needed
q	every
qd	once daily
q.i.d.	four times daily
qod	every other day
$\bar{s}$	without
sig.	label
ss	one-half
stat	at once
t.i.d.	three times daily
ung	ointment
ut dict.	as directed

Mathematic conversions

Abbreviations

kg = kilograms	ng = nanograms	mEq = milliequivalent
g = grams	m = meter	μm = micron
mg = milligrams	cm = centimeter	L = liter
μg = micrograms	mm = millimeter	ml = milliliter

Metric system

WEIGHT

1 kilogram	= 1000 grams
1 gram	= 1000 milligrams
1 milligram	= 1000 micrograms
1 microgram	= 0.001 milligram
1 milligram	= 0.001 gram
1 gram	= 0.001 kilogram

VOLUME

1 deciliter	= 100 milliliters
1 liter	= 1000 milliliters
1 milliliter	= 0.001 liter
1 deciliter	= 0.1 liter

LENGTH

1 centimeter	= 10 millimeters
1 decimeter	= 10 centimeters
1 meter	= 10 decimeters
1 kilometer	= 1000 meters
1 millimeter	= 0.1 centimeter
1 centimeter	= 0.1 decimeter
1 decimeter	= 0.1 meter
1 meter	= 0.001 kilometer

Common system

APOTHECARY WEIGHT

1 scruple (℈)	= 20 grains (gr)
60 grains	= 1 dram (ʒ)
8 drams	= 1 ounce (℥)
1 ounce	= 480 grains
12 ounces	= 1 pound

AVOIRDUPOIS WEIGHT

1 ounce (oz)	= 437.5 grains
1 pound (lb)	= 16 ounces

APOTHECARY VOLUME

60 minims (♏)	= 1 fluidram (fl℥)
8 fluidrams	= 1 fluid ounce (fl℥)
1 fluid ounce	= 480 minims
16 fluid ounces	= 1 pint (pt)

LENGTH

12 inches	= 1 foot
36 inches	= 1 yard
3 feet	= 1 yard
5280 feet	= 1 mile
1760 yards	= 1 mile

Metric and common system equivalents

MILLIGRAMS	GRAMS	GRAINS		
.1	.0001	1/600	1 gram	= 15.4 grains
.2	.0002	1/300	1 grain	= 64.8 milligrams
.3	.0003	1/200	1 ounce (℥)	= 31.1 grams
.4	.0004	1/150	1 ounce (oz)	= 28.3 grams
.5	.0005	1/120	1 pound (lb)	= 453.6 grams
.6	.0006	1/100	1 kilogram (kg)	= 2.2 pounds
1.0	.001	1/60	1 milliliter (ml)	= 16.23 minims
			1 minim (♏)	= 0.06 ml
			1 fluid ounce	= 29.5 ml
			(fl℥)	
2.0	.002	1/30	1 pint	= 473 ml
10	.01	1/6	1 meter	= 39.3 inches
15	.015	1/4	1 kilometer	= .6 mile
30	.03	1/2	1 mile	= 1.6 mile
45	.045	3/4	1 inch	= 2.54 cm
60 (65)	.06	1	1 foot	= 30 cm
300 (330)	.3	5	1 yard	= .9 meter
600 (650)	.6	10		
1000	1.0	15		
2000	2.0	30		
3000	3.0	45		

Approximate household measurements

1 teaspoonful		5 ml
1 dessertspoonful		10 ml
1 tablespoonful	½ fl oz	15 ml
1 jigger	1½ fl oz	45 ml
1 wineglassful	2 fl oz	60 ml
1 teacupful	4 fl oz	120 ml
1 glassful (tumblerful)	8 fl oz	240 ml

Temperature conversion table

F	C	F	C	F	C
95.0	35.0	98.4	36.9	101.8	38.7
.2	35.1	.6	37.0	102.0	38.8
.4	35.2	.8	37.1	.2	38.9
.6	35.3	99.0	37.2	.4	39.1
.8	35.4	.2	37.3	.6	39.2
96.0	35.5	.4	37.4	.8	39.3
.2	35.6	.6	37.5	103.0	39.4
.4	35.7	.8	37.6	.2	39.5
.6	35.9	100.0	37.7	.4	39.6
.8	36.0	.2	37.8	.6	39.7
97.0	36.1	.4	37.9	.8	39.8
.2	36.2	.6	38.1	104.0	40.0
.4	36.3	.8	38.2	.2	40.1
.6	36.4	101.0	38.3	.4	40.2
.8	36.5	.2	38.4	.6	40.3
98.0	36.6	.4	38.5	.8	40.4
.2	36.7	.6	38.6	105.0	40.5

$C° = \frac{5}{9} (F° - 32°)$; $F° = \frac{9}{5} C° + 32°$

Weight conversion table

lb	kg	lb	kg	lb	kg
5	2.3	105	47.7	210	95.5
10	4.5	110	50	220	100
15	6.8	115	52.3	230	104.5
20	9.1	120	54.5	240	109
25	11.4	125	56.8	250	113.6
30	13.6	130	59	260	118.2
35	15.9	135	61.4	270	122.7
40	18.1	140	63.6	280	127.2
45	20.4	145	66	290	131.8
50	22.7	150	68.1	300	136.4
55	25	155	70.5	310	140.9
60	27.3	160	72.7	320	145.5
65	29.5	165	75	330	150
70	31.8	170	77.3	340	154.5
75	34.1	175	79.5	350	159
80	36.4	180	81.8	360	163.6
85	38.6	185	84.1	370	168.2
90	40.9	190	86.4	380	172.7
95	43.2	195	88.6	390	177.2
100	45.4	200	90.9	400	181.8

1 lb = 0.454 kg; 1 kg = 2.2 lb

Formulas for the calculation of infants' and children's dosages

Children's dosages

Bastedo's rule:

$$\text{Child's approximate dose} = \frac{\text{age in years} + 3}{30} \times \text{adult dose}$$

Clark's rule:

$$\text{Child's approximate dose} = \frac{\text{weight of child (lb)}}{150} \times \text{adult dose}$$

Cowling's rule:

$$\text{Child's approximate dose} = \frac{\text{age (on next birthday)}}{24} \times \text{adult dose}$$

Dilling's rule:

$$\text{Child's approximate dose} = \frac{\text{age (in years)}}{20} \times \text{adult dose}$$

Young's rule:

$$\text{Child's approximate dose} = \frac{\text{age of child (in years)}}{\text{age} + 12} \times \text{adult dose}$$

Infants' dosages (younger than 1 year of age)

Fried's rule:

$$\text{Infant dose} = \frac{\text{age (in months)}}{150} \times \text{adult dose}$$

Pediatric emergency drug dosages

Drug	Dosage	10 lb (4.5 kg)	20 lb (9.1 kg)	30 lb (13.6 kg)	40 lb (18.2 kg)	50 lb (22.7 kg)	60 lb (27.3 kg)	Reference
Atropine sulfate 0.4 mg/1 ml ampules	0.01 mg/kg/dose IV (maximum, 0.4 mg)	0.045 mg (0.11 ml)	0.09 mg (0.22 ml)	0.14 mg (0.35 ml)	0.18 mg (0.45 ml)	0.23 mg (0.58 ml)	0.27 mg (0.68 ml)	Shirkey Schwerman
Calcium chloride (10%) solution 100 mg/ml-10 ml ampules; contains 270 mg Ca^{2+}/10 ml	0.2 ml/kg IV (equivalent to 5 mg Ca^{2+}/kg) (maximum, 1 ml/5 kg) Administer at rate of 1 ml/min	22.5 mg (0.90 ml)	45.0 mg (1.82 ml)	68.0 mg (2.70 ml)	91.0 mg (3.64 ml)	113.5 mg (4.54 ml)	136.5 mg (5.46 ml)	Schwerman AHA Nelson
Calcium gluconate 100 mg/ml-10 ml ampules; contains 97 mg Ca^{2+}/10 ml	1.0 ml/kg IV (equivalent to 10 mg Ca^{2+}/kg) (maximum, 10 ml) (100 mg/kg/dose) Inject at 1 ml/min	22.5 mg (2.34 ml)	45.0 mg (4.68 ml)	68.0 mg (7.02 ml)	91.0 mg (9.36 ml)	97 mg (10.0 ml)	97 mg (10.0 ml)	Schwerman Kempe

Continued.

Pediatric emergency drug dosages

Drug	Dosage	10 lb (4.5 kg)	20 lb (9.1 kg)	30 lb (13.6 kg)	40 lb (18.2 kg)	50 lb (22.7 kg)	60 lb (27.3 kg)	Reference
Digoxin (Lanoxin) IM, IV 0.5 mg/2 ml ampules	Premature: 0.015 mg/kg STAT, then 0.0075 mg/kg every 12 hr × 2 doses	0.068 mg/ 0.27 ml then 0.034 mg/ 0.14 ml						Shirkey
	2 weeks to 2 years: 0.02 mg/kg STAT, then 0.01 mg/kg every 12 hr × 2 doses	0.09 mg/ 0.36 ml then 0.045 mg/ 0.18 ml	0.18 mg/ 0.72 ml then 0.09 mg/ 0.36 ml	0.27 mg/ 1.08 ml then 0.135 mg/ 0.54 ml	0.36 mg/ 1.44 ml then 0.18 mg/ 0.72 ml	0.45 mg/ 1.80 ml then 0.23 mg/ 0.9 ml	0.54 mg/ 2.16 ml then 0.27 mg/ 1.08 ml	
Phenytoin (Dilantin) IV 50 mg/ml in a 2 ml syringe	Anticonvulsant dose: 1 to 5 mg/kg/24 hr Single dose or divide into 2 doses Give IV slowly (50 mg/min) NOTE: Values given are for single dose	4.5 mg/ 0.09 ml to 22.5 mg/ 0.45 ml	9.1 mg/ 0.18 ml to 45.0 mg/ 0.9 ml	13.5 mg/ 0.27 ml to 67.5 mg/ 1.35 ml	18.2 mg/ 0.36 ml to 90 mg/1.8 ml	22.7 mg/ 0.45 ml to 112.5 mg/ 2.25 ml	27.3 mg/ 0.54 ml to 135 mg/ 2.70 ml	Shirkey Kempe

Epinephrine hydrochloride (1:1000) SC 1 ml ampules	0.01 ml/kg/dose (maximum, 0.5 ml) May repeat at 15 min intervals, 2 to 3 times NOTE: Dose given in ml rather than mg	0.045 ml	0.09 ml	0.14 ml	0.18 ml	0.23 ml	0.27 ml	Shirkey
Epinephrine (1:10,000) IV Add 9.0 ml of normal saline to 1.0 ml ampule of epinephrine 1:1000; resultant solutions is 1:10,000 conc. for IV use	0.1 ml/kg/dose Repeat every 3 to 5 min. to have persistent effect NOTE: Dose given in ml rather than mg	0.45 ml	0.91 ml	1.36 ml	1.82 ml	2.27 ml	2.73 ml	Shirkey
Isoproterenol hydrochloride (Isuprel hydrochloride) 1.0 mg/5 ml ampules	NOT GIVEN DIRECT IV Add 1.0 mg isoproterenol to 250 ml of D5W; this provides a solution containing	NOT RECOMMENDED FOR DIRECT IV INJECTION FOR CHILDREN GIVE BY IV INFUSION						Schwerman Kempe

Continued.

Pediatric emergency drug dosages

Drug	Dosage	10 lb (4.5 kg)	20 lb (9.1 kg)	30 lb (13.6 kg)	40 lb (18.2 kg)	50 lb (22.7 kg)	60 lb (27.3 kg)	Reference
Isoproterenol hydrochloride—cont'd	4 µg per ml of isoproterenol HC1; attach a Mini-Dripper to the IV set and administer at an initial rate of 5 µgtts/min							
Levarterenol bitartrate (Levophed) IV 4 ml ampules containing 0.2% levarterenol bitartrate (equiv. to 0.1% base) 1 ml of solution = 1 mg of base	Place 2 ml of 0.2% solution (as supplied by ampule) in 500 ml D₅W; administer at 0.5 ml/min to give 2 µg (base/min); titrate with blood pressure To prevent sloughing and necrosis in areas in which extravasation has taken place, infiltrate *as soon as possible* with 10 to 15 ml of normal	DO NOT GIVE DIRECTLY IV, BUT RATHER BY IV INFUSION						Shirkey

		4.5 mg 0.23 ml	9.1 mg 0.46 ml	13.6 mg 0.69 ml	15.0 mg 0.75 ml	15.0 mg 0.75 ml	25.0 mg 1.2 ml	
	to 10 mg phentolamine (Regitine)							
Lidocaine hydrochloride IV 2% solution in ampules (100 mg/5 ml)	1 mg/kg (maximum, up to 15 mg, if under 55 lb) (maximum, up to 25 mg, if above 55 lb)	4.5 mg 0.23 ml	9.1 mg 0.46 ml	13.6 mg 0.69 ml	15.0 mg 0.75 ml	15.0 mg 0.75 ml	25.0 mg 1.2 ml	Shirkey Schwerman
			GIVE DIRECTLY IV — IV INFUSION NOT RECOMMENDED FOR PEDIATRICS					
Naloxone (Narcan) IM, IV 0.4 mg/ml ampules	0.01 mg/kg initially; may repeat at 2 to 3 min intervals × 2 or 3 doses. Indicated for treatment of diphenoxylate hydrochloride (Lomotil) poisoning. Also indicated for treatment of propoxyphene hydrochloride (Darvon) overdosage and narcotic analgesic overdoses; response is diagnostic for narcotic analgesic use	0.05 mg 0.12 m	0.09 mg 0.23 ml	0.14 mg 0.35 ml	0.18 mg 0.45 ml	0.22 mg 0.55 ml	0.28 mg 0.7 ml	Shirkey Rumack

Pediatric emergency drug dosages

Drug	Dosage	10 lb (4.5 kg)	20 lb (9.1 kg)	30 lb (13.6 kg)	40 lb (18.2 kg)	50 lb (22.7 kg)	60 lb (27.3 kg)	Reference
Phenobarbital sodium 130 mg/1 ml (Dosette) (Ready for use)	Anticonvulsant dose 3.5 mg/kg/dose IM IF GIVEN IV: DILUTE WITH NORMAL SALINE AND GIVE SLOWLY	15.8 mg (0.12 ml)	31.6 mg (0.24 ml)	47.4 mg (0.36 ml)	63.2 mg (0.48 ml)	79.0 mg (0.6 ml)	94.8 mg (0.72 ml)	Shirkey
Procainamide hydrochloride (Pronestyl) 100 mg/ml 10 ml vials	2 mg/kg/dose IV (maximum, 100 mg) Diluted and given over a period of 5 min IV, and the dose is repeated every 10 to 15 min until the arrhythmia is controlled (maximum total dose is 1.0 g)	9 mg	18.2 mg	27.2 mg	36.4 mg	45.4 mg	54.6 mg	Shirkey Kempe

Drug	Administration	Dose							Reference
Sodium bicarbonate 50 ml syringe containing 1 mEq/ml	Administration must be continuously monitored by EKG and frequent blood pressures	2 mEq/kg/dose IV Dose may be repeated in 8 to 10 min, but further doses should depend on blood gases	9.0 mEq (9.0 ml)	18.2 mEq (18.2 ml)	27.2 mEq (27.2 ml)	36.4 mEq (36.4 ml)	45.4 mEq (45.4 ml)	50.0 mEq (50.0 ml)	Schwerman Nelson
Diazepam (Valium) 10 mg/2 ml ampules		0.1 to 0.2 mg/kg/dose Because of varied responses to CNS drugs, initiate therapy with lowest dose NOT FOR USE IN CHILDREN UNDER 6 MONTHS OF AGE DO NOT MIX OR DILUTE WITH OTHER FLUIDS OR DRUGS		0.9 mg/ 0.18 ml to 1.8 mg/ 0.36 ml	.36 mg/ 0.27 ml to 2.72 mg/ 0.54 ml	1.82 mg/ 0.36 ml to 3.64 mg/ 0.72 ml	2.27 mg/ 0.45 ml to 4.54 mg/ 0.9 ml	2.73 mg/ 0.55 ml to 5.46 mg/ 1.09 ml	Shirkey

REFERENCES

American Heart Association: Standards for cardiopulmonary resuscitation (CPR) and cardiac care (ECC), JAMA **227**:837-868, Feb. 18, 1974.

Kempe, C.H., et al.: Current pediatric diagnosis and treatment, ed. 3, Los Altos, Calif., 1974, Lange Medical Publications.

Nelson, W.E., et al., editors: Textbook of pediatrics, ed. 11, Philadelphia, 1979, W.B. Saunders Co.

Rumack, B.H., and Temple, A.R.: Lomotil poisoning, Pediatrics **53**:495, 1974.

Schwerman, E., et al.: The pharmacist as a member of the cardiopulmonary resuscitation team, Drug Intell. Clin. Pharm. **7**:298-308, July, 1973.

Shirkey, H.C., editor: Pediatric therapy, ed. 6, St. Louis, 1980, The C.V. Mosby Co.

Drugs excreted in human milk

Agent	Significance
Alcohol	Moderate amounts have little if any effect
Aloe	May cause diarrhea
Amantadine (Symmetrel)	May cause urinary retention, vomiting, skin rash
Ampicillin (Penbritin, Polycillin, Amcill, Omnipen)	a*
Aspirin	May cause a bleeding tendency by interfering with the function of the infant's platelets or by decreasing the amount of prothrombin in the blood
Atropine sulfate (ingredient in many prescription and nonprescription products)	Inhibits lactation; may cause atropine intoxication in the infant
Barbiturates	a; high doses may cause sedation; may cause induction of drug metabolizing enzymes
Bromides	Reactions include rash and drowsiness
Bromocriptine (Parlodel)	Inhibits prolactin levels
Calciferol (Vitamin D)	May result in hypercalcemia
Carbenicillin (Pyopen, Geopen)	a
Carisoprodol (Soma)	Concentrated in breast milk; may cause CNS depression and gastric upset
Cascara	Increases gastric motility in infant
Chloral hydrate (Noctec, Somnos)	a

Adapted from O'Brien, T.E.: Excretion of drugs in human milk, Am. J. Hosp. Pharm. **31**:846-853, Sept., 1974. Copyright © 1974, American Society of Hospital Pharmacists, Inc. All rights reserved.
*a = Not significant in therapeutic doses to affect infant.

Continued.

Agent	*Significance*
Chloramphenicol (Chloromycetin)	Infant has underdeveloped enzyme system, immature liver and renal function; may not have glycuronide system adequately developed to conjugate chloramphenicol; caution advised
Chlorazepate (Tranxene)	May cause drowsiness
Chlordiazepoxide (Librium)	a
Chlorpromazine (Thorazine)	a; may cause galactorrhea
Codeine	a
Contraceptives (oral)	May inhibit lactation if administered during first postnatal weeks; possible gynecomastia in male infants
Cyanocobalamin (Vitamin B_{12})	a
Cyclophosphamide (Cytoxan)	Nursing should be discontinued
Dextrothyroxine	a
Diazepam (Valium)	Infant reported lethargic and experienced weight loss; may cause hyperbilirubinemia
Diphenhydramine (Benardryl)	a
Ergot (Cafergot)	Symptoms range from vomiting and diarrhea to weak pulse and unstable blood pressure
Erythromycin (Ilosone, E-Mycin, Erythrocin)	Greater concentrations in milk than in plasma
Fluoxymesterone (Halotestin, Ultandren)	Used to suppress lactation
Folic acid	a
Gallium citrate	Significant exposure to radioactive compound
Guanethidine (Ismelin sulfate)	a
Heroin	Not enough to prevent withdrawal in addicted infants
Hexachlorobenzene	Severe skin disease, porphyria, death
Hydrochlorothiazide (Hydro-Diuril, Esidrix)	To be avoided based on manufacturer's recommendation
Indomethacin (Indocin)	a
Iodides	May affect infant's thyroid gland
Iopanoic acid (Telepaque)	a

Agent	*Significance*
Iron (maternal vitamins)	Do not need additional supplementation in pediatric vitamins
Isoniazid (INH)	Monitor closely for toxicity
Kanamycin (Kantrex)	Monitor closely for toxicity
Lincomycin (Lincocin)	a
Lithium carbonate (Eskalith, Lithane)	Monitor closely for toxicity
Mefenamic acid (Ponstel)	a
Meperidine (Demerol)	a
Meprobamate (Equanil)	Present in milk at 2 to 4 times maternal plasma level; monitor for toxicity
Mesoridazine (Serentil)	a
Mestranol	*see* Contraceptives
Methenamine	a
Methocarbamol (Robaxin)	a
Metronidazole (Flagyl)	Apparently not significant in therapeutic doses
Morphine	a
Nalidixic acid (NegGram)	a
Nicotine	No effect with less than 20 cigarettes per day
Norethindrone (Norlutin)	*see* Contraceptives
Norethynodrel (Enovid)	*see* Contraceptives
Oxyphenbutazone (Tandearil)	a
Penicillin G (All penicillins)	May sensitize infant to penicillin
Phenformin (DBI)	a
Phenindione	Possible hemorrhage
Phenobarbital (Luminal)	*see* Barbiturates
Phenytoin	Cyanosis, methemoglobinemia
Phytonadione (Vitamin K_1, Aquamephyton)	a
Piperacetazine (Quide)	Unknown
Potassium iodide	May affect infant's thyroid
Primidone (Mysoline)	May cause undue drowsiness
Prochlorperazine (Compazine)	a
Propoxyphene (Darvon)	a
Pyrimethamine (Daraprim)	Unknown
Quinine sulfate	a
Reserpine (Serpasil)	May produce galactorrhea
Salicylates	a

Continued.

Agent	*Significance*
Sulfisoxazole (Gantrisin) (all sulfonamides)	May cause kernicterus; to be avoided during first 2 weeks postpartum
Technecium TC 99 m	Significant exposure to radioactivity
Tetracycline hydrochloride (all tetracyclines)	Theoretically may cause discoloration of teeth
Thiamine	Necessary for normal development
Thiazides (Diuril, Hydro-Diuril) (all thiazides)	To be avoided based on manufacturer's recommendation
Thiopental (Pentothal)	a
Thioridazine hydrochloride (Mellaril)	a
Thiouracil	Higher concentrations in milk than serum; may cause goiter or agranulocytosis in nursing infant; to be avoided
Thyroid	a
Tolbutamide (Orinase)	a
Tranylcypromine sulfate (Parnate)	a
Trifluoperazine hydrochloride (Stelazine)	a
Trimeprazine tartrate (Temaril)	a
Warfarin (Coumadin)	Infant should be monitored along with mother

Agents that discolor the feces

Agent	Color
Aluminum hydroxide preparations	Whitish discoloration or speckling
Antibiotics, oral	Greenish gray color caused by undigested material
Barium	Clay, putty
Bismuth compounds	Black
Charcoal	Black
Iron	Black
Lead	Bloody or black caused by presence of lead sulfide
Phenylbutazone (Butazolidin, Azolid)	Black caused by intestinal bleeding
Pyrvinium pamoate (Povan)	Red
Rifampin (Rifadin)	Orange-red
Salicylates	Pink to red to black resulting from internal bleeding
Senna	Yellow, yellow-greenish cast
Warfarin (Coumadin)	Pink to red to black caused by internal bleeding

---

Adapted from Baran, R.B., and Rowles, B: Factors affecting coloration of urine and feces, J.A.Ph.A. NS **13:**139-142, 155, March 1973.

Agents that discolor the urine

Agent	Color
Amitriptyline hydrochloride (Elavil)	Blue-green
Azuresin (Diagnex Blue)	Blue or green
Cascara	Red in alkaline urine
Chloroquine (Aralen)	Rust-yellow or brown
Deferoxamine mesylate (Desferal)	Red
Furazolidone (Furoxone)	Brown, orange-brown
Indigo blue	Green or blue
Indigo carmine	Green or blue
Indomethacin (Indocin	Green caused by biliverdinemia
Iron IV	Blackening
Levodopa (Dopar, Larodopa)	Darkening of urine on standing
Methocarbamol (Robaxin)	Brown to black to green on standing
Methyldopa (Aldomet)	Red to black caused by standing in a hypochloride solution
Methylene blue	Bluish green, green
Metronidazole (Flagyl)	Darkened urine
Nitrofurantoin (Furadantin, Macrodantin)	Rust-yellow or brownish
Phenacetin	Dark brown to black on standing
Phenazopyridine hydrochloride (Pyridium)	Red or orange
Phenolphthalein	Red in alkaline urine
Phenolsulfonphthalein (PSP)	Red in alkaline urine
Phenothiazines	Pink to red or red-brown
Phensuximide (Milontin)	Pink to red to red-brown
Phenytoin (Dilantin)	Pink or red to red-brown
Primaquine phosphate	Darkening of the urine
Quinacrine hydrochloride (Atabrine)	Yellow
Quinine	Brown to black
Resorcinol	Dark green
Riboflavin (Vitamin B_2)	Yellow
Rifampin (Rifadin, Rimactane)	Bright red-orange
Sulfasalazine (Azulfidine)	Orange-yellow in alkaline urine
Sulfonamides	Rust-yellow or brownish
Triamterene (Dyrenium)	Pale blue fluorescence
Warfarin sodium (Coumadin sodium)	Orange

Adapted from Baran, R.B., and Rowles, B.: Factors affecting coloration of urine and feces, J.A.Ph.A. NS **13**:139-142, 155, March 1973.

Contents of general emergency cart

Quantity	Medication	Concentration	Size
2	Aminophylline	25 mg/ml	10 ml
2	Amyl nitrite perles		0.3 ml
5	Atropine sulfate injection*	0.5 mg/ml	1 ml
6	Bretylium tosylate	50 mg/ml	10 ml
2	Calcium chloride 10%	100 mg/ml	10 ml
1	Deslanoside (Cedilanid-D)	0.2 mg/ml	4 ml
1	Dextrose 50% injection*	500 mg/ml	50 ml
1	Dexamethasone injection	4 mg/ml	5 ml
2	Digoxin (Lanoxin)	0.25 mg/ml	2 ml
2	Diphenhydramine hydrochloride (Benadryl)	50 mg/ml	1 ml
4	Dobutamine hydrochloride	12.5 mg/ml	20 ml
4	Dopamine hydrochloride (Intropin)	40 mg/ml	5 ml
6	Epinephrine hydrochloride 1:1000*	1 mg/ml	1 ml
4	Epinephrine hydrochloride 1:10,000* (intracardiac needle)	0.1 mg/ml	10 ml
10	Furosemide (Lasix)	10 mg/ml	10 ml
2	Glucagon injection	1μ/ml	10 ml
4	Isoproterenol 1:5000 (Isuprel)	0.2 mg/ml	5 ml
4	Levarterenol (Levophed)	2 mg/ml	4 ml
1	Lidocaine hydrochloride 2% (anesthetic)		20 ml
1	Lidocaine hydrochloride (drip infusion)	40 mg/ml	50 ml
3	Lidocaine hydrochloride (bolus infusion)*	20 mg/ml	5 ml
4	Metaraminol bitartrate (Aramine bitartrate)	10 mg/ml	10 ml
3	Naloxone (Narcan)	0.4 mg/ml	1 ml
1	Normal saline		20 ml
2	Phentolamine (Regitine)	5 mg/ml	1 ml

Available as a prefilled syringe.   *Continued.*

Quantity	Medication	Concentration	Size
4	Physostigmine salicylate (Antilirium)	0.5 mg/ml	2 ml
4	Phenytoin (Dilantin)*	50 mg/ml	5 ml
1	Procainamide hydrochloride (Pronestyl)	100 mg/ml	10 ml
4	Propranolol (Inderal)	1 mg/ml	1 ml
1	Quinidine gluconate	80 mg/ml	10 ml
4	Sodium bicarbonate*	44 mEq/50 ml	50 ml
2	Sterile water for injection		30 ml

	IV solutions		
1	Dextrose 5% in 0.2% sodium chloride		1000 ml
4	Dextrose 5% in water		1000 ml
1	Normal saline		500 ml
1	Lactated Ringer's		1000 ml

*Available as a prefilled syringe.

Emergency tray contents

Quantity	Medication	Concentration	Size
2	Aminophylline	25 mg/ml	10 ml
4	Atropine sulfate injection*	0.5 mg/ml	1 ml
6	Bretylium tosylate	50 mg/ml	10 ml
2	Calcium chloride 10%	100 mg/ml	10 ml
1	Dextrose 50% injection*	500 mg/ml	50 ml
2	Diphenhydramine hydrochloride (Benadryl)*	50 mg/ml	1 ml
4	Dobutamine hydrochloride	12.5 mg/ml	20 ml
4	Dopamine hydrochloride (Intropin)	40 mg/ml	5 ml
4	Epinephrine hydrochloride 1:1000*	1 mg/ml	1 ml
2	Epinephrine hydrochloride 1:10,000* (intracardiac needle)	0.1 mg/ml	10 ml
2	Isoproterenol 1:5000 (Isuprel)	0.2 mg/ml	5 ml
4	Levarterenol (Levophed)	2 mg/ml	4 ml
3	Lidocaine hydrochloride (bolus infusion)*	20 mg/ml	5 ml
2	Metaraminol bitartrate (Aramine bitartrate)	10 mg/ml	10 ml
3	Naloxone (Narcan)	0.4 mg/ml	1 ml
2	Phentolamine (Regitine)	5 mg/ml	1 ml
2	Phenytoin (Dilantin)*	50 mg/ml	5 ml
1	Procainamide hydrochloride (Pronestyl)	100 mg/ml	10 ml
4	Propranolol (Inderal)	1 mg/ml	1 ml
4	Sodium bicarbonate*	44 mEq/50 ml	50 ml
1	Sterile water for injection		30 ml

*Available as a prefilled syringe.

Nomogram for calculating the body surface area of adults and children

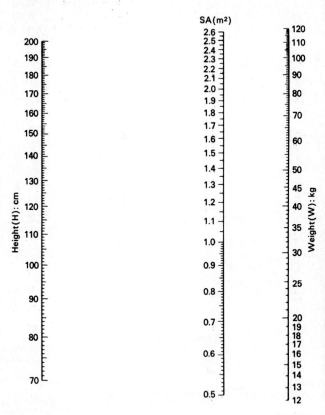

Align a ruler with the height and weight. The point at which the center line is intersected gives the corresponding value for surface area (SA). (From Haycock, G.B.: J. Pediatr. **93**:62-66, July 1978.)

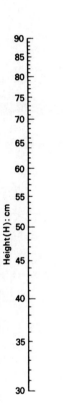

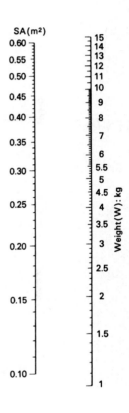

Bibliography

Aladjem, S., editor: Obstetrical practice, St. Louis, 1980, The C.V. Mosby Co.

American Academy of Pediatrics: Report of the Committee on Infectious Diseases, ed. 18, Evanston, Ill., 1977, American Academy of Pediatrics.

Bergerson, B.S.: Pharmacology in nursing, ed. 14, St. Louis, 1979, The C.V. Mosby Co.

Boedeker, E.C., and Dauber, J.H., editors: Manual of medical therapeutics, ed. 21, Boston, 1974, Little, Brown & Co.

Brunner, L., and Suddarth, D.S.: Lippincott manual of nursing practice, Philadelphia, 1974, J.B. Lippincott Co.

Goodman, L.S., and Gilman, A., editors: The pharmacological basis of therapeutics, ed. 6, New York, 1980, Macmillan, Inc.

Goth, A.: Medical pharmacology: principles and concepts, ed. 11, St. Louis, 1984, The C.V. Mosby Co.

Govani, L.E., and Hayes, J.E.: Drugs and nursing implications, ed. 3, New York, 1978, Appleton-Century-Crofts.

Greenwald, E.S.: Cancer chemotherapy, ed. 2, Flushing, 1973, Medical Examination Publishing Co., Inc.

Hansten, P.D.: Drug interactions, ed. 4, Philadelphia, 1979, Lea & Febiger.

Hansten, P.D., editor: Drug interactions newsletter, San Francisco, 1981-1983, Applied Therapeutics, Inc.

Hatcher, R.A., et al.: Contraceptive technology, 1978-1979, ed. 9, New York, 1978, Irvington Publishers.

Herfindal, E.T., and Hirschman, J.L., editors: Clinical pharmacy and therapeutics, ed. 2, Baltimore, 1979. The Williams & Wilkins Co.

Johns, M.P.: Pharmacodynamics and patient care, St. Louis, 1974, The C.V. Mosby Co.

Katcher, B., Young, L., and Koda-Kimble, M.A., editors: Applied therapeutics, ed. 3, San Francisco, 1983, Applied Therapeutics, Inc.

Kimble, M.A., and Young, L.Y., editors: Applied therapeutics for clinical pharmacists, Oakland, Calif., 1975, Applied Therapeutics, Inc.

Knoben, J.E., et al.: Handbook of clinical drug data, ed. 5, Hamilton, Ill., 1983, Drug Intelligence Publications.

Lichtiger, M., and Moya, F., editors: Introduction to the practice of anesthesia, ed. 2, New York, 1978, Harper & Row Publishers, Inc.

Lilly Research Laboratories: Diabetes mellitus, ed. 7, Indianapolis, 1973, Lilly Research Laboratories.

Loebl, S., et al.: The nurse's drug handbook, ed. 2, New York, 1980, John Wiley & Sons, Inc.

McEvoy, G., editor: American hospital formulary service, Washington, D.C., 1983, American Society of Hospital Pharmacists, Inc.

Melmon, K.L., and Morrelli, H.F., editors: Clinical pharmacology, basic principles in therapeutics, ed. 2, New York, 1978, MacMillan, Inc.

Metheny, N.M., and Snively, W.D., Jr.: Nurses handbook of fluid balance, ed. 2, Philadelphia, 1974, J.B. Lippincott Co.

Modell, W., editor: Drugs of choice, 1984-1985, St. Louis, 1984, The C.V. Mosby Co.

Pagliaro, L.A., et al.: Pediatric drug therapy, Hamilton, Ill., 1979, Drug Intelligence Publications, Inc.

Petersdorf, R.G., et al.: Principles of internal medicine, ed. 10, New York, 1983, McGraw-Hill Book Co.

Physician's desk reference, Oradell, N.J., 1983, Medical Economics Co.

Squire, J.E., and Clayton, B.D.: Basic pharmacology for nurses, ed. 7, St. Louis, 1981, The C.V. Mosby Co.

Vickers, M.D., et al.: Drugs in anesthetic practice, ed. 5, Boston, 1978, Butterworth & Co.

Index